Study Guide for

Fundamentals of Nursing: Active Learning for Collaborative Practice

Study Guide for

Fundamentals of Nursing: Active Learning for Collaborative Practice

Patricia A. Castaldi, DNP, RN, ANEF
Director
Practical Nursing & Allied Health Programs
Union County College
Plainfield, New Jersey

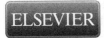

3251 Riverport Lane
St. Louis, Missouri 63043

STUDY GUIDE FOR FUNDAMENTALS OF NURSING:
ACTIVE LEARNING FOR COLLABORATIVE PRACTICE   ISBN: 978-0-323-35853-8

Executive Content Strategist: Tamara Myers
Content Development Manager: Jean Fornango
Senior Content Development Specialist: Laura Selkirk
Publishing Services Manager: Hemamalini Rajendrababu
Project Manager: Kamatchi Madhavan
Design Direction: Gopalakrishnan Venkatraman

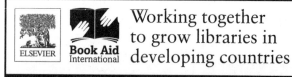

Printed in United States

Last digit is the print number: 9 8 7 6 5 4 3 2 1

This is dedicated to my family who have always been there for me.
For my husband and son who brighten my life and bring me coffee while I'm writing.
For my wonderful in-laws who made me part of their family from the very beginning.
For my nursing and allied health colleagues for their support.
This is for you.

Introduction and Preface

This guide is designed to correspond, chapter by chapter, to *Fundamentals of Nursing,* 1e. Each chapter in this guide contains study questions to assist in learning and applying the theoretical concepts from the text.

The chapter review sections allow you the opportunity to evaluate your own level of comprehension after reading the text. Use of the study group questions with fellow students may help in your overall understanding of the nursing content, as well as provide a way to further evaluate your familiarity with that content. There are also more short-answer, priority order and multiple-response questions to promote your preparation for classroom examinations and the alternate-format items on the NCLEX® examination. Answers are available printed in the back of the book for all of the questions and activities contained within this study guide.

The following is a summary of some of the major concepts and terms that are found in the text. You may encounter these prior to the chapter where they are discussed in more detail. Referring to this summary before you read through the text should help you to recognize the information. It is strongly recommended that you also have a medical dictionary and an anatomy and physiology text available for additional reference.

Concept/Terminology	Summary Description
Nursing	Nursing involves independent and collaborative care for individuals across the life span within families and communities, in a variety of health care settings. Nurses function in many roles each day to care for their patients. Nurses have various responsibilities within each role that relate to promotion of health, prevention of illness, and alleviation of suffering.
Caring	Caring encompasses the nurse's ability to be a good listener, nonjudgmental, compassionate, empathetic, available, and knowledgeable advocate.
Nursing process	The nursing process is a systematic and dynamic approach to patient care. It involves the continuous use of critical thinking skills to provide high quality care. There are five stages that are part of the nursing process, including: • Assessment- observation and communication to collect data • Nursing Diagnosis- identification of the primary areas of concern • Planning- identifying goals/outcomes and actions to take • Implementation- performance of nursing interventions • Evaluation- determination of goal achievement
Evidence-based practice	Nursing practice supported by research incorporates the clinical expertise of health care professionals, patient needs, and high quality, cost-effective care.
Delegation	Delegation is the assignment of responsibility or authority to another person, while still maintaining the ultimate accountability for the task.
Communication	All interactions with patients are a combination of verbal and nonverbal communication. How a nurse responds and reacts, in words and action, sets the tone for the entire professional relationship. Professional communication is at a different level than that between family members and friends.
Standards of care	Standards of care are the minimum requirements for providing safe nursing care. Federal and state laws, rules and regulations, accreditation standards, and institutional policies and procedures are used to formulate nursing standards of care. Institutional policies and procedures must be consistent with state laws, rules, and regulations, which in turn must comply with federal law. Accountability may be defined as the concept of being answerable for one's actions.
Ethical practice	Maintaining a standard of moral conduct within the profession is accomplished through honesty, respect, integrity, unbiased caring and advocacy.
Patient teaching	Providing necessary information to patients and families helps to prevent illness, avoid complications, and achieve an optimum level of health.
Vital signs	Vital signs a nurse must be able to accurately assess include temperature, pulse, respirations, blood pressure, pulse oximetry, and pain assessment.

Concept/Terminology	Summary Description
Physical assessment skills	Key assessment skills include: • Inspection- the use of vision and smell to assess physical characteristics • Palpation- the use of touch to assess body organs and skin texture, temperature, moisture, turgor (tension due to fluid content), tenderness, and thickness. • Percussion- tapping on the skin to determine the character of the sound and the density of the underlying area • Auscultation- listening to sounds made by body organs or systems such as the heart, blood vessels, lungs, and abdominal cavity, with and without the assistance of a stethoscope.
Six Rights	The Six Rights for medication administration are: • Right Drug • Right Dose • Right Time • Right Route • Right Patient (always use at least 2 identifiers!) • Right Documentation
QSEN competencies	Quality and Safety Education for Nurses (QSEN) competencies for nursing include: • Patient-Centered Care • Teamwork & Collaboration • Evidence-Based Practice • Quality Improvement • Safety • Informatics
National Patient Safety Goals	The Joint Commission National Patient Safety Goals 2014 include: • Identify patients correctly • Use medicines safely • Use alarms safely • Prevent infection • Identify patient safety risks • Prevent mistakes in surgery
Informatics	Informatics deal with the resources, devices, and methods required for the acquisition, storage, retrieval, and use of information in health and biomedicine. In addition to computers, informatics tools in health care include clinical guidelines, formal medical terminologies, and information and communication systems.
Safety	Common sense guidelines to improve safety include: • Always listen to and observe the patient carefully • Never force anything into or onto the patient • WASH YOUR HANDS! • Get help when you need it • Ask questions • Remember the 'triple check' • Never stop reading about quality care measures • If it does not seem right- DO NOT DO IT!
Reporting	Be factual, concise, honest and accurate. Use SBAR for hand-off communication: • Situation • Background • Assessment • Recommendation Never record what you have not yet done!

General Study Tips

While Reading

- Read before the scheduled class: Highlight key points or outline content in the text that will be covered in the classroom. Don't highlight everything! Clarify with your instructor(s) what the expected readings are for your class. Tables and boxes in the text can help to summarize critical information.
- Look up definitions: Find the meanings of words you do not recognize while you are going through the text. It helps to have a medical dictionary and a regular dictionary handy!
- Make notes: Write down a list of topics that you do not understand while you are reading so that you may clarify them with the instructor.
- Compare notes: Use notes taken from the book and in class to create a complete picture of the content.
- Use study/comparison charts: Put facts and ideas in an organized form so that you can refer to them easily at a later point, such as when studying for an examination.
- Use references: Go back to texts and notes used in other courses (such as anatomy and physiology) to help in understanding new material.

In the Classroom

- Make notes: Do not try to write everything down. Note the essential information from the class. Use the margins of notebook paper or type in your mobile device any questions that you may have as you go along so that you remember to ask them at some point. Before the end of the class, note any areas that you need to clarify with the instructor.
- Ask questions: Remember to take advantage of the expertise of the instructor. Do not go away from the class without trying to clear up areas of confusion!
- Digital recordings/Audiotape: Make recordings of classroom discussions, only with instructor permission, if:
  1. There is time to listen to them at some point (such as in the car).
  2. There are positive results from this process, with better understanding of the material and improved examination grades.

On Your Own

- Use available resources: Take advantage of all of the resources at the school, such as the library, computer laboratory, and skill laboratory. Make time to practice nursing techniques, watch DVDs or videos, and complete computer learning programs.
- Join/create a study group: Get together with other students in your class to review material. Study groups offer an opportunity to share information, challenge one another, and provide mutual support.
- Use time management techniques: Use available time as efficiently as possible. For example, the time that is spent waiting for an appointment or riding on public transportation may be used to read over materials or complete assignments.

Before an Examination

- Try to remain calm: Easy to recommend, but hard to do! Learn and use relaxation skills. Do not jump immediately into the examination. Relax and get focused first, then start the test.
- Be prepared: check with the instructor to be sure you have covered the content that will be on the examination. Bring the right materials: Pencils, pens, erasers, computer passwords, and so on. Leave enough time to get to the examination area so that there is no last-minute "rushing in."

During the Examination

- Read the questions carefully: Determine what the question is asking. Stay focused on the actual question without reading into the situations. If allowed to mark on the examination paper, underline key words or cross out unnecessary information to assist in getting to the heart of the question.
- Do not keep changing your answers: Most of the time, the first answer selected is correct. Do not change an answer unless you have remembered the correct response.
- Stay focused: Take brief moments during the examination, if necessary, to stop and use relaxation techniques to compose yourself.
- For multiple response (Select All That Apply), approach each answer as being True or False in relation to the question.
- When doing math of pharmacology, think about the answer that you obtain to see if it makes sense. How often would you give 10 tablets or 10 mL IM? If the answer does not seem realistic, re-calculate!

General Suggestions for Classroom-Based and Online Courses

- Review the syllabus in advance to identify the course requirements and expectations.
- Make a calendar to keep track of dates for examinations, quizzes, and assignments.
- Schedule time to study or complete assignments, especially if you are working.
- Connect with other students in the course electronically, by telephone, or in person.

- Take advantage of all of the available resources, such as online or on-campus tutorial programs.
- If your study habits are leading to positive results in the class, then don't make major changes. If, however, you are finding that you are not passing or just getting by in the course, you should talk with an instructor about how to change your approach in order to be more successful. Don't wait until it is too late to make a difference in your grade!
- Keep in contact with the instructor! Do not forget to ask questions.
- Maintain professional behavior with your instructors and classmates.

Contents

1 Nursing, Theory, and Professional Practice

CHAPTER REVIEW

Match the description/definition in Column A with the correct term in Column B.

Column A

_____ 1. Standards of right and wrong behavior

_____ 2. Treating the patient's physical, mental, emotional, spiritual, and social self

_____ 3. Learning the theory and skills for the nursing role

_____ 4. Process of entrusting or transferring the responsibility for certain tasks to other personnel

_____ 5. Statement about the beliefs and values of nursing in relation to a specific phenomenon, such as health

Column B

a. Delegation

b. Philosophy

c. Ethics

d. Holistic

e. Socialization

Complete the following:

6. Identify at least three common concepts from the definitions of nursing from the American Nurses Association, International Council of Nurses, and Virginia Henderson.

7. Identify the different nursing roles (e.g., advocate) that are indicated with the following situations:
   a. Patients need to be informed about their medications, procedures, diagnostics, and health promotion measures.
   b. Nurses provide direction and purpose to others, build a sense of commitment toward common goals, communicate effectively, and assist with addressing challenges.
   c. RNs, UAPs, LPNs, primary care providers, social workers, clergy, and therapists all interact productively to provide quality patient care.
   d. Nurses determine care concerns and ask questions about nursing practices.

8. Identify the following nurses:
   a. Founder of modern nursing _____
   b. Head of the U.S. Sanitary Commission _____
   c. Practiced nursing in the Civil War and established the American Red Cross _____
   d. America's first trained nurse _____

9. Identify the four general concepts that are addressed in a conceptual model for nursing.

10. What is the difference between a conceptual model and a theory?

11. Identify at least one concept included in the theories from each of the following nurse theorists:

Nurse Theorist	Theoretic Concept(s)
a. Nightingale	
b. Roy	
c. Rogers	
d. Orem	
e. Watson	

12. Indicate the levels in Maslow's hierarchy of needs pyramid.

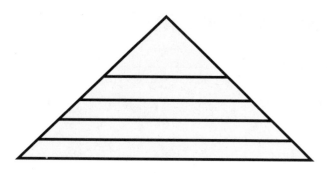

13. Identify at least three of the criteria that identify a profession.

14. Indicate the standard of care being demonstrated in practice or performance for each of the following:
    a. The RN admits the patient to the unit and collects comprehensive data on his health status.
    b. The nurse attends a conference and attends workshops on new techniques for patients with cardiac pathology.
    c. The primary nurse discusses the goals of treatment with the patient, family, and respiratory therapist.
    d. The RN documents the care provided to the patient and gives a report to the nurse on the next shift.
    e. Care is taken by the nurse to open and use only the supplies necessary for the dressing change.

15. Which of the following are core beliefs of individuals' perceptions in Rosenstock's health belief model? *Select all that apply.*
    a. Perceived susceptibility of their risk of getting the condition. _____
    b. Perceived anxiety over the treatment plan. _____
    c. Perceived severity of the seriousness of the condition. _____
    d. Perceived conflict with the health care providers. _____
    e. Perceived benefits of the positive consequences of adopting the behavior. _____

16. What is the primary purpose of a state's nurse practice act?

17. Identify two differences between the licensed practical nurse and the registered nurse.

18. How does certification differ from licensure?

19. Which of the following are being observed in society? *Select all that apply.*
    a. A majority of countries indicate that they are experiencing a nursing and midwifery shortage. _____
    b. The 65-year-old and older population is rapidly increasing. _____
    c. Developing countries are seeing the largest population growth. _____
    d. People worldwide are living longer and healthier lives. _____
    e. Nursing faculty numbers are remaining constant. _____
    f. Health care requirements of the world population are decreasing. _____

20. For the specified National Patient Safety Goals, indicate an example of how nurses can achieve each goal.
    a. Identify patients correctly.
    b. Prevent infection.
    c. Prevent mistakes in surgery.

21. Characteristics of collaboration among health care professionals include:

22. Provide an example of cultural competency for the nurse who is working with the following patients in the hospital:
    a. The patient speaks a different language.
    b. There are specific preferences for meals.

Select the best answer for each of the following questions:

23. According to the Agency for Healthcare Research and Quality, low health literacy is associated with which of the following?
    a. Increased hospitalizations
    b. Reduced emergency care use
    c. Greater use of diagnostic procedures, such as mammography
    d. Less hesitancy to receive vaccines

24. Which of the following actions indicates the act of refreezing in Lewin's change theory?
    a. A patient overcomes inertia and changes her mind set.
    b. There is a time of transition and confusion when change takes place.
    c. Change is completed, reinforced, and accepted.
    d. The right environment is created for change.

25. Florence Nightingale's theory focuses on which of the following?
    a. Environmental adaptation
    b. Interpersonal processes
    c. Energy fields
    d. Levels of systems

26. In reviewing the history of nursing, advances in health care and the role of nurses have been associated with which of the following?
    a. Weather disasters
    b. Military conflicts
    c. Women's rights movements
    d. Economic growth periods

Practice situation

Your neighbor asks you what kind of education is necessary to become a registered nurse. He says that the nurse in the clinic does much of what the doctor used to do for him, including writing his prescription.
a. What is your response regarding the education needed for registered nursing?
b. What educational preparation does the nurse in the clinic appear to possess?

REVIEW QUESTIONS

- How is nursing defined, and what are the commonalities in its definitions?
- What are the functions and roles of the nurse?
- Who are some of the major nursing theorists and what are the key components of their theories?
- What non-nursing theories influence nursing practice?
- What are the criteria for a profession, and how are they demonstrated in nursing?
- How are practice standards incorporated into the nursing profession?
- How does a state's nurse practice act influence care?
- How do nurses become socialized into the profession and nursing role?
- How can an individual become a nurse, and what are the role distinctions between the educational levels?
- Which nursing organizations exist, and what are their primary purposes?
- How can a nurse become certified?
- What are the current and future trends in society and health care?

2 Values, Beliefs, and Caring

CHAPTER REVIEW

Match the description/definition in Column A with the correct term in Column B.

Column A

_____ 1. Enduring ideas about what an individual considers is good, best, and the right thing to do

_____ 2. Belief about an individual, a group, or an event that is thought to be typical of all others in that category

_____ 3. A dysfunctional relationship in which the individual who wants to help acts in a manner that enables harmful behavior by another individual

_____ 4. A mental representation of reality or an individual's perceptions about what is right, true, or real, or what the individual expects to happen in a given situation

_____ 5. Broad statement or idea about people or things

_____ 6. Having concern or regard for that which affects the welfare of another

Column B

a. Beliefs

b. Generalization

c. Codependency

d. Values

e. Caring

f. Stereotype

Complete the following:

7. Provide an example of a value conflict that a nurse may have in caring for a patient.

8. Identify the appropriate interventions for the nurse who is assisting a patient through values clarification. *Select all that apply.*
   a. Being aware of the potential influence of the professional role. _____
   b. Identifying the nurse's values in the situation. _____
   c. Providing advice in difficult circumstances. _____
   d. Sharing information to assist in decision making. _____
   e. Avoiding direct confrontation and serious conflict. _____
   f. Using a very stern and serious approach to identify consequences. _____

9. The nurse is working with a patient who does not speak English. An interpreter is contacted and brought to the unit to relay information. Which of the following are appropriate interventions when an interpreter is used for patient communication? *Select all that apply.*
   a. It is best to use an interpreter whose age, gender, and background fit best with the patient or family. _____
   b. Do not brief the interpreter with information before the face-to-face translation. _____
   c. During face-to-face translation, be sure to look at the patient and not at the interpreter when speaking. _____
   d. Have the interpreter speak to the patient by starting with, "The nurse says... ." _____
   e. Use short sentences and stop often to allow time for the interpreter to translate. _____
   f. Ask the interpreter to paraphrase or abbreviate what the patient says. _____

10. Identify the main concept for each of the following theorists on caring and a real-life example of how the concept may be implemented by the nurse:

Theorist	Concept	Practice Example
a. Madeline Leininger		
b. Jean Watson		
c. Joyce Travelbee		
d. Kristen Swanson		

11. What behaviors are associated with codependency?

12. Identify an example for each of the following caring behaviors:
    a. Presence
    b. Consistency and predictability
    c. Touch

13. In a study conducted by Lohri-Posey (2005), the development of compassion was found to be related to several factors. Identify one of these factors.

14. Provide examples for diversity considerations for the following areas:
    a. Life span _____
    b. Cultural, ethnicity, and religion _____
    c. Disability _____

15. First-order beliefs are derived from _____
    _____.

Select the best answer for each of the following questions:

16. A subdimension of Swanson's process of caring, Knowing, involves which of the following?
    a. Sharing feelings with the patient
    b. Performing thorough assessments
    c. Focusing on the patient's experiences
    d. Offering realistic optimism

17. A patient expresses to the nurse that she is fearful of the upcoming surgery. Which caring behavior is being used by the nurse at this time?
    a. Listening
    b. Touch
    c. Predictability
    d. Consistency

18. The nurse has delegated the hygienic care of a patient to the nursing assistant. It is important to the nurse that the assistant treats the patient in a caring manner. Additional instruction is required if the nurse observes the nursing assistant doing which of the following?
    a. Asking the patient what preferences he has for personal care
    b. Having the patient assist with parts of the bath, as able
    c. Leaving the patient uncovered while the bath water is discarded
    d. Telling the patient that she will return shortly with new linens

Practice Situation

You have been assigned to the same patient each day you have worked during the past week. You have developed a good relationship with the patient. When you walk into the room to tell the patient that you will once again be caring for her during this shift, the patient does not seem to be her normal self. You ask the patient if she is okay.
a. What type of caring process/behavior are you demonstrating?

b. What will you do next in this situation?

REVIEW QUESTIONS

- What are the differences between beliefs and values, and how do they develop?
- How is the values clarification process used to deal with a values conflict?
- How do the beliefs of nurses and patients influence health care?
- What are the major concepts of four nursing theories of caring?
- How do nurses develop into caring professionals?
- What behaviors demonstrate caring?

3 Communication

CHAPTER REVIEW

Match the description/definition in Column A with the correct term in Column B.

Column A	Column B
_____ 1. The method of communication	a. Message
_____ 2. An event or thought initiating the communication	b. Assertiveness
_____ 3. Translate their thoughts and feelings into communication with a receiver	c. Sender
_____ 4. To sort out the meaning of what is being communicated	d. Proxemics
_____ 5. The person who initiates and encodes the communication	e. Encode
_____ 6. The study of the spatial requirements of humans and animals	f. Receiver
_____ 7. The response of the receiver	g. Channel
_____ 8. The person who receives and decodes, or interprets, the communication	h. Decode
_____ 9. The actual content transmitted during communication	i. Feedback
_____ 10. The ability to express ideas and concerns clearly while respecting the thoughts of others	j. Referent

Complete the following:

11. Interpretation of nonverbal communication may require further validation with the patient. Which of the following should prompt further physical assessment and/or discussion? The patient: *Select all that apply.*
    a. grimaces. _____
    b. ambulates independently and purposely. _____
    c. pulls away when touched. _____
    d. responds incongruently to questions asked. _____
    e. sits with the head down and shoulders slumped. _____
    f. maintains eye contact and nods during instruction. _____

12. Identify what emotions can be conveyed by patients through inflection.

13. Provide an example of how the nurse can use positive self-talk for a patient.

14. Per Quality and Safety Education for Nurses (QSEN), effective interdisciplinary communication is critical. Which communication and collaborative strategies can be implemented to promote patient safety?

15. Which of the following actions fall within accepted ethical guidelines? *Select all that apply.*
    a. Sharing personal information with the patient _____
    b. Posting photos of the patient on a social media site _____
    c. Refusing to provide health information on a patient to a caller from a newspaper _____
    d. Meeting with the patient for a social event after his or her hospitalization _____
    e. Speaking with other members of the health care team about the patient's status _____
    f. Telling the patient's roommate about the outcome of the patient's surgical procedure _____

16. What are the essential components of professional nursing communication?

17. What happens at each point of the helping relationship?
    a. Orientation phase

    b. Working phase

    c. Termination phase

18. Identify how each of the following factors can influence communication with patients and how the nurse can eliminate or reduce each one.
    a. Location

    b. Pain

19. Identify an example of how each of the following statements made by the nurse can become therapeutic communication.
    a. "I don't know why you don't take your medication, Mrs. Jones."

    b. "Try not to forget to use the call button if you need me."

    c. "Don't be concerned. I'm sure that the test results will be fine."

    d. "Honey, it's time for your bath."

20. For the acronym SOLER, identify what actions/skills are used.
    S—
    O—
    L—
    E—
    R—

21. How would you describe the location of the food on this plate to a visually impaired patient?

22. Identify communication strategies that may be used for a patient with expressive aphasia.

23. For the widely accepted method of hand-off communication, SBAR, identify what the acronym means.
    S—
    B—
    A—
    R—

24. Provide examples of nonverbal communication.

25. Which of the following statements made by the nurse are therapeutic? *Select all that apply.*
    a. "Everything will be okay." _____
    b. "I don't agree with what you want to do." _____
    c. "It's for your own good." _____
    d. "Have you made a decision about accepting the treatment?"

    _____
    e. "You seem happy about being discharged today." _____
    f. "So, there are two areas that you want more information about—your medications and diet." _____

26. What was identified as one of the top three causes of sentinel events from 2011–2013?

Select the best answer for each of the following questions:

27. The nurse tells the patient that he will stay until the physician comes back with the results of the diagnostic tests. This is an example of which communication technique?
    a. Using focused comments
    b. Providing general leads
    c. Validating
    d. Offering self

28. Which of the following statements is an example of reflecting?
    a. "Tell me more about how you feel."
    b. "What is your biggest concern?"
    c. "Your surgery is scheduled for 10 a.m. tomorrow morning."
    d. "You feel like the world is closing in on you and making it hard to breathe?"

29. During the storming phase of group development, the group leader:
    a. determines ground rules.
    b. works with members to resolve conflicts.
    c. encourages participation by all members.
    d. identifies the achievement of goals.

30. Which of the following behaviors is associated with the defense mechanism of displacement?
    a. After having a hard time at work, an individual comes home and yells at his spouse.
    b. The patient refuses to speak about the problem with the nurse.
    c. The individual takes on more responsibility at home.
    d. The patient does not believe that he has an addiction.

31. In the working phase of the helping relationship, the nurse expects to:
    a. observe and assess the patient.
    b. establish professional role boundaries.
    c. implement the care plan or contract.
    d. evaluate the outcomes achieved.

32. Which of the following actions are appropriate to use during communication with a patient who is hearing impaired?
    a. Facing the patient
    b. Standing over the patient
    c. Turning 3/4 away from the patient
    d. Raising the voice significantly

Practice Situation

You observe the new staff nurse and see that her uniform is wrinkled and soiled, her hair is unkempt, and she is wearing a lot of makeup and perfume.
a. How may this nurse's appearance influence communication with her patients?

b. What communication strategy would you use in this situation?

REVIEW QUESTIONS

- What are the key components of the communication process?
- What are examples of verbal and nonverbal modes of communication?
- How can the nurse interact with the patient without verbally communicating?
- How is the nursing process implemented within the nurse-patient helping relationship?
- Which factors affect the timing of patient communication?
- How are respect, assertiveness, collaboration, delegation, and advocacy incorporated in professional nursing communication?
- What are examples of social, therapeutic, and nontherapeutic communication techniques?
- What defense mechanisms may be used by patients while communicating, and how can they be recognized by the nurse?
- How can communication methods be adapted for patients with special needs?

4 Critical Thinking in Nursing

CHAPTER REVIEW

Match the description/definition in Column A with the correct term in Column B.

Column A

_____ 1. Uses specific facts or details to make conclusions and generalizations; proceeding from specific to general

_____ 2. A mutually supporting and sensible combination of combined thoughts, whereby the conclusion follows from presented facts

_____ 3. To focus on facts and ideas directly related and pertinent to the subject at hand

_____ 4. Using critical thinking, knowledge, and experience to develop solutions to problems and make decisions in a clinical setting

_____ 5. Gathering information to determine whether the information or data collected are factual and true

Column B

a. Clinical reasoning

b. Validation

c. Inductive reasoning

d. Logic

e. Relevance

Complete the following:

6. Identify at least four essential traits of critical thinking.

7. How does the nurse use *information gathering* in the critical thinking process?

8. Which critical thinking error is present in the following situations?
   a. Refusing to alter the procedure to accommodate the patient's preference for hygienic care

   b. Performing a treatment without knowing about the technique

   c. Deciding that the parents of a pediatric patient will be very meddlesome

   d. Making an incorrect connection between the patient's respiratory problems and their cause

9. How can critical thinking be used to meet the Quality and Safety Education for Nurses standard for patient safety?

10. What is the role of each of the following in improving critical thinking?
    a. Concept maps

    b. Simulation

    c. Discussion with colleagues

11. How is critical thinking used in the following steps of the nursing process?
    a. Assessment

    b. Implementation

Select the best answer for each of the following questions:

12. Which assessment question should the nurse use for the intellectual standard of clarity?
    a. "What are the most important things you need to know about your diet?"
    b. "Am I correct that you take two medications at home for your blood pressure?"
    c. "Have we talked about all of the issues that you have with wound care?"
    d. "Can you be more specific about the location of the discomfort?"

13. Which essential critical thinking trait is the nurse using when he/she tries out a new way to do a dressing?
    a. Curiosity
    b. Discipline
    c. Creativity
    d. Perseverance

14. The nurse on the surgical unit has a multiple-patient assignment. Upon beginning the shift, the nurse determines that the first patient to see in the morning is the individual who:
    a. has a blood pressure of 90/50.
    b. requires instruction for wound care.
    c. needs to be transferred from the bed to the chair.
    d. received pain medication 10 minutes ago.

15. For the process of reflection, the nurse asks himself or herself which of the following?
    a. "How should I report the increased blood pressure reading?"
    b. "Why is the patient having pain now?"
    c. "Did the patient's respiratory status just change?"
    d. "How should I have taught the patient to do self-injection more efficiently?"

16. The nurse is using the critical thinking trait of integrity when he or she does which of the following?
    a. Feels certain about being able to perform the skill
    b. Provides factual and honest information to the patient
    c. Considers all of the information before moving forward with the plan of care
    d. Follows an orderly approach to completing the required interventions

17. The nurse keeps working with the patient to help him ambulate, motivating him to reach his goal of being independent. The nurse is demonstrating which critical thinking trait?
    a. Confidence
    b. Humility
    c. Perseverance
    d. Fairness

Practice Situation

You have just come on to the unit and been given a multiple-patient assignment. Many medications and treatments have been ordered.
a. How can you apply critical thinking to this assignment?

b. What specific actions will you take to maintain patient safety?

REVIEW QUESTIONS

- What is the relationship between critical thinking and clinical reasoning?
- How do theories of critical thinking apply to professional nursing practice?
- What are the intellectual standards of critical thinking?
- What are the critical-thinking components and attitudes?
- How can critical thinking be applied in nursing practice?
- How can critical thinking be applied to provide safe patient care and avoid errors?
- What methods can be used to improve critical thinking in nursing?

5 | Introduction to the Nursing Process

CHAPTER REVIEW

Match the description/definition in Column A with the correct term in Column B.

Column A

_____ 1. Includes initiating specific nursing interventions and treatments

_____ 2. Determination of whether the patient's goals are met, examination of the effectiveness of interventions

_____ 3. Patient care data are gathered through observation, interviews

_____ 4. A listing of behaviors or observable items that indicate attainment of a goal

_____ 5. Data are analyzed, validated, and clustered to identify patient problems

Column B

a. Assessment

b. Nursing diagnosis

c. Outcome identification

d. Implementation

e. Evaluation

Complete the following:

6. How is the nursing process defined?

7. What are the characteristics of the nursing process?

8. Who is the primary source of data?

9. For the following, indicate which are examples of objective data. *Select all that apply.*
   a. Patient tells the nurse, "I feel hungry." _____
   b. Blood pressure 140/90 _____
   c. Rash noted on lower right abdomen _____
   d. Patient informs the nurse that he did not eat breakfast _____
   e. Uneven gait on ambulation _____
   f. Potassium level noted in electronic medical record as 4.3 _____

10. What are the components of actual, risk, and health promotion diagnoses?

11. Who may be involved in collaborative care for a patient?

12. Identify the essential qualities of patient goals.

13. What are clinical pathways and protocols/standing orders, and how are they used by the nurse?

14. For the following patient assessments, identify possible nursing diagnoses:
    a. The patient is not drinking enough fluids and has dry mucous membranes and poor skin turgor.

    b. The patient has difficulty emptying the bladder following lower abdominal surgery.

    c. With an inner ear problem, the patient has been experiencing some dizziness during ambulation.

15. Revise the following in order to meet the criteria for patient goals:
    a. The patient will report feeling more comfort.

    b. Urinary output will be satisfactory.

16. What would be an outcome identification for the following goal?

    The pressure ulcer will be free of infection during the healing and treatment.

17. How would you evaluate the patient's achievement of the goal on the basis of the observations noted?

    Goal—Patient will report a pain level of 2 to 3 out of 10 during a.m. care within 24 hours.

    During a.m. care, the patient indicated that the pain level was about 5 on a scale of 10. It was noted that he was protecting the surgical site and his apical pulse was 108 bpm.

Select the best answer for each of the following questions:

18. The patient tells the nurse that she is not confident with self-injection of insulin. The nurse should use which of the following to validate this information from the patient?
    a. Ask the family how the patient performed the self-injection.
    b. Confer with the other staff members to see how the technique was taught to the patient.
    c. Determine what insulin was prescribed by the provider.
    d. Observe the patient giving the insulin injection.

19. For a patient who has chronic obstructive pulmonary disease with an excess of secretions in the bronchioles, which nursing diagnosis is most appropriate?
    a. Ineffective airway clearance
    b. Altered respiratory pattern
    c. High risk of asphyxia
    d. Difficulty maintaining spontaneous ventilation

20. Which of the following nursing interventions is most clearly stated and will assist other staff members to provide safe care?
    a. Provide extra fluids.
    b. Increase ambulation in hallway.
    c. Reinforce use of incentive spirometer t.i.d.
    d. Complete physical assessment with patient in the a.m.

21. The nurse is working with a patient who has the following signs and symptoms: weight gain, edema to the lower extremities, increased blood pressure, and abdominal distention. On the basis of this information, which of the following is the most appropriate nursing diagnosis?
    a. Altered nutrition: intake exceeds the body's needs
    b. Excess fluid volume
    c. Urinary retention
    d. High risk of trauma

22. In planning for the patient assignment, the nurse prioritizes a schedule on the basis of the patient's needs and conditions. In reviewing the nursing diagnoses, which of the following patients should be seen first in the morning?
    a. Urinary, impaired elimination
    b. Altered sleep pattern
    c. Decreased cardiac output
    d. Self-care deficit: grooming

23. Which of the following is the best example of a measurable patient goal? The patient will:
    a. ambulate independently at least 20 feet in the hallway by the end of the week.
    b. be seen by the nurse for regular monitoring of blood pressure.
    c. increase intake of potassium-rich foods.
    d. have less pain and anxiety.

24. The nurse asks a colleague to look at the care plan that has been developed with the patient. The colleague suggests that the best risk-oriented nursing diagnosis statement is:
    a. Risk for knowledge deficit
    b. Risk for increased weight gain
    c. Risk for airway problems related to having had a stroke
    d. Risk for injury with lower-extremity weakness

25. For the patient with a nursing diagnosis of *high risk of aspiration,* the nurse anticipates that there will be goals and interventions related to safety observations during:
    a. feeding.
    b. bathing.
    c. ambulating.
    d. transferring.

26. Which of the following is the best example of a measurable patient goal? The patient will:
    a. sit out of bed in the chair.
    b. eat low-sodium foods.
    c. verbalize feelings about surgery at some point.
    d. identify the five major drug side effects before discharge tomorrow.

Practice Situation

Your patient has been recently diagnosed with diabetes mellitus type 2. With no prior history in his family, he is unfamiliar with the diet and treatments. He will require an oral hypoglycemic medication, as well as information about the prescribed diet.
a. What other information may be important to assess for this patient?

b. Start a care map for this patient.

REVIEW QUESTIONS

- How is the *nursing process* defined?
- What is the historical development and significance of the nursing process?
- What are the characteristics of the nursing process?
- What are the steps in the nursing process?
- How is the nursing process cyclic and dynamic in nature?
- How are nursing diagnoses, goals/outcomes, and nursing interventions decided on and written?
- What is the purpose of a care plan?

Chapter **5** **Introduction to the Nursing Process**

6 Assessment

CHAPTER REVIEW

Match the description/definition in Column A with the correct term in Column B.

Column A

_____ 1. The use of touch to assess body organs and skin texture, temperature, moisture, turgor, tenderness, and thickness

_____ 2. A subjective indication of a disease or a change in condition as perceived by the patient

_____ 3. Information shared by family members, friends, or other members of the health care team

_____ 4. The use of vision, hearing, and smell to closely scrutinize physical characteristics of a whole person and individual body systems

_____ 5. Conclusions

_____ 6. Includes all pertinent information that can guide the development of a patient-centered plan of care

_____ 7. A technique of listening, with the assistance of a stethoscope, to sounds made by organs or systems such as the heart, blood vessels, lungs, and abdominal cavity

_____ 8. Tapping the patient's skin with short, sharp strokes that cause a vibration to travel through the skin and to the upper layers of the underlying structures

Column B

a. Symptom

b. Percussion

c. Inferences

d. Health history

e. Palpation

f. Inspection

g. Secondary data

h. Auscultation

Complete the following:

9. What are the different methods that may be used by the nurse for patient assessment?

10. For each of the senses, identify what information the nurse can gather.
   a. Sight

   b. Hearing

   c. Touch

   d. Smell

11. The nurse is asking the patient about the family medical history. What information will the nurse want to obtain?

12. How can the nurse arrange the environment so that a patient interview will be most effective?

13. What are the usual components of a health history?

14. The nurse wants to know if there is fluid in the abdominal cavity. What physical assessment technique(s) should be used?

15. What should the nurse do to prepare the patient and environment for the physical assessment?

16. In an emergency assessment, the nurse will pay particular attention to:

17. The patient is unconscious following a motor vehicle accident. How does the nurse obtain information on this patient?

18. Along with physical data, the nurse will collect information from the patient about:

19. Which of the following are included in the orientation/ introductory phase of the patient interview? *Select all that apply.*
    a. Establishing the name by which the patient prefers to be called _____
    b. Providing personal information to the patient _____
    c. Using all open-ended questions _____
    d. Being seated at eye level with the patient _____
    e. Avoiding maintaining eye contact _____
    f. Asking all of the family members to remain _____

20. Provide an example of a question that could be used during a review of systems.

21. How does the nurse prepare for a physical assessment?

22. What are the three kinds of physical assessments that can be performed by the nurse and when are they usually conducted?

23. The patient tells the nurse that she feels lightheaded when she goes from lying down to sitting up. What further information will the nurse want to obtain to validate this finding?

24. In a body systems model for data organization, identify how the following signs and symptoms should be organized:
    a. Episodes of chest pain

    b. Decreased range of motion to the left knee

    c. Periodic epigastric distress after eating

25. The nurse observes that the patient is unable to independently move to the examination table. What action should be taken by the nurse?

26. Provide an example of a question that a nurse can ask to determine the patient's level of knowledge about the medical diagnosis.

27. Which of the following are demographic data? *Select all that apply.*
    a. Gender _____
    b. Medications _____
    c. Educational level _____
    d. Spiritual preferences _____
    e. Date of last tuberculosis test _____
    f. Use of tobacco and alcohol _____

Select the best answer for each of the following questions:

28. Which of the following information is classified by the nurse as subjective data from the patient?
    a. "I feel dizzy."
    b. There is a red area on the abdomen.
    c. An oral temperature reading is 99° F.
    d. The hematocrit is below the expected level.

29. The new nursing staff member is observed by the unit manager during a patient interview. Which of the following behaviors should the manager identify to the new nurse to *avoid?*
    a. Using a moderate tone of voice
    b. Sitting close and leaning toward the patient
    c. Asking open-ended questions
    d. Tapping her pen on the bedside table

30. During the termination phase of the patient interview, the nurse does which of the following?
    a. Prepares the environment
    b. Performs the physical examination
    c. Sets goals with the patient for care
    d. Summarizes and validates information from the patient

31. For Baby Boomers, which of the following is a generational factor that may influence behavior?
    a. Being slow to warm up
    b. Expecting detailed information
    c. Being very technologically literate
    d. Having very short attention spans

32. Which of the following actions can be safely delegated to unlicensed assistive personnel?
    a. Assessment of a patient who has just had surgery
    b. Determination of the patient's level of stability when using crutches
    c. Measurement of vital signs on a stable patient
    d. Provision of analgesic medications

33. In a five-tier triage system, what finding is designated as Level 2—Emergent?
   a. Cardiac arrest
   b. Severe pain
   c. Dehydration
   d. Abrasion

Practice Situation

You have performed an assessment on the patient and found the following:

   The patient has an active social life, spending time with friends after work. His caloric intake is appropriate for his size. He has no difficulty with breathing and no cardiovascular symptoms. His vision and hearing are acute.
• Organize the data according to functional health patterns.

REVIEW QUESTIONS

• What are the methods used during the assessment phase of the nursing process?
• What techniques are used by the nurse during a physical assessment?
• What are the three types of physical assessment?
• Which types of data are collected during the assessment process?
• How does the nurse validate patient assessment data?
• How can data be organized according to established theoretical frameworks?

7 | Nursing Diagnosis

CHAPTER REVIEW

Match the description/definition in Column A with the correct term in Column B.

Column A

_____ 1. The identification of actual or potential health problems/life processes and responses to a problem

_____ 2. Identified from the North American Nursing Diagnosis Association International (NANDA-I) list of approved diagnostic statements

_____ 3. A unified language classification system

_____ 4. Clustered supporting data

_____ 5. Organizing patient assessment data into groupings with similar etiologies

Column B

a. Clustering

b. Defining characteristics

c. Diagnosis label

d. Nursing diagnosis

e. Taxonomy

Complete the following:

6. What are the three types of nursing diagnoses?

7. How does a nursing diagnosis differ from a medical diagnosis?

8. What is NANDA and what is its role?

9. For the following patient information, identify how they may be clustered into a diagnostic label:
   - States, "I am very thirsty"
   - Reports weight loss of 5 lbs over the past 3 days
   - Complains of feeling tired
   - Has increased hematocrit and creatinine
   - Has decreased blood pressure with a slight increase in body temperature

10. Identify the errors that the nurse should avoid when formulating nursing diagnoses.

11. For the label of Impaired Gas Exchange, indicate which defining characteristics are most appropriate to include in the diagnostic statement. *Select all that apply.*
    a. Emphysema _____
    b. Diminished lung sounds to R lower lung base _____
    c. Pulse oximetry of 89% _____
    d. Weight gain—5% in 2 weeks _____
    e. Pain in lower R leg on ambulation _____
    f. Crackles heard on auscultation _____

Select the best answer for each of the following questions:

12. Nursing diagnoses are primarily used in order to:
    a. make all of the patient's problems easier to solve.
    b. assist the medical provider to determine care.
    c. meet accreditation requirements.
    d. facilitate clear communication of patient needs.

13. Which of the following actual nursing diagnoses best meets the criteria for a diagnostic statement?
    a. Impaired physical mobility R/T reduced range of motion as manifested by slow, unsteady gait.
    b. Excess fluid volume R/T loss of body weight.
    c. Risk for constipation R/T fluid intake and movement.
    d. Readiness for enhanced learning R/T knowledge deficit.

14. The nurse is concerned that the patient has developed atelectasis following surgery. Which of the following is an appropriate diagnostic label for this problem?
    a. Ineffective airway clearance
    b. Impaired gas exchange
    c. Decreased cardiac output
    d. Impaired spontaneous ventilation

17

15. For the nursing diagnosis, *Altered speech related to recent neurological disturbances as evidenced by an inability to speak coherently,* the etiology is:
    a. altered speech.
    b. as evidenced by.
    c. recent neurological disturbances.
    d. inability to speak coherently.

16. Which of the following nursing diagnoses best meets the criteria for a diagnostic statement?
    a. Risk for diarrhea with the risk factor of the possible side effect of antibiotic therapy
    b. Risk for heart disease with the risk factor of smoking
    c. Risk for urinary retention following catheter removal
    d. Risk for pneumonia

17. For the health-promotion nursing diagnosis of *Readiness for enhanced nutrition,* which of the following is the most appropriate defining characteristic?
    a. Inability to feed self
    b. Diminished oral intake
    c. Reduction in body mass and strength
    d. Identification of healthy food choices

18. For the patient with the nursing diagnosis of *Activity Intolerance,* the nurse expects that the patient will specifically demonstrate:
    a. elevated body temperature.
    b. disinterest in diversional activities.
    c. dyspnea on exertion.
    d. erythema.

Practice Situation

Your patient has been recently diagnosed with diabetes mellitus type 2. With no prior history in his family, he is unfamiliar with the diet and treatments. He will require an oral hypoglycemic medication, as well as information about the prescribed diet. He tells you, "I don't have any idea of what I will have to do."
a. What are the key pieces of data in this patient's assessment?

b. Identify at least one nursing diagnosis for this patient.

REVIEW QUESTIONS

- What are the steps in the formulation of nursing diagnoses?
- How were NANDA-I and the nursing taxonomy developed?
- What are the differences among the three types of nursing diagnostic statements?
- How are actual, risk, and health-promotion nursing diagnoses accurately written?
- How can the nurse avoid common problems associated with the diagnostic process?
- How does the nursing diagnosis contribute to the individualized care of patients?

8 Planning

CHAPTER REVIEW

Complete the following:

1. Identify the difference between long- and short-term goals.

2. What is the first step in the planning phase of the nursing process?

3. How does involving the patient and/or family in planning help to improve goal attainment?

4. Place the following examples of patient needs in priority order (first to fifth), according to Maslow's hierarchy:
   a. Autonomy _____
   b. Compassion of care provider _____
   c. Oxygen level _____
   d. Ability to perform role functions _____
   e. Physical safety _____

5. What are the ABCs of life support?

6. Provide an example of how the nurse and patient may have conflicting priorities for care.

7. Describe the characteristics that make goals most effective.

8. Revise the following goal statements to make them more precise, time oriented, and measurable.
   a. Temperature will be normal.

   b. The patient will walk more.

   c. The diet will be understood.

9. For the revised goal statements in the previous question, identify the outcome indicators.

10. What are the five key elements that are considered for nursing interventions?

11. Provide examples for each type of nursing interventions.
    a. Independent (nurse initiated)

    b. Dependent

    c. Collaborative

12. When should discharge planning begin for the patient in acute care?

13. What effect could a patient's disability have in determining goals?

14. In writing goal statements, it is important to use measurable verbs. Identify the verbs that are best to use in developing measurable and patient-oriented goal statements. *Select all that apply.*
    a. Understand _____
    b. Verbalize _____
    c. Know _____
    d. Perform _____
    e. Think _____
    f. List _____

15. What is one of the major challenges that nurses face in providing health information to patients?

16. On the basis of the following nursing diagnoses, identify a goal and outcome indicator(s) for each.
    a. Nutrition, imbalanced: more than body requirements

    b. Pain related to surgical incision

Select the best answer for each of the following questions:

17. Which one of the following is associated with specifically meeting the Quality and Safety Education for Nurses Teamwork and Collaboration competencies?
    a. Providing the patient with the schedule for diagnostic testing
    b. Assessing the patient's level of pain
    c. Engaging the patient in conversation
    d. Working with the patient and nutritionist

18. The nurse receives the patient assignment in the morning. Which one of the patients should be seen first? The patient who:
    a. takes a hypnotic medication at bedtime.
    b. has fluctuations in blood sugar readings.
    c. needs assistance with morning care.
    d. has an order for a daily dressing change.

19. The patient works in a tailor shop and is having surgery to correct bilateral cataracts. If all of the following are realistic, what is the long-term goal for this patient?
    a. Return to his occupation
    b. Prevention of ocular infection
    c. Independent performance of hygienic care
    d. Self-administration of eye drops postoperatively

20. A goal for a patient who is hypertensive is a return to expected limits. Which one of the following outcome indicators is most appropriate?
    a. Patient expresses decreased discomfort q3h
    b. Patient identifies two things that reduce stress
    c. Patient will not experience headaches
    d. Patient's blood pressure is between 120/80 mm Hg and 130/90 mm Hg

21. Which one of the following interventions is considered independent or nurse initiated?
    a. Teaching the patient about the therapeutic diet
    b. Giving an enema in preparation for radiologic testing
    c. Providing analgesics for postoperative discomfort
    d. Administering wound care

22. Which one of the following best meets the criteria for a goal statement?
    a. Respiratory rate will remain within 20-24 breaths per minute through discharge
    b. Patient will ambulate in the hallway frequently
    c. Treatment regimen will be understood
    d. Patient will describe activity restrictions

Practice Situation

Your patient has been recently diagnosed with diabetes mellitus type 2. With no prior history in his family, he is unfamiliar with the diet and treatments. He will require an oral hypoglycemic medication, as well as information about the prescribed diet. He expresses to you that he does not know how he will manage the diabetes.
a. On the basis of these data, identify a nursing diagnosis. You may use the one that you formulated for Chapter 7.

b. Specify at least one short-term goal for the nursing diagnosis selected.

REVIEW QUESTIONS

- What nursing actions occur during the planning process?
- How does the nurse prioritize patient care?
- What is included in the development of goals?
- How are outcome identification and goal attainment related?
- What are the different formats in which patient-centered plans of care can be developed?
- What are the three different types of nursing interventions?
- How is planning an important process throughout all of patient care?

9 Implementation and Evaluation

CHAPTER REVIEW

Complete the following:

1. What actions are involved in implementing the nursing process?

2. Provide examples of direct and indirect nursing care.

3. Safe practice requires that the nurse check the patient's identity. What two methods are commonly used to identify patients?

4. What is the purpose of continual patient reassessment?

5. Identify the tasks that are included in activities of daily living (ADLs).

6. Provide at least three examples of what a nurse may teach a patient and/or family.

7. What circumstances can lead the nurse to refer a patient to a specialized service?

8. What resources are available to nurses to obtain evidence-based practice information?

9. How can the nurse be a patient advocate?

10. What are the five rights of delegation?

11. Provide examples of prevention-oriented nursing interventions.

12. Which of the following are independent nursing interventions? *Select all that apply.*
    a. Administering an IV antibiotic _____
    b. Cleaning a wound and applying a dressing _____
    c. Providing emotional support _____
    d. Administering oxygen _____
    e. Performing oral care _____
    f. Repositioning the patient in bed _____

13. Carrying out standing orders limits the responsibility of the nurse.

    True _____   False _____

14. For the outcomes, which patient information indicates that the goal was achieved? *Select all that apply.*

a. Pain level less than 5 on a 0-10 scale	An expression of pain of 6 out of 10
b. Urinary output of 100 mL/hour	Output of 600 mL in 8-hour shift
c. Reduction in pressure ulcer to 3-5 cm	Pressure ulcer 4.2 cm
d. Ambulate independently tid.	Ambulated without assistance at 11 a.m., 3 p.m., and 8 p.m.
e. Demonstrate colostomy care technique	Able to identify necessary supplies, unable to prepare the skin and apply the bag
f. Anxiety level of less than 2+ preoperatively	1+ anxiety noted

15. If a patient achieves the identified goals, the nurse should continue to address them in the care plan.

   True _____   False _____

16. How do the following influence patient care?
   a. Life span

   b. Gender

   c. Culture

17. What is an advantage of the electronic health record (EHR) in planning and implementing care?

Select the best answer for each of the following questions:

18. Which of the following actions is considered indirect patient care?
   a. Providing assistance with ambulation
   b. Starting an IV line
   c. Making a change-of-shift report
   d. Teaching the patient about the prescribed medications

19. For a patient with a nursing diagnosis of *Impaired physical mobility related to bilateral arm casts,* the nurse should select which of the following direct care interventions?
   a. Counseling
   b. Teaching
   c. Reassessment
   d. Assisting with ADLs

20. The patient is seen in the clinic for her first prenatal visit. It is determined that, by the next visit, the patient should be able to identify five symptoms that indicate a possible problem with the pregnancy. On her return to the clinic, the patient can state three symptoms. The evaluation for this patient goal is which of the following?
   a. Goal met; patient able to state sufficient symptoms
   b. Goal partially met; patient able to state three of five symptoms
   c. Goal not met; patient unable to state all five symptoms
   d. Goal not met; patient identifies three of the symptoms

21. The nurse is working with a postoperative patient on the surgical unit. Which aspect of care demonstrates a manipulation of the patient's environment?
   a. Providing wound care
   b. Administering analgesic medication
   c. Making sure that the room is warm enough
   d. Measuring the patient's vital signs

22. An antibiotic medication is administered to the patient. Shortly afterward, the patient develops itching and redness of the skin. If an antihistamine is given to the patient to counteract the antibiotic's effect, then the nurse is:
   a. compensating for adverse reactions.
   b. preparing for a special procedure.
   c. assisting with ADLs.
   d. using preventive measures.

Practice Situations

Your patient has been recently diagnosed with diabetes mellitus type 2. With no prior history in his family, he is unfamiliar with the diet and treatments. He will require an oral hypoglycemic medication, as well as information about the prescribed diet.
   a. On the basis of these data, identify a nursing diagnosis. You may use the one that you formulated for Chapter 7.

   b. Specify at least one short-term goal for the nursing diagnosis selected.

   c. Indicate which intervention(s) you will implement to meet the goal.

Another nurse does not accurately document that the patient is allergic to a medication.
   a. What is a possible consequence of this omission?

   b. What should have been done and when?

REVIEW QUESTIONS

- What is the significance of implementation and evaluation in the nursing process?
- What are the different types of direct-care interventions?
- What are various forms of indirect-care interventions?
- What are examples of independent nursing interventions?
- How are dependent nursing interventions different from independent interventions?
- What is the significance of documentation within the implementation step?
- How are evaluation principles applied within the nursing process?
- What is the relationship between care plan modification and quality improvement?

10 Documentation, Electronic Health Records, and Reporting

CHAPTER REVIEW

Complete the following:

1. Identify the meaning of each of the following acronyms.
   a. APIE
   b. MAR
   c. EHR
   d. SBAR
   e. HIPAA
   f. BCMA
   g. POMR

2. What is the purpose of documentation?

3. Identify the guidelines for documenting.

4. Describe the advantages and disadvantages of paper and electronic health records.

5. What are the major components of the electronic health record?

6. Indicate the ways in which patient data can be put into the electronic health record.

7. Select an appropriate Quality and Safety Education for Nurses competency and describe the relationship of documentation and reporting to the competency/focus.

8. What is meant by point-of-care documentation?

9. How does the nurse maintain confidentiality of electronic health records?

10. Do-not-use abbreviations can be a threat to patient safety. The nurse is reviewing patients' records and sees the following abbreviations. Which of these should not be used? *Select all that apply.*
    a. QOD _____
    b. tid. _____
    c. IU _____
    d. mL _____
    e. MS _____
    f. hs _____

11. Explain charting by exception.

12. How can the following notations be corrected or improved?
    a. The patient ate well.

    b. The patient's mood was poor.

    c. VS were normal.

13. What information is usually included in an admission and discharge note?

14. Documenting within a legal and ethical framework is critical. Identify which of the following actions are within the guidelines for documentation. *Select all that apply.*
    a. Completely erasing or deleting any errors _____
    b. Charting as soon as care is completed _____
    c. Documenting personal opinions about the patient _____
    d. Making sure that the patient is unable to see the record. _____
    e. Dating and signing each written entry. _____
    f. Allowing a co-worker to use your electronic health record password. _____

15. In accordance with HIPAA, what are the only uses for protected health information?

16. What are the different types of handoff reports, and what is their purpose?

17. What is the ANTICipate Model?

18. What are the guidelines for taking telephone and verbal orders?

19. When is an incident report completed?

Select the best answer for each of the following questions:

20. Which of the following is the best information to put in a flow sheet format?
    a. Admission note
    b. Diagnostic test results
    c. Provider's orders
    d. Vital sign measurements

21. It is the current belief that patient handoffs can be improved with which of the following actions?
    a. Use of standardized bedside shift reports
    b. Recorded messages left for oncoming staff
    c. Application of DAR recording
    d. Sharing written documents

22. The use of telephone and verbal orders has been reduced as a result of which of the following?
    a. More standing orders for patients in acute care environments
    b. The use of computerized order entry for the electronic health record
    c. The requirement for all orders to be in writing
    d. Staffing issues

23. For a patient-related incident report, which of the following is correct?
    a. The report is included in the patient's record.
    b. Only subjective information from the patient is included.
    c. Possible causes of the incident are identified.
    d. The nurse includes how the patient was found.

24. Which one of the following is the most correct notation for the nurse to make in the record?
    a. "Dr. Green made an error in the amount of medication to administer, so re-calculation was done."
    b. "Verbalized sharp pain to lower right side of the abdomen."
    c. "Nurse Barber spoke with the patient about the diet."
    d. "The patient was upset with the respiratory therapist."

Practice Situations

The patient has just been diagnosed with hypertension. He was anxious about learning how to manage his blood pressure medications and new diet restrictions. The patient told you that he has never had to take medications regularly and does not really understand the diet. You discuss the patient's treatment regimen with him and his spouse. A referral is made to the nutritionist. At the next clinic visit, the patient can accurately discuss his diet and medications.
a. Document the patient situation using a problem, intervention, and evaluation and/or data, action, and response format.

At the end of your shift, you have identified a nursing diagnosis of *Fluid Volume, Excess*. The patient is on fluid restrictions and a reduced-sodium diet and takes a diuretic.
a. On the basis of the information provided, what information will you need to include in a handoff report?

REVIEW QUESTIONS

- What are the standards for effective documentation by nurses?
- What are the functions of the medical record, including the electronic health record?
- How should nursing documentation be completed in the electronic and medical records?
- How do *privacy* and *confidentiality* relate to information in a medical record?
- Which standardized formats are used for handoffs and change-of-shift reports?
- How does the nurse accept and confirm verbal and telephone orders?
- What is the proper use and documentation of incident reports?

Ethical and Legal Considerations

CHAPTER REVIEW

Match the description/definition in Column A with the correct term in Column B.

Column A

_____ 1. Civil law

_____ 2. Assault

_____ 3. Slander

_____ 4. Felony

_____ 5. Malpractice

_____ 6. Accountability

_____ 7. Tort

_____ 8. Libel

_____ 9. Battery

_____ 10. Negligence

Column B

a. Creating a risk of harm to others by failing to do something that a "reasonable person" would ordinarily do or doing something that a "reasonable person" would ordinarily not do

b. Actual physical harm caused to another person

c. Wrongs committed against another person that do not involve a contract

d. A threat of bodily harm or violence

e. The concept of being answerable for one's actions

f. Governs unjust acts against individuals, rather than federal or state crimes

g. Written forms of defamation of character

h. Negligence committed by a person functioning within a professional role

i. A more serious crime that results in the perpetrator being imprisoned in a state or federal facility for more than 1 year

j. Oral defamation of character

Complete the following:

11. What are ethics, and how are they developed?

12. Identify a major concept of the following ethical theories:
    a. Deontology _____
    b. Utilitarianism _____

13. For the following ethical concepts, provide an example of how each one has an impact on nursing care:
    a. Advocacy _____
    b. Autonomy _____
    c. Beneficence _____
    d. Confidentiality _____
    e. Veracity _____

14. A nurse who makes a medication error demonstrates accountability when he or she does what?

15. Identify examples of situations where the concept of non-maleficence may be in direct conflict with health care practice.

16. A student finds out that a peer in the class has plagiarized a large part of her research paper. What should the student do?

17. What are the roles of an ethics committee?

18. What are key concepts of civility?

19. Identify and define the four major sources of law that have an impact on professional nursing.

20. What are some general expectations for nurses based on the professional Code of Ethics?

21. What are some specific ethical considerations for nursing students?

22. Identify at least two bioethical challenges in health care today.

23. Provide examples of felonies that are specific to nursing.

24. What are the four components ("four D's") of negligence?

25. Indicate at least two ways that nurses avoid charges of malpractice.

26. Students are automatically covered by a school's malpractice insurance.

    True _____   False _____

27. Which of the following are professional boundary violations? *Select all that apply.*
    a. Documenting punctually _____
    b. Intervening in personal patient relationships _____
    c. Following legal guidelines _____
    d. Keeping secrets with a patient _____
    e. Spending excessive time with one patient _____
    f. Maintaining confidentiality _____

28. What are other examples of nursing practice misconduct?

29. Which of the following patients are *not* able to give consent? *Select all that apply.*
    a. An adult patient who has received preoperative medications _____
    b. The legal guardian _____
    c. A mentally competent adult _____
    d. A married 16-year-old _____
    e. An intoxicated adult _____
    f. The health care proxy _____

30. Indicate at least two documentation errors that can be legal violations.

31. What are some legal considerations for organ donation?

32. Identify some of the general patient expectations in the Patient's Bill of Rights.

33. The three documents that are part of advance directives are:

34. Health Insurance Portability and Accountability Act (HIPAA) seeks to limit access of protected health information (PHI). What is PHI?

35. Answer the following questions regarding standards of care:
    a. What are they?

    b. How are they developed?

    c. Which organization identifies them for nursing?

36. What is the difference between licensure and certification?

37. Part of HIPAA is the Privacy Rule, the purpose of which is:

38. Identify which of the following are accurate in regard to Good Samaritan Acts. *Select all that apply.*
    a. All 50 states have enacted these laws. _____
    b. Protection is provided if a fee is charged for services. _____
    c. Care given needs to be within the scope of knowledge of the provider. _____
    d. Permission for treatment may be necessary before providing care. _____
    e. Health care professionals in some states are required to provide assistance. _____
    f. Negligence is overlooked in emergency situations. _____

39. What are the two criteria for establishing a patient's death?

40. How do Natural Death Acts differ from assisted suicide or euthanasia?

41. Individuals who are protected under the Americans with Disabilities Act (ADA) include:

42. The nurse goes to apply a restraint to a patient. What does the nurse need to do to be in line with legal guidelines?

43. Which of the following are principles from HIPAA? *Select all that apply.*
    a. Patients must be offered a notice of their rights under this act. _____
    b. Provisions are made only for electronic health records. _____
    c. Patient names cannot be posted or released. _____
    d. Discussions cannot be held about patients. _____
    e. Individual facilities must have specific policies and procedures in place. _____
    f. Access passwords can be shared among unit staff. _____

Select the best answer for each of the following questions:

44. Which one of the following actions specifically demonstrates that the nurse is practicing the ethical principle of fidelity?
    a. Calling the patient in for the clinic appointment at the arranged time
    b. Telling the patient about the complications of the surgical procedure
    c. Learning about the technique for an unfamiliar patient care skill
    d. Reporting on the patient's concerns regarding a medication

45. The nurse goes into the room to give the patient an intramuscular medication. The patient refuses, but the nurse proceeds with the injection. The nurse is committing which of the following?
    a. Assault
    b. Defamation
    c. Battery
    d. Invasion of privacy

46. A competent adult patient wants to leave the medical center, but the nurses believe that would be detrimental to the patient's health. If the patient is not allowed to leave, the nurses should:
    a. restrain the patient.
    b. call for a security officer.
    c. contact the agency's legal representative.
    d. have the patient sign an against-medical-advice form.

47. A nurse goes to another unit to see a friend who has been admitted. The nurse goes to look at her friend's medical record. This is an example of which of the following?
    a. Invasion of privacy
    b. Malpractice
    c. Incivility
    d. Liability

48. The nurse enters a patient's room to obtain the informed consent and discovers that the patient has no idea about the possible complications of the surgery. The nurse should:
    a. continue having the patient sign the consent form.
    b. explain the possible complications of the surgery.
    c. request that the physician come and speak to the patient.
    d. document the information in the patient's record.

49. A living will serves to:
    a. identify a patient's wishes for distribution of property after death.
    b. specify desires for end-of-life care.
    c. designate a person to have decision-making authority.
    d. limit medical care that will be provided.

50. A patient has been diagnosed with cancer, but the primary care provider is hesitant to share the information with her. The nurse encourages the provider to tell the patient so that she can make decisions about her care. The nurse is using the ethical principle of:
    a. justice.
    b. fidelity.
    c. veracity.
    d. nonmaleficence.

51. Patient advocacy is best demonstrated by the nurse:
    a. learning how to do a new procedure safely.
    b. returning to speak with the patient at an agreed-upon time.
    c. preparing the patient's room for comfort and privacy.
    d. supporting the patient's right to refuse treatment.

52. Which one of the following statements is accurate in regard to end-of-life issues?
    a. A competent adult may refuse treatment.
    b. Assisted suicide is a constitutional right.
    c. Passive euthanasia is illegal throughout the United States.
    d. Organ donation must be attempted if it is a life-saving act.

53. A patient was in an accident, is unconscious, and needs emergency surgery. His wife speaks a different language and there is no interpreter readily available to explain the surgery. Which of the following is the best action in this situation?
    a. Wait for an interpreter to arrive before moving the patient to surgery.
    b. Explain as much as possible and proceed with the surgery.
    c. Look for a friend of the family or another relative to give consent.
    d. Have two licensed health professionals sign the consent on behalf of the patient.

54. There is a long waiting time in the emergency department and a patient believes that he has been left longer because he does not have insurance. The ethical principle involved in this situation is:
    a. justice.
    b. autonomy.
    c. beneficence.
    d. accountability.

55. Nurses may be held liable for actions that are considered unintentional torts. Which one of the following actions is an example of this type of tort?
    a. Restraining a patient who refuses care and wants to leave the hospital
    b. Taking photos of a patient's surgical wound to post on a website
    c. Leaving the side rails down, leading to the patient falling and becoming injured
    d. Discussing the patient's sexually transmitted disease while riding in the elevator with visitors

Practice Situations

The patient has been diagnosed with a malignant form of cancer that has been unresponsive to treatment. The provider has started a new type of treatment that is making the patient very ill and keeping her bedridden. In discussion with the oncologist, you discover that there is very little hope for this treatment to work.
a. Identify the ethical principle(s) involved in this situation.

b. How can this be an ethical dilemma for you?

c. What should you do in this situation?

You have been asked by the primary care provider to administer a medication to the patient, but the dosage ordered is twice the normal amount. The provider tells you that this is the amount that the patient should receive.
a. How should you proceed?

b. Who is liable in this situation?

REVIEW QUESTIONS

- What are the key ethical theories that have an impact on nursing practice?
- How are ethical concepts applied to professional nursing practice?
- How does the American Nurses Association Code of Ethics for Nurses apply to nursing education and practice?
- What role does ethics play in genetic, biomedical, and end-of-life health care decision making?
- What are the legal implications of nursing practice?
- How do constitutional, statutory, regulatory, and case law differ in their relationship to professional nursing practice?
- What are the various types of statutory law, including intentional and unintentional torts, and their potential impact on nurses providing patient care?
- Which liability issues, such as professional boundaries, delegation, and documentation, are pertinent to nursing practice?
- What are the legal issues that guide patient care?
- Which specific federal and state laws have an impact on nursing practice?

12 Leadership and Management

CHAPTER REVIEW

Match the description/definition in Column A with the correct term in Column B.

Column A

_____ 1. Employs methods that inspire people to follow their lead

_____ 2. Believes that employees are motivated by internal means and want to participate in decision making

_____ 3. Uses reward and punishment to gain the cooperation of followers

_____ 4. Exercises strong control over subordinates

_____ 5. Provides little or no direction to followers

Column B

a. Autocratic leader

b. Democratic leader

c. Laissez-faire leader

d. Transactional leader

e. Transformational leader

Complete the following:

6. What is the difference between leadership and management?

7. For the following leadership theories, identify the major concept:
   a. Trait theory——

   b. Behavioral theory——

   c. Situational theory——

8. How would individuals with the following leadership styles do patient assignments on a unit?
   a. Autocratic——

   b. Democratic——

   c. Laissez-faire——

9. Provide an example of how the nurse can exhibit each of the following leadership qualities:
   a. Integrity——

   b. Dedication——

   c. Magnanimity——

   d. Humility——

   e. Openness——

   f. Creativity——

10. What is the difference between formal and informal leadership?

11. What are the functions of management?

12. In Mintzberg's Contemporary management model, there are different levels. For the People Level, the actions that the manager focuses on are: *Select all that apply.*
    a. Communicating _____
    b. Linking _____
    c. Controlling _____
    d. Doing tasks _____
    e. Obtaining resources _____
    f. Motivating _____

13. Identify at least three competencies of effective managers.

14. McGregor (1960) identified that managers have either Theory X or Theory Y characteristics. Which of these styles is more conducive to productivity and why?

15. Describe the following nursing leadership roles:
    a. Patient advocate——

    b. Case manager——

16. How does the nurse manager use business skills?

17. In regard to delegation:
    a. Where can the nurse find resources about delegation?

    b. What are the primary principles of delegation?

18. What are some of the benefits of becoming a magnet institution?

19. What are ways that the cultural phenomena should be considered when delegating to a diverse staff?
    a. Communication——

    b. Time——

    c. Environmental factors——

Select the best answer for each of the following questions:

20. An emergency situation has occurred on the medical unit. Which is the best leadership style to employ in this circumstance?
    a. Laissez-faire
    b. Democratic
    c. Bureaucratic
    d. Autocratic

21. Which of the following is an example of the management function of directing?
    a. The charge nurse coordinates patient admissions.
    b. The nurse works with the family on discharge plans.
    c. The RN delegates care to the LPNs and unlicensed staff members.
    d. The case manager evaluates the patient's progress toward his or her goals.

22. The new nurse manager is delegating tasks to the staff. What is a requirement for the nurse manager in the delegation process?
    a. Working alongside the staff to observe and evaluate their care
    b. Communicating the work assignment in understandable terms
    c. Acquiring the employees' voluntary acceptance of the assignment
    d. Releasing personal accountability for the tasks

Practice Situation

You are the staff nurse working with an unlicensed assistive personnel (UAP) to provide patient care. In reviewing the assignment, you identify the following:
- The UAP is new to the unit and you have not worked with her before.
- The assignment includes some patients who have experienced fluctuations in their vital signs, with one patient who has a changing level of consciousness.
- A new admission is coming to the unit.

With this information in mind, indicate how you will apply the five rights of safe delegation.

REVIEW QUESTIONS

- What are the differences between leadership and management?
- What are the styles of leadership and qualities of effective leaders?
- How are management theories applied?
- What are the qualities of effective managers?
- How is leadership demonstrated in nursing and the health care delivery system?
- What are the underlying principles of delegation in health care?

13 Evidence-Based Practice and Nursing Research

CHAPTER REVIEW

Match the description/definition in Column A with the correct term in Column B.

Column A

_____ 1. Identifies data and characteristics about the population or phenomenon

_____ 2. Used to explore a relationship between two variables

_____ 3. Deriving a theory from the data collected in the research

_____ 4. Examines a causal relationship between variables but may not meet strict guidelines

_____ 5. Studies documents to determine an accurate picture of a past event or time period

_____ 6. Examines a specific causal relationship between variables

_____ 7. Testing the application of theories in different situations with different populations

_____ 8. Used when testing theories about the effectiveness of interventions

_____ 9. Conducted to generate theories

_____ 10. Exploring the lived experiences of a specific group of people experiencing a similar event in their lives

Column B

a. Applied research

b. Basic research

c. Clinical research

d. Correlational research

e. Descriptive research

f. Experimental research

g. Grounded theory research

h. Historical research

i. Phenomenological research

j. Quasi-experimental research

Complete the following:

11. What is evidence-based practice?

12. How is research different from evidence-based practice?

13. What is the difference between quantitative and qualitative research?

14. Put the following components of the research process in the usual order of completion.
    a. Data collection _____
    b. Dissemination of outcomes _____
    c. Literature review _____
    d. Data analysis _____
    e. Identification of the problem _____
    f. Application to practice _____

15. A hypothesis is:

16. What are the expectations of nurses for participating in research?

17. On the basis of the following information, identify the independent variable, dependent variable, and control group. The nurse is participating in a research study about the effect of a new medication to reduce skin itching from dryness or rashes. Group A will receive the medication, but Group B will only receive a placebo.

18. What are the ethical principles that need to be included in research?

19. In a research project that involves human subjects, how does the nurse protect the participants?

20. The nurse has conducted a research study that resulted in findings that could be used in clinical practice. How can the nurse share (disseminate) this information?

21. What is the primary role of an institutional review board (IRB)?

22. How does the nurse usually perform data analysis for quantitative and qualitative research studies?

23. a. Filtered resources include:

    b. Unfiltered resources include:

24. Identify which of the following is consistent with a study that has internal validity. *Select all that apply.*
    a. The study addresses a clearly focused issue. _____
    b. Participants were hand-selected to the control group on the basis of their ethnicity and finances. _____
    c. Measures used were objective. _____
    d. Data collection methods were not clear. _____
    e. Participants were aware of who had been assigned to the control group. _____
    f. Subjects were provided with an explanation of the study, and informed consent was obtained. _____

25. Identify at least one of the criteria for Magnet designation.

26. Which of the following individuals are considered as vulnerable subjects and may not be able to participate in a research study? *Select all that apply.*
    a. Children _____
    b. Experiencing an emergency _____
    c. Mentally disabled person _____
    d. Competent adult _____
    e. Incarcerated adult _____
    f. Literate individual _____

27. How is evidence-based practice incorporated into delegation?

Select the best answer for each of the following questions:

28. A study that can be applied to other settings has:
    a. deductive reasoning.
    b. experimental findings.
    c. external validity.
    d. stakeholder approval.

29. The Health Information Portability and Privacy Act (HIPAA) influences nursing research primarily in the area of:
    a. the cost of the study.
    b. how the data will be protected.
    c. what type of research method can be used.
    d. where the study may be published.

30. The nurse researcher distributed an explanatory brochure to participants in the study. Which of the following principles is the researcher using?
    a. Informed consent
    b. Freedom from harm
    c. Confidentiality of data
    d. Selection of the control group

31. After identifying the problem to be investigated for the research project, the next step is to:
    a. obtain review board approval.
    b. identify the data collection instrument.
    c. select the population to participate.
    d. complete a literature review.

32. A nurse on an orthopedic unit reads a case study about the potential positive effects of a new type of exercise to promote ambulation. Which of the following should be a priority consideration before the research results are used by the nurse?
    a. Similarity of the case study patients to those on the unit
    b. Integration of ethical principles in the study
    c. Publication of the case study in other journals
    d. Cost of the case study

Practice Situation

You are working in a clinic and notice that some adult patients with diabetes mellitus are not able to follow their diabetic diets, while others have less difficulty. You want to conduct evidence-based research to see if there is a difference in the way in which the patients are taught about the diet.
a. Using the evidence-based research model, identify how you would set up the study, including the formulation of the research question.

REVIEW QUESTIONS

- What are the various types of nursing research?
- How do quantitative and qualitative research methods differ?
- What are the steps involved in the research process?
- How is research related to evidence-based practice?
- What are the steps required in conducting evidence-based research?
- What are the considerations for implementing research in nursing practice?
- How is hospital Magnet status related to nursing research and practice?

14 Health Literacy and Patient Education

CHAPTER REVIEW

Complete the following:

1. What is health literacy?

2. Identify the components/purposes of patient education.

3. Provide at least two examples of how the gap between the health care information provided and the health literacy of the patient/caregiver can adversely influence patient safety.

4. What are some of the expected competencies for patients and health literacy?

5. What is the difference between teaching and learning?

6. Identify the three domains of learning and give an example of each domain.

7. Indicate ways in which the following factors influence patient education.
   a. Age

   b. Environment

   c. Timing

8. What are some indications that the patient may have inadequate health literacy?

9. Write a nursing diagnosis, goal, and nursing intervention for a patient who needs to learn how to perform wound care.

10. Provide examples of possible teaching strategies to use for patient education.

11. Indicate how the Quality and Safety Education for Nurses (QSEN) competency of teamwork and collaboration are related to patient education.

12. After teaching the patient, what needs to be documented by the nurse?

13. Which of the following are accurate principles for patient teaching? *Select all that apply.*
    a. Teaching multiple concepts at once. _____
    b. Keeping sessions short. _____
    c. Continuing if the patient becomes fatigued. _____
    d. Providing positive feedback to the patient. _____
    e. Starting with familiar material and progressing to new information. _____
    f. Reviewing key points at the end of the session. _____

14. How do learning styles influence patient teaching?

Select the best answer for each of the following questions:

15. An occupational health nurse is going to provide a workshop to employees on body mechanics. In planning the presentation, what information would be most helpful for the nurse to obtain in advance of the presentation?
    a. Specific ages of all of the employees
    b. Names of the employees
    c. Names of the managers
    d. Number of participants

16. Which of the following strategies is the most appropriate for teaching a toddler about a hospital procedure?
    a. Discussion
    b. Pictures
    c. Role-playing
    d. Independent learning

17. The nurse assesses the patient's readiness to learn wound care. What is the most important factor for the nurse to determine first?
    a. Intelligence level of the patient
    b. Willingness to learn the technique
    c. Financial resources available to the patient
    d. Support from the patient's family

18. Which one of the following examples is an evaluation of a psychomotor skill?
    a. Patient is able to discuss side effects of medications
    b. Patient maintains eye contact with nurse
    c. Patient has planned menu within therapeutic diet
    d. Patient uses walker correctly

19. When teaching an older adult patient, the nurse should incorporate which teaching strategy into the plan?
    a. Keep the teaching sessions short.
    b. Teach in the later evening.
    c. Include as many concepts as possible.
    d. Focus on teaching the family members.

20. Which of the following statements by the patient indicates that he may not be ready to learn at this time?
    a. "I'll call and make an appointment with the physical therapist for follow-up on the exercises."
    b. "I want to know more about the side effects of the medications."
    c. "There's no sense in talking about this now. I don't feel very well."
    d. "Let me know if I am doing this dressing the right way."

21. Which one of the following examples is an evaluation of cognitive learning? The patient:
    a. explains the use of the incentive spirometer.
    b. looks at the site of the amputation.
    c. uses the crutches to go up and down the stairs.
    d. completes hygienic care independently.

22. In the affective domain of learning, the patient exhibits the ability to do which of the following?
    a. Perform self-catheterization
    b. Provide information on dialysis
    c. Return demonstrate blood pressure measurement
    d. Verbalize feelings about how to manage arthritis pain

23. To promote a patient's cognitive learning, the nurse decides to use which teaching strategy?
    a. Demonstrating a procedure
    b. Modeling appropriate ways to interact
    c. Showing a DVD about the disease process
    d. Discussing personal thoughts about surgery

Practice Situation

You are working with a patient who has a new colostomy and needs to learn how to manage the care. You suspect that the patient does not understand English well. There are members of the family who are more fluent in English and visit frequently.
    a. What questions can you ask to determine the patient's comfort with English?
    b. What adaptations will you need to make to ensure that the patient understands how to do the colostomy care?
    c. How will you evaluate the patient's knowledge about and ability to perform the colostomy care?

REVIEW QUESTIONS

- What is *health literacy?*
- What is the role of health literacy in nursing and patient education?
- What strategies can the nurse use to provide patient education?
- Where can patient education occur?
- What are the differences between the three domains of learning?
- How do learning styles affect patient teaching?
- What are the factors that affect health literacy and patient teaching?
- How can you assess the patient's health literacy and education needs?
- Which nursing diagnoses are appropriate for utilization with patient education?
- Which goals and outcome criteria are applicable to patient education?
- How can you implement teaching plans and evaluate their effectiveness?

15 Nursing Informatics

CHAPTER REVIEW

Complete the following:

1. What are informatics and nursing informatics?

2. How can nursing informatics enhance patient care?

3. Identify the technological advances/tools that are being used for health/patient data collection and sharing.

4. What is *telehealth* nursing?

5. Indicate specific patient safety benefits from the use of computerized resources.

6. What is the difference between an electronic medical record (EMR) and an electronic health record (EHR)?

7. Identify the specific advantages of electronic record management.

8. The nurse at the level of informatics competencies specifically exhibits which of the following abilities? *Select all that apply.*
   a. Identify and collect relevant data. _____
   b. Develop new software. _____
   c. Suggest system improvement. _____
   d. Conduct research and generate theories. _____
   e. Use keyboarding skills. _____
   f. Make judgments on trends and data patterns. _____

9. How does information literacy differ from computer literacy?

10. What is the purpose of standardizing nursing terminology?

11. How can networks and social media be used effectively by nurses?

12. Identify the specific informatics concerns in the eHealth Code of Ethics.

Select the best answer for each of the following questions:

13. Which nursing action demonstrates the category of utility in the informatics competency classification system?
    a. Computer and software use
    b. Maintenance of privacy
    c. Critical thinking and evidence-based practice
    d. Application of accountability and quality assurance

14. Which of the following is the biggest advantage of mobile technology in the health care setting?
    a. Improvement in research awareness
    b. Advancement of computer skills
    c. Increased job satisfaction
    d. Prevention of medication errors

Practice Situation

A patient has an uncommon pathology that reduces platelet production (idiopathic thrombocytopenia). A thorough search of the nursing and medical databases provided substantiated data on the topic. You are now using the Internet to collect information that is available to health care consumers. Before recommending a site to a patient or family, you need to do a website evaluation.
a. What are the steps that you will use to evaluate the website?

b. Identify a site that is available on this topic area.

REVIEW QUESTIONS

- What are *nursing informatics*?
- How is technology used in health care?
- How can informatics benefit patient care?
- How do the competency levels of nursing informatics differ?
- What is the importance of using standardized terminologies in EHRs?
- How is information technology used to obtain health information for consumers and in educating nurses?
- What are potential ethical issues related to the use of health care information technology?
- What are possible future directions for nursing informatics?

16 Health and Wellness

CHAPTER REVIEW

Match the description/definition in Column A with the correct term in Column B.

Column A

_____ 1. Promotion of human welfare

_____ 2. Confidence in one's ability to take action

_____ 3. Risk of disease expression based on hereditary factors

_____ 4. Concepts focus on the interrelatedness of the physical body and the mind, with aspects of spirituality, emotional security, and the environment

_____ 5. Physiologic disease or mental disorder

_____ 6. A state of complete physical, mental, and social well-being and not merely the absence of disease or infirmity

Column B

a. Health

b. Genetic vulnerability

c. Humanistic

d. Illness

e. Self-efficacy

f. Holistic health

Complete the following:

7. Identify an ethical consideration related to the cost of health care.

8. The nurse wants to use holistic health strategies with the patient. What types of interventions will be investigated by the nurse?

9. Identify the levels of prevention for the following:
   a. Showing a patient how to use a cane

   b. Teaching new parents about the use of a car seat

   c. Having a colonoscopy

   d. Receiving nutrition information

10. For the following health models, identify the primary concept.

Theory/Model	Primary Concept
Basic Human Needs	
Health Belief Model	
Holistic Health	

11. Identify at least three health promotion activities that the nurse can discuss with a patient.

12. Provide an example of a risk-factor reduction activity.

13. *Healthy People 2020* is designed to track which specific personal risk behaviors?

14. In relation to illness:
    a. What factors influence an individual's response to illness?

    b. What type of responses may be exhibited by the patient?

15. Identify all of the following behaviors that are associated with stage IV in the Stages of Illness model. *Select all that apply.*
    a. Recognition that something is wrong _____
    b. Resumption of usual tasks _____
    c. Acceptance of the sick role _____
    d. Performance of treatments _____
    e. Validation of the illness _____
    f. Requirement of emotional support _____

16. Indicate whether the following are classified as acute or chronic illnesses.
    a. Appendicitis

    b. Multiple sclerosis

    c. Diabetes mellitus

    d. Arthritis

    e. Influenza

17. For chronic illness:
    a. How do individuals with chronic illnesses need to adapt their lives?

    b. What general strategies should the nurse employ when helping patients with chronic illnesses?

18. For the following factors, identify an example of how each one can influence health.
    a. Age _____

    b. Gender _____

    c. Lifestyle _____

    d. Environment _____

19. Self-concept is the way individuals see themselves in relation to:

20. How can a patient's cultural practices have an influence on health and illness behaviors?

21. How is health care access a challenge to people in rural areas?

Select the best answer for each of the following questions:

22. In the Stages of Illness model, stage II is characterized by the individual:
    a. accepting medical treatment.
    b. seeking medical advice.
    c. deciding that care is necessary.
    d. recognizing that something is wrong.

23. Which one of the following is a main goal of *Healthy People 2020*?
    a. Health care cost reduction
    b. Access to health services
    c. Elimination of intrinsic risk factors
    d. Identification of morbidity rate thresholds

24. Which of the following is an example of tertiary prevention?
    a. Providing information on immunizations
    b. Screening a family for a hereditary disease
    c. Presenting a class on hand hygiene to an elementary school class
    d. Working with a patient who is paraplegic to prevent musculoskeletal complications

25. Assessment of the patient reveals some negative health behaviors. Which of the following indicates a lifestyle risk factor?
    a. Hypertension
    b. Sunbathing
    c. Overcrowded living conditions
    d. Manufacturing-based occupation

26. In Rosenstock's Health Belief Model, focus is placed on which of the following?
    a. Basic human survival needs
    b. Functioning of the individual in all dimensions
    c. Relationship of perceptions and compliance
    d. Multidimensional nature of patients in the environment

27. The nurse is working with a patient to modify his risk factors. Which one of the following areas can be addressed by the nurse?
    a. Diet
    b. Family history
    c. Developmental level
    d. Gender-oriented susceptibility

28. An example of a holistic measure that can be incorporated into the patient's care plan is the use of:
    a. analgesic medication.
    b. therapeutic touch.
    c. wound debridement.
    d. passive range of motion.

29. According to the Health Promotion model, one of the focus points is:
    a. complementary therapy.
    b. basic survival requirements.
    c. interrelationship of the mind and body.
    d. behavior-specific knowledge.

Practice Situation

You are visiting a friend who has experienced a heart attack. You notice that he is reacting differently than usual, being quiet and withdrawn. He tells you that, "I have to change my whole life—my diet, medicine, and cardiac rehab." He follows by saying that he is not happy about any of it.
    a. Using the Stages of Illness, in which stage would you place this individual? What behaviors support this assessment?

    b. As a nurse, how would you assist this individual to cope with his illness and need to adapt his lifestyle?

REVIEW QUESTIONS

- What are the concepts of *health* and *wellness* in an individual and a corporate context?
- What are the similarities and differences between the theoretical models of health and wellness that provide the basis for nursing practice?
- How does health promotion relate to wellness?
- What are the three levels of preventive care and the nursing interventions associated with each?
- What are the key aspects of each type of illness and the stages of illness behavior?
- Which factors influence health and have an impact on illness?

17 Human Development: Conception Through Adolescence

CHAPTER REVIEW

Match the description/definition in Column A with the correct term in Column B.

Column A

_____ 1. Enables older children and adults to change direction in their thinking to return to the starting point

_____ 2. Use of a new object in the same way that more familiar objects are used

_____ 3. Form of learning based on reinforcement or punishment

_____ 4. Ability to recognize that objects remain the same even if they change in appearance

_____ 5. Process of adjusting schemes in response to stimuli within the environment

_____ 6. Ability to store the information that was given attention for later recall

_____ 7. Changes the pattern of behavior when encountering new similar objects

_____ 8. Something still exists when it is out of sight

_____ 9. Focusing on only one aspect of an object

_____ 10. Ability to arrange things in a logical order

Column B
a. Seriation

b. Accommodation

c. Centration

d. Object permanence

e. Retention

f. Reversibility

g. Operant conditioning

h. Assimilation

i. Adaptation

j. Conservation

Complete the following:

11. Explain the difference between growth and development.

12. What is the meaning of "nature versus nurture"?

13. Identify the key concept in each of the following theories:

14. What are teratogens?

15. For new parents, what information can the nurse provide to help them to become more confident in the care of their infant?

Theorist	Type of Theory*	Major Concept(s)
Freud		
Erikson		
Piaget		
Kohlberg		
Westerhoff		

*Psychosocial, cognitive, etc.

16. To reduce the occurrence of sudden infant death syndrome (SIDS), the nurse instructs the parents to:

17. Care must be taken that infants and toddlers do not choke. Which foods are hazardous to give to children of this age?

18. For each of the following age groups, indicate at least two characteristics of growth and/or development:
    a. Newborn _____

    b. Infant _____

    c. Toddler _____

    d. Preschool _____

    e. School age _____

    f. Adolescent _____

19. Place the following developmental steps in their order of occurrence from earliest to latest.
    a. Fetus _____
    b. Embryo _____
    c. Implantation _____
    d. Fertilization _____
    e. Zygote _____

20. The parents tell you that they are going away on vacation and will be renting a car. They will be taking their two children, ages 2 and 4. For their safety, the nurse reminds them to:

21. The patient comes in for the initial prenatal examination. Provide at least two examples of questions that the nurse will ask to determine lifestyle risk factors.

22. Identify two of the screening tests that are done to determine fetal abnormalities or defects.

23. Although children can progress at different rates, there are some expectations for infant behavior. Which of the following are expectations for development at 4 to 6 months? *Select all that apply.*
    a. Passing toys from one hand to another. _____
    b. Trying to stand up. _____
    c. Rolling from the back to the side. _____
    d. Sitting unassisted. _____
    e. Reaching for objects held in front of him/her. _____
    f. Playing games like peek-a-boo. _____

24. A 4-year-old child is in the clinic for a regular checkup. The mother tells the nurse that he has been hitting the other children in the day care center. What does the nurse suggest to the mother that may reduce this behavior?

25. For an adolescent patient:
    a. What is the Freudian stage and the behavior associated with this age group?
    b. What does Erikson see as the psychosocial stage and behavior?
    c. How does puberty affect the physical appearance?
    d. What are some of the general challenges faced by adolescents?

26. Although children can progress at different rates, there are some expectations for behavior. Which of the following are expectations for development by age 2? *Select all that apply.*
    a. Riding a tricycle _____
    b. Hopping on one foot _____
    c. Drawing letters _____
    d. Grasping small objects _____
    e. Walking up and down stairs _____
    f. Dropping small objects into a container _____

27. For a toddler in the hospital, what can the nurse do to support ritualistic behavior?

28. An example of magical thinking by the preschooler is:

29. The nurse suspects that the child is a victim of abuse. What are some of the signs that would lead the nurse to this assessment?

Select the best answer for each of the following questions:

30. The nurse recognizes that additional teaching is necessary if the new parents indicate that they will:
    a. remove pillows from the crib.
    b. perform hand washing before infant feedings.
    c. take small objects away from the baby.
    d. place the baby on its stomach to sleep.

31. Screening for Tay-Sachs disease would most likely be recommended for a female of:
    a. Jewish descent.
    b. African descent.
    c. Mediterranean descent.
    d. Southeast Asian descent.

32. Which of the following responses from the mother about her infant should be investigated further by the nurse?
    a. He was born 1 day before the due date.
    b. He doesn't react to loud noises.
    c. He sleeps through the night.
    d. He smiles when he sees me.

33. Which of the following are expectations for development of a preschool age child?
    a. Talking in sentences
    b. Playing a game of baseball
    c. Riding a two-wheel bicycle
    d. Playing apart from other children

34. The nurse recognizes that using pictures to explain a procedure to a 3-year-old child coincides with which one of Piaget's stages?
    a. Sensorimotor
    b. Preoperational
    c. Concrete operational
    d. Formal operational

35. For an 8-month-old girl, the nurse expects that the parents will identify which behaviors have been observed?
    a. Getting to a sitting position without help
    b. Crawling forward on her belly
    c. Responding to her own name
    d. Saying two words clearly

36. Erikson's developmental stage for a toddler, Autonomy versus Shame, coincides with which of the following concepts in Piaget's theory?
    a. Having no sense of "good" or "bad" behavior
    b. Realizing own actions can cause reactions in others
    c. Seeing the viewpoints of others
    d. Thinking about the way that others think

37. Which of the following is a general recommendation for infant nutrition?
    a. Start Vitamin D in the first week
    b. Provide iron supplements between 4 and 6 months
    c. Give whole milk after 6 months
    d. Add honey to the infant formula

38. Which one of the following children is most likely to enjoy starting a collection of seashells and rocks? A child who is:
    a. 2 years old.
    b. 4 years old.
    c. 8 years old.
    d. 17 years old.

39. A 5-year-old child is admitted to the surgical center for a tonsillectomy. In caring for children of this age, the nurse plans to:
    a. have the child do the hygienic care before the procedure.
    b. allow the child to handle the equipment while taking his blood pressure.
    c. leave the child alone to relax before the surgery.
    d. provide magazines and puzzles.

40. A parent of a 3-year-old tells the nurse he is concerned that his son, who was toilet trained, now refuses to use the toilet and wants a diaper again while in the hospital. On the basis of her knowledge of behavior, which of the following is the nurse's best response?
    a. "Children often lose the ability to use the toilet when they are hospitalized."
    b. "Your son was probably not fully toilet trained before he was admitted."
    c. "He is probably feeling neglected because you aren't staying with him all night."
    d. "This is not uncommon when children are in unfamiliar environments and situations."

41. The nurse is teaching the parents of a 3-month-old about basic infant safety for this age group. The nurse will emphasize which of the following?
    a. The use of gates at stairways
    b. Keeping the bathroom door closed
    c. Giving only large pieces of food
    d. Removing bibs at bedtime

42. Which of the followings snacks should the nurse recommend to the parent of a 9-year-old?
    a. Bite-size candy
    b. Plain popcorn
    c. Diet soda
    d. Potato chips

43. A 6-year-old is hospitalized for asthma. To help the child deal with the hospitalization, the nurse should provide a:
    a. needle and thread for sewing.
    b. baseball to throw in the room.
    c. 1000-piece jigsaw puzzle to complete.
    d. coloring book and crayons.

44. A 16-year-old comes to the clinic to get birth control supplies. To obtain the most information, the nurse should ask which of the following questions?
    a. "Have you told your parents that you are sexually active?"
    b. "Are your friends having sexual relations?"
    c. "What can you tell me about your sexual activity?"
    d. "Are you protecting yourself?"

43

45. The patient is in her fourth month of the pregnancy and asks the nurse what is happening with the baby now. The nurse responds by telling her that the:
    a. heart has just begun to develop.
    b. neural tube is forming.
    c. weight is about 1/2 pound.
    d. eyes first appear.

46. In planning a health care presentation for 17-year-old students, the nurse wants to incorporate the most common cause of injuries for this age group. Which of the following does the nurse focus on in her discussion?
    a. Falls
    b. Poisoning
    c. Drug overdose
    d. Motor vehicle accidents

Practice Situation

You are a visiting nurse going to the home of a family with two parents and two children, ages 3 years and 16 years. When you walk into the home, you identify the following: cleaning supplies in lower cabinets, no gates by the stairs, prescription medications in the medicine cabinet, fast food wrappers in the garbage, soda, and snack foods with low nutritional value.
a. On the basis of your assessment, what are your priorities for teaching this family and what will you include in your teaching plan?

b. What will you want to ask the adolescent about?

REVIEW QUESTIONS

- What are the major theories of human development?
- What is the process of human development from conception to birth?
- What are the primary developmental tasks for newborns?
- Which developmental milestones are important for infants?
- How does the toddler develop physically, psychosocially, and cognitively?
- How do children in the preschool years grow and develop?
- What development occurs during the school-age years?
- How do adolescents develop physically, psychosocially, and cognitively?

18 Human Development: Young Adult Through Older Adult

CHAPTER REVIEW

Match the description/definition in Column A with the correct term in Column B.

Column A

_____ 1. Biological process of aging influenced by genetics

_____ 2. Represents basic information-processing skills (i.e., the ability to detect relationships among stimuli, the speed with which information is analyzed, and the capacity of working memory)

_____ 3. Situation where children are living with the grandparents and not the parents.

_____ 4. Skills that depend on accumulated knowledge, experience, good judgment, and mastery of social conventions

_____ 5. Move from viewing truth in absolute terms of right and wrong (obtained from "good" or "bad" authorities) to recognizing multiple, conflicting versions of "truth" representing legitimate alternatives

_____ 6. Cognitive development past Piaget's formal operational stage

_____ 7. Reaching out to others in ways that guide and give to the next generation

_____ 8. Thought is more responsive to context and less constrained by the need to find only one answer to a question

_____ 9. People place their own comfort and security above challenges that include other people

_____ 10. Dividing information, values, and authority into right and wrong, good and bad, we and they

Column B

a. Crystallized intelligence

b. Relativist thinking

c. Stagnation

d. Adaptive cognition

e. Dualistic thinking

f. Generativity

g. Senescence

h. Skipped generation

i. Fluid intelligence

j. Postformal thought

Complete the following:

11. Which of the following changes are associated with the normal aging process? *Select all that apply.*
    a. Decreased bone density _____
    b. Presbycusis _____
    c. Enhanced ability to smell _____
    d. Weaker respiratory effort _____
    e. Reduced peristalsis _____
    f. Slower immune response _____

12. What are some of the challenges for young adults?

13. What is the difference between delirium and dementia?

14. What are the most common causes of death in older adults?

15. There are many myths about aging and older adults. Identify which of the following are facts about aging. *Select all that apply.*
    a. Most older adults have Alzheimer's disease. _____
    b. A majority are unemployed or retired. _____
    c. Independence is often related to financial status. _____

d. Sexuality and sexual activity lose importance. _____
e. A large number live in institutional settings. _____
f. This population is becoming more racially diverse. _____

16. Classification of adults is as follows:
    a. Young adults are ages:

    b. Middle adults are ages:

    c. Older adults are above age:

17. For the following theories on aging, identify the major concept(s):

Theory	Concept(s)
Wear and Tear	
Cross-Linking Theory	

18. What is meant by the term "emerging adulthood"?

19. What should lifestyle assessment of the younger adult include?

20. Provide examples of developmental tasks and health risks:

	Developmental Tasks	Health Risks
Young adult		
Middle adult		
Older adult		

21. Which screenings are important for adults?
    a. Young adults

    b. Middle adults

    c. Older adults

22. How does exercise benefit adult health?

23. Which mental health disorder is being seen more commonly in adults of all ages?

24. Which of the following statements are accurate for middle adults? *Select all that apply.*
    a. The majority of adults live in families. _____
    b. Cardiovascular disease is a leading cause of death. _____
    c. This period is for "launching children and moving on." _____
    d. This age group has the worst financial status. _____
    e. Positive social relationships can promote well-being. _____
    f. About one third have achieved a bachelor's degree or higher. _____

25. The number of older adults in America is predicted to double by 2030.

    True _____   False _____

26. What does primary prevention for the older adult include?

27. Identify signs and symptoms that are associated with adult pathology in the following systems:
    a. Cardiovascular

    b. Respiratory

    c. Endocrine

28. What should be done by the nurse to assess and respond to evidence of domestic violence?

29. Which behaviors are associated with anxiety disorders in adults?

30. To help the patient reduce the incidence of the following, which information should the nurse include in the teaching plan?
    a. Sexually transmitted disease

    b. Cancer

31. How is the QSEN competency of teamwork and collaboration exhibited in the home environment?

32. Identify the recommendations for exercise for adults.

33. Identify which of the following commonly abused drugs is associated with respiratory depression. *Select all that apply.*
    a. Marijuana _____

    b. Oxycontin _____

    c. Cocaine _____

    d. Flunitrazepam (GBH) _____

    e. LSD _____

    f. Nicotine _____

Select the best answer for each of the following questions:

34. According to Gould's theory of adult development, individuals aged 22-28 years of age are in the stage of:
    a. leaving the parents' world.
    b. getting into the adult world.
    c. questioning and reexamination.
    d. reconciliation and mellowing.

35. To promote positive health habits for young and middle adults, the nurse will:
    a. tell individuals to abstain from all alcohol consumption.
    b. demonstrate blood pressure measurement.
    c. assist in determining effective daily exercise plans for stress reduction.
    d. describe the usual types of medications used for common disorders.

36. In reviewing the developmental patterns of young adults, the nurse is aware that individuals at this point in their lives are generally expected to do which of the following?
    a. Continue their physical growth
    b. Experience severe illnesses
    c. Ignore physical symptoms
    d. Experience a diminished physical condition

37. Following a physical assessment of an older adult, the nurse compares the results with what is expected for individuals in this age group. An expected finding is:
    a. dry eyes.
    b. hepatomegaly.
    c. a decrease in blood pressure.
    d. a better ability to hear high-pitched sounds.

38. A nurse is preparing an education program for a group of young adults. On the basis of the leading cause of mortality and morbidity for this age group, the nurse will focus on which of the following?
    a. Birth control
    b. Occupational hazards
    c. Motor vehicle safety
    d. Prevention of sports injuries

39. As a health nurse in the local college, the primary population is young adults. An important part of the nurse's assessment specific to the risks of this age group is which of the following?
    a. Marital status
    b. Leisure activities
    c. Experience with chronic disease
    d. History of childhood accidents

40. The nurse is performing a physical examination for a 58-year-old patient. The nurse will most likely find which of the following physiological changes related to normal aging?
    a. Rapid pupillary response
    b. Palpable thyroid lobes
    c. Decreased skin turgor
    d. Extended range of motion

41. The nurse recognizes that one of the major stressors having a major influence on young adults in today's world is the:
    a. need to adapt to cognitive changes.
    b. responsibility for aging parents.
    c. adjustment to physiological changes.
    d. pursuit of a satisfying occupation.

42. A patient has been diagnosed with Alzheimer disease. In teaching the family, which of the following statements accurately explains the prognosis of this disease?
    a. "Many individuals can be cured, if the disease is identified early."
    b. "Some new drugs can slow the progression of the disease."
    c. "The life expectancy is rarely more than 2 years."
    d. "Diet and exercise are effective strategies to reverse the dementia."

43. Which of the following is the most common cause of long-term disability in the adult population?
    a. Cancer
    b. Stroke
    c. Accidents
    d. Pulmonary disease

44. An older patient has been placed on anticoagulant medication. What specifically should the nurse teach the caregiver about this medication?
    a. Be alert to bleeding.
    b. Double the dosage if one is missed.
    c. Make sure to take the pulse before administering.
    d. Give the medication with a large volume of water.

45. The nurse is speaking with older adults at an assisted living facility. The participants have a number of questions about their medications. The nurse responds most appropriately by saying:
    a. "Don't worry about the names of the medications. They all sound very similar."
    b. "Feel free to check with the doctor about the medications that are prescribed for you."
    c. "Remember that it usually takes a while for the hepatic system to deal with the pharmacological effects of your medication."
    d. "Unless you have serious side effects from your medications, you shouldn't be concerned about minor changes in how you feel."

46. In planning to discharge an older adult patient from the hospital, the nurse is aware that the majority of older adults:
    a. require nursing home care.
    b. have no social or family support.
    c. are unable to afford any health care.
    d. are capable of managing their own lives.

47. An older adult patient asks the nurse why she has hypertension. The nurse explains that this is often experienced as a result of which of the following?
    a. Myocardial damage
    b. Reduction in physical activity
    c. Ingestion of large amount of processed foods
    d. Stiffening of the blood vessels, which impairs blood flow

48. To assist older adults to meet their needs for sexuality, the nurse should recognize that:
    a. safe sex practices are no longer necessary.
    b. the sexual drive becomes more intense.
    c. medications can have an influence on function.
    d. physiologic changes do not have a significant effect.

49. Skeletal function is improved for the older adult with an increase in which of the following?
    a. Protein
    b. Vitamin A
    c. Vitamin B
    d. Fiber

50. Which of the following is a positive choice for adults?
    a. Grilled chicken and broccoli
    b. Hamburger and fried potatoes
    c. Hot dog and sauerkraut
    d. Baked potato with sour cream and bacon bits

51. An older adult is semi-independent but requires assistance with meals and laundry. Which of the following is the best living arrangement option?
    a. Palliative care
    b. Long-term care
    c. Adult day care
    d. Assisted living

52. Which information is accurate to share with an adult group in regard to HPV (human papillomavirus)?
    a. All sexually active individuals will have genital HPV at some point.
    b. There is one definitive strain of HPV.
    c. High-risk HPV can lead to cancer.
    d. Vaccination is most effective after sexual contact occurs.

Practice Situation

You are the nurse on the unit working with a middle adult patient who has just been diagnosed with type 2 diabetes. In your assessment of the patient, you find that she is a single parent who has three children at home, as well as responsibility for her 78-year-old mother. Her mother fell last month, fractured her hip, had surgery, and is now living with her while she goes through rehabilitation. The patient is unsure if her mother will be able to return to her own home because there are many stairs.
a. On the basis of your assessment, what are your concerns for this patient when she goes home?

b. How can you provide support to this patient?

REVIEW QUESTIONS

- What are the theories on aging and adult development?
- How does the body change through the aging process?
- What are the physiologic, cognitive, emotional, and social changes that impact the young adult?
- What are the health risks and concerns for the young adult?
- What are the physiologic, cognitive, emotional, and social changes that occur in the middle-adult age group?
- How do the health risks and concerns differ for the middle adult in comparison with the young adult?
- What are the physiologic, cognitive, emotional, and social changes that impact the older adult?
- How do the risks and concerns for the older adult differ from those of the middle adult?

19 Vital Signs

CHAPTER REVIEW

Match the description/definition in Column A with the correct term in Column B.

Column A

_____ 1. Difficult, labored breathing

_____ 2. Peak of the pressure wave on arterial walls

_____ 3. A bluish discoloration of the skin and mucous membranes

_____ 4. A slow heart rate

_____ 5. Absence of breathing

_____ 6. Presence of a fever

_____ 7. Apical pulse exceeds the radial pulse

_____ 8. Increased respiratory rate

_____ 9. Difficulty in breathing in positions other than upright

_____ 10. Lowest pressure on arterial walls, occurs when the heart rests

Column B

a. Systolic pressure

b. Apnea

c. Pulse deficit

d. Dyspnea

e. Diastolic pressure

f. Orthopnea

g. Cyanosis

h. Tachypnea

i. Bradycardia

j. Febrile

Complete the following:

11. Identify which of the following vital signs are within the expected range for a 40-year-old patient, assuming that these are consistent readings. *Select all that apply.*
    a. Temperature 98° F _____
    b. Blood pressure 110/70 mm Hg _____
    c. Pulse 140 bpm _____
    d. Temperature 39° C _____
    e. Pulse 50 bpm _____
    f. Respiration 18/min _____

12. Which landmarks are used to locate the site for the apical pulse?

13. Identify which of the following can cause tachycardia. *Select all that apply.*
    a. Hypothermia _____
    b. Head injury _____
    c. Fever _____
    d. Hypoxia _____
    e. Stress _____
    f. Use of beta-blocker medications _____

14. Indicate on the model where the following pulses should be palpated:
    a. Carotid
    b. Brachial
    c. Radial
    d. Apical
    e. Popliteal
    f. Dorsalis pedis

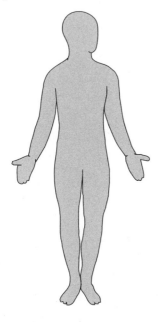

15. Indicate on the aneroid scale where the following blood pressure reading should be noted:

    Korotkoff I sound heard at 142 mm Hg and Korotkoff V heard at 88 mm Hg

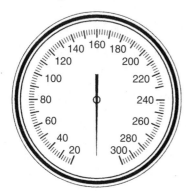

16. For a patient with an IV in the left arm and a mastectomy on the right side, the blood pressure needs to be monitored in which site?

17. What can affect the accuracy of pulse oximetry?

18. Which of the following are signs of hyperthermia (fever)? *Select all that apply.*
    a. Bradypnea _____
    b. Malaise _____
    c. Pale skin _____
    d. Shivering _____
    e. Decreased muscle coordination _____
    f. Tachycardia _____

19. What is the correct procedure for a tympanic temperature measurement?

20. Identify a nursing diagnosis, goal, and intervention for the following individuals:
    a. A patient with a fever

    b. A patient with shortness of breath

21. Which of the following are accurate for pulse measurement? *Select all that apply.*
    a. The brachial artery is used for children in emergency situations. _____
    b. Bilateral carotid pulses are measured simultaneously. _____
    c. The most definitive site to use is the radial pulse. _____
    d. Peripheral circulation can be evaluated by checking the posterior tibial arteries. _____
    e. Auscultation is required for the apical site. _____
    f. A pulse deficit is measured by two nurses at once. _____

22. When are rectal temperatures contraindicated?

23. How frequently is vital sign assessment done for stable patients?

24. Which factors can lead to hypoventilation?

25. When should an electronic blood pressure device not be used?

26. Identify general guidelines for measurement of vital signs.

27. What steps are included in assessment of pain?

28. What are nonverbal indications that a patient is experiencing pain?

29. Where is the correct location for the temporal artery temperature measurement?

30. Irregular and apical pulses should be counted for _____ (time).

31. Place the steps for pulse oximetry in the correct order. It has already been prepared for safe use.
    a. Turn on the oximeter. _____
    b. Remove probe. _____
    c. Clean probe with alcohol. _____
    d. Place probe on site. _____
    e. Explain the procedure. _____
    f. Observe reading. _____

32. What is the pulse used for blood pressure measurement in the lower extremity?

33. What is the correct order of steps for the two-step manual blood pressure measurement?
    a. Close valve and inflate cuff. _____
    b. Place stethoscope diaphragm over brachial pulse. _____
    c. Position the cuff. _____
    d. Palpate brachial pulse and note reading. _____
    e. Palpate the brachial and radial pulses. _____
    f. Deflate cuff and wait 2 minutes. _____
    g. Inflate cuff, release valve, and auscultate blood pressure. _____

34. What does the nurse need to do before using a Doppler ultrasound to obtain a pulse?

35. To prevent hypothermia in an older adult patient, the nurse instructs the patient to do what?

36. For the use of a dual-head stethoscope:
    a. How should it be cleaned?

    b. Which side of the dual head is used for higher-pitched sounds?

37. Nurses can be held liable for not monitoring vital signs appropriately.

    True _____   False _____

38. How is orthostatic hypotension assessed?

Select the best answer for each of the following questions:

39. Which of the following factors will result in a decrease in a patient's blood pressure?
    a. Pain
    b. Head injury
    c. Hemorrhage
    d. Use of oral contraceptives

40. The patient has difficulty seeing and is complaining of pain. It is most appropriate to use which of the following pain scales?
    a. Faces Scale
    b. A large-print Faces Scale
    c. Numeric Pain Assessment Scale
    d. Multiple Language Pain Assessment Scale

41. The patient has been on the floor for 2 days with a diagnosis of asthma. She has been stable and her discharge is planned for tomorrow. She uses her call bell and complains of feeling anxious but denies difficulty breathing and cannot verbalize the cause of her anxiety. Which of the following would be the best intervention at this point?
    a. Check the electronic record to see if she has an order for an antianxiety medication.
    b. Reassure her that she is probably anxious about being discharged tomorrow.
    c. Check her temperature to make sure she does not have an infection.
    d. Perform a pulse oximetry measurement.

42. The nurse documents Cheyne-Stokes respirations for the patient who has which of the following?
    a. Rhythmic respiration, from very deep to very shallow to apneic periods
    b. Abnormally deep and rapid respirations
    c. Shallow, slow respirations
    d. Shallow, rapid respirations

43. The nurse instructs the aide that a falsely low blood pressure reading will be obtained by which of the following methods?
    a. Using a cuff that is too narrow
    b. Releasing the pressure valve too slowly
    c. Assessing the blood pressure after the patient exercises
    d. Placing the arm above the level of the heart

51

44. A patient with a 2+ pulse volume has a pulse that is:
    a. absent.
    b. weak.
    c. normal.
    d. bounding.

45. A patient comes to the emergency department after having been in the sun all day. The nurse also determines that the patient is taking a diuretic. Heat stroke is suspected, and the nurse observes for which of the following?
    a. Diaphoresis
    b. Confusion
    c. Temperature of 35° C to 37° C
    d. Decreased heart rate

46. The nurse is taking vital signs on a 6-year-old child who has just finished a grape popsicle. Which of the following is an appropriate action?
    a. Wait 30 minutes to take the oral temperature.
    b. Proceed to take a tympanic temperature reading.
    c. Take a rectal temperature measurement.
    d. Have the child rinse out the mouth and take the oral temperature.

47. The adult patient is seen in the 24-hour medicenter for heat exhaustion. The nurse anticipates that treatment will include which of the following?
    a. Fluid replacement
    b. Antibiotic therapy
    c. Hypothermia wraps
    d. Tepid water baths

48. Which site should the nurse use to assess the pulse in a 2-year-old child?
    a. Radial
    b. Femoral
    c. Apical
    d. Pedal

49. On entering the room, the nurse observes that the patient appears to be tachypneic. The nurse should:
    a. ask if there have been visitors.
    b. have the patient lie flat.
    c. take the radial pulse.
    d. measure the respiratory rate.

50. The patient is experiencing pain and asks for medication, which has been ordered by the provider. The nurse first assesses the vital signs and finds them to be: blood pressure 144/82, pulse 88/min, and respirations 24/min. The nurse should:
    a. give the medication as ordered.
    b. check again that the patient has pain.
    c. withhold the medication.
    d. wait 20 minutes and check the vital signs again before giving the medication.

51. For a patient who needs the blood pressure measured in the lower extremities, the nurse knows that the measurement will be:
    a. the same as the upper extremity.
    b. 20 mm Hg lower than in the brachial artery.
    c. 20 mm Hg higher than in the brachial artery.
    d. 40 mm Hg higher than in the brachial artery.

52. For a 72-year-old patient, which of the following vital sign measurements is within the expected range?
    a. BP 80/40, P 110, R 40
    b. BP 100/70, P 72, R 20
    c. BP 84/60, P 80, R 26
    d. BP 90/60, P 110, R 16

53. The nurse has taken vital signs on a 34-year-old patient. Which of the following findings should be reported as outside of the expected range for this age group?
    a. T 98° F
    b. P 140 bpm
    c. R 22/min
    d. BP 120/78

54. The patient had abdominal surgery this morning. When the nurse checks the vital signs, the findings are as follows: BP 110/60, P 110, and R 32/min. What should the nurse do first?
    a. Retake the vital signs in 15 minutes.
    b. Continue with the care as planned.
    c. Check the surgical dressing.
    d. Administer the medication for pain.

55. The patient gets out of bed to go to the bathroom and tells the nurse that he "feels dizzy." The nurse should first:
    a. go for help.
    b. take the blood pressure.
    c. help the patient to sit down.
    d. have the patient take deep breaths.

56. A teenage patient with the flu is febrile and needs the body temperature reduced. The nurse anticipates that treatment will include which of the following?
    a. Ice packs to the axilla and groin
    b. A cooling blanket
    c. An ice water bath
    d. Aspirin

57. When measuring vital signs, the nurse is aware that blood pressure is usually lower in the presence of or following:
    a. anxiety.
    b. exercise.
    c. cigarette smoking.
    d. diuretic administration.

58. A patient asks the nurse about whether her blood pressure is too high. The nurse informs the patient that the blood pressure associated with stage I hypertension is:
    a. 120/70.
    b. 130/80.
    c. 140/90.
    d. 160/100.

59. The nurse is taking temperature readings in the newborn nursery. The site that is most often used for healthy newborns is the:
    a. oral site.
    b. axillary site.
    c. rectal site.
    d. tympanic site.

60. An emergency department nurse receives a call about a person who has been exposed to extreme cold after a snowboarding accident. The nurse instructs the caller to take care of the hypothermia by giving the victim:
    a. sips of brandy.
    b. a cup of hot coffee.
    c. a bowl of warm soup.
    d. extra hot compresses.

61. A primary concern for a patient with orthostatic hypotension is the:
    a. risk of injury.
    b. fluid overload.
    c. oxygen demand.
    d. mental confusion.

Practice Situation

For the case study patient in the chapter, Mr. Donley, complete the following areas in the care map:
- Admission Diagnoses/Chief Complaint
- Assessment Data
- Treatments
- Lab Values/Test Results
- Past Medical History
- Medications

REVIEW QUESTIONS

- Why are vital signs measured?
- What are the techniques for obtaining accurate temperature measurement?
- What are the common assessment sites and techniques for assessing pulse?
- How are respirations and blood oxygenation assessed?
- How is blood pressure measured?
- How is pain assessment conducted in diverse populations?

CHAPTER REVIEW

Complete the following:

1. Define the following terms:
   a. Alopecia:

   b. Atelectasis:

   c. Bruit:

   d. Cerumen:

   e. Diplopia:

   f. Ecchymosis:

   g. Erythema:

   h. Jaundice:

   i. Paresthesia:

   j. Pruritus:

   k. Tortuosity:

   l. Vertigo:

2. How does the nurse promote comfort for the patient during a physical examination/assessment?

3. When may a third person be present in the room during a physical examination?

4. The nurse tells the patient during the examination, "That's nice to know, Mrs. J, but we really need to get through all of these questions."
   a. How might the patient respond to this statement?

   b. How can the nurse refocus the patient in a better way?

5. Which equipment is needed for the following?
   a. Vital sign measurement:

   b. Oral examination:

   c. Weber test:

6. Identify the following positions for a patient during a physical examination.

   a.

   b.

   c.

   d.

7. Describe the four assessment techniques that are used during a comprehensive physical examination.
   a. Inspection—

   b. Palpation—

   c. Percussion—

   d. Auscultation—

   What is the order of the performance of these techniques for an abdominal assessment?

8. The nurse is trying to auscultate heart and lung sounds but cannot hear them clearly. What should the nurse do?

9. What is included in the general survey?

10. The patient has an open wound on the skin. To perform the assessment, what should the nurse obtain?

11. For an assessment of the skin, identify all of the **expected** findings. *Select all that apply.*
    a. Pallor _____
    b. Cyanosis _____
    c. Supple to touch _____
    d. Uniform tone _____
    e. Purpura _____
    f. Even coloration _____

12. Identify the following skin lesions:

a.

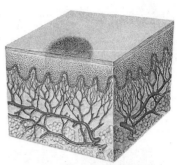

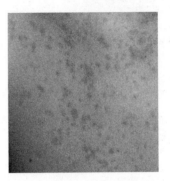

b.

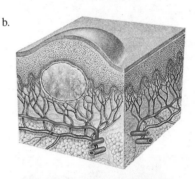

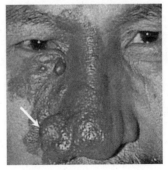

c.

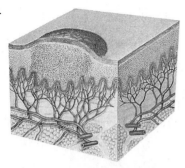

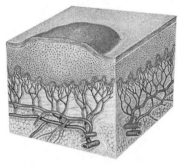

d.

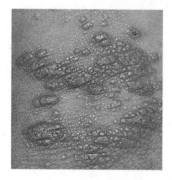

13. Identify which of the following are accurate palpation techniques. *Select all that apply.*
    a. Deep palpation is performed first, then followed by light palpation. _____
    b. The presence of lumps or masses can be determined. _____
    c. Tender areas are palpated first. _____
    d. The surface of the fingers is used to determine the shape of an organ. _____
    e. Palpation is not done over vascular structures. _____
    f. Turgor can be determined. _____

14. For an assessment of the hair and nails, which are **expected** findings? *Select all that apply.*
    a. Nailbed light pin to reddish brown tinged _____
    b. 160-degree angle between the nail and nail plate _____
    c. Alopecia _____
    d. Pruritus _____
    e. Capillary refill of 10 seconds _____
    f. Dry, brittle hair _____

15. Changes in hair growth are usually indications of:

16. Areas assessed in the head include:

17. For the assessment of the eyes, identify the **expected** findings. *Select all that apply.*
    a. Strabismus _____
    b. Ptosis _____
    c. Hordeolum _____
    d. Periorbital edema _____
    e. Xanthelasma _____
    f. Transparent, glossy cornea _____

18. The nurse notes that the patient's pupils are less than 2 mm in size and do not dilate. What does the nurse suspect?

19. When PERRLA is documented it means:

20. For assessment of visual acuity:
    a. What are the instructions for the patient?

    b. If the patient reads the line that says 20/100, what does that indicate?

    c. The patient does not read. What should the nurse do?

21. During assessment of the nose and ears, the nurse documents **unexpected** findings. *Select all that apply.*
    a. Erythema around the nares _____
    b. Small amount of cerumen _____
    c. Translucent, pearly gray eardrum _____
    d. Auricles aligned with the corner of the eyes _____
    e. Septum deviated from midline _____
    f. Tragus sensitive to palpation _____

22. What safety measure needs to be taken when administering the Romberg test?

23. During assessment of the mouth, throat, and neck, the nurse documents **unexpected** findings. *Select all that apply.*
    a. Oral membranes pale-pink _____
    b. Able to clench the teeth and smile _____
    c. White patches on pharynx _____
    d. Nonpalpable lymph nodes _____
    e. Distended jugular veins at 45 degrees _____
    f. Cheilitis _____

24. How are the carotid arteries assessed?

25. Identify on the graphic how the assessment of lung sounds will proceed.

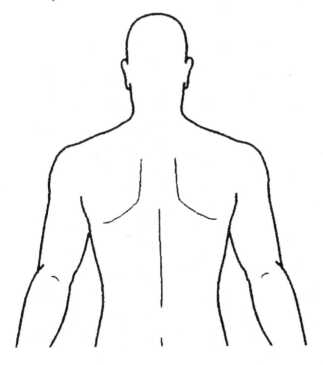

26. During assessment of the thorax, the nurse documents **expected** findings. *Select all that apply.*
    a. AP diameter is less than transverse diameter _____
    b. Quiet breathing _____
    c. Accessory muscles used for breathing _____
    d. Tactile fremitus present across chest _____
    e. Tripod posture observed _____
    f. Symmetrical lung excursion _____

27. Identify on the graphic where the nurse should listen for the apical pulse.

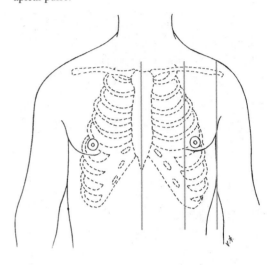

28. Identify three unexpected cardiac findings for an adult patient older than 30 years old.

29. A peripheral pulse that is faint but detectable is documented by the nurse as:

30. How does the nurse assess for phlebitis in the lower extremities?

31. Identify which of the pulses are being assessed.

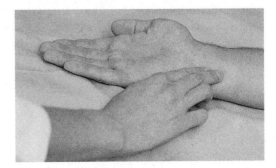

Chapter **20**   **Health History and Physical Assessment**

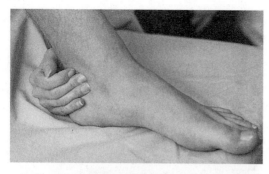

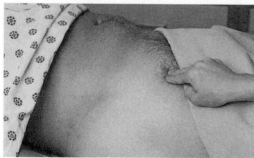

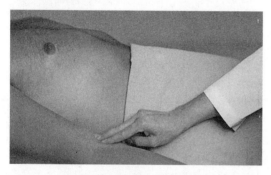

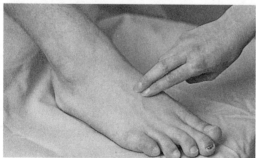

34. During assessment of the musculoskeletal system, the nurse documents **unexpected** findings. *Select all that apply.*
    a. Hypotonicity _____
    b. Full range of motion to upper extremities _____
    c. Muscles firm _____
    d. Clonus noted _____
    e. Symmetrical leg strength _____
    f. Slight muscle hypertrophy to dominant side _____

35. The patient is assessed as follows:
    Eye Opening: Opens eyes to verbal command
    Verbal: Confused but able to answer questions
    Motor: Obeys commands
    What is the Glasgow Coma Scale score? Is it within the range for a responsive patient?

36. What questions are asked to determine the patient's orientation and mental status?

37. How can a patient's long-term memory be tested?

38. Identify on the graphic where discomfort in the lower right quadrant would be noted.

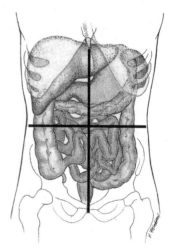

32. How is an Allen test performed and what is the purpose of this test?

33. What are the first clinical signs of osteoporosis?

39. During assessment of the abdomen, the nurse documents **expected** findings. *Select all that apply.*
    a. Visible protrusion by the umbilicus _____
    b. Flat abdomen _____
    c. Palpable firmness above the pubis symphysis _____
    d. Bowel sounds to all quadrants every 2-5 seconds _____
    e. Rebound tenderness to lower right side _____
    f. Borborygmi _____

Chapter **20**   **Health History and Physical Assessment**

40. To maintain asepsis during a female genital examination, the nurse should:

41. During assessment of the female and male genitalia, the nurse documents **expected** findings for a young adult. *Select all that apply.*
    a. Perineal skin color slightly darker than surrounding skin _____
    b. Hemorrhoids _____
    c. Purulent drainage noted at urethral meatus _____
    d. Nodules noted on palpation of labia majora _____
    e. Smooth, pliable testes _____
    f. Coarse, thick pubic hair _____

42. Identify community resources for public and home health services.

43. What are the preventive strategies that the nurse can teach the patient about in relation to:
    a. Cataracts—

    b. Glaucoma—

44. In teaching a young adult woman about reducing her risk of breast cancer, the nurse includes information about:

45. During the physical examination, the patient begins to experience respiratory distress. The nurse should:

Select the best answer for each of the following questions:

46. During an inspection of the patient's skin, the nurse finds a tan-brown, flat lesion with irregular borders. The nurse suspects that this may be:
    a. melanoma.
    b. squamous cell carcinoma.
    c. basal cell carcinoma.
    d. an area of old scar tissue.

47. The adolescent patient is found to have an S-shaped curvature of the spine. The nurse documents this finding as:
    a. lordosis.
    b. kyphosis.
    c. scoliosis.
    d. stenosis.

48. To test fine motor skills, the nurse will ask the patient to:
    a. walk.
    b. stand on one foot.
    c. bend over and touch the toes.
    d. turn pages one at a time.

49. The nurse is examining a patient with dark skin. In assessing for jaundice, the nurse will specifically look at the:
    a. dorsal surface of the hands.
    b. buccal mucosa.
    c. ear lobe.
    d. sclera.

50. A female patient is seen in the outpatient clinic for numerous cuts, bruises, and apparent burns. In a discussion with the patient, the nurse finds that the injuries are inconsistent with the stated cause. The patient also states that she is having trouble sleeping and she appears anxious. On the basis of these findings, the nurse suspects that the patient may be experiencing:
    a. substance abuse.
    b. domestic violence.
    c. vascular disease.
    d. mental illness.

51. In preparing to conduct a physical examination on a patient, the nurse plans to:
    a. perform painful procedures at the end of the examination.
    b. take long, detailed notes of all the findings during the examination.
    c. keep the TV or radio on to distract the patient throughout the examination.
    d. assess the dominant side of the body only during the examination.

52. The nurse is auscultating the patient's lungs and notes normal vesicular sounds as:
    a. medium-pitched blowing sounds with inspiration equalling expiration.
    b. loud, high-pitched, hollow sounds with expiration longer than inspiration.
    c. soft, breezy, low-pitched sounds with longer inspiration.
    d. sounds created by air moving through small bronchial airways.

53. The nurse suspects that the patient may have vascular disease. During the examination, the nurse is alert to the patient's specific complaints of:
    a. diplopia, floaters, and headaches.
    b. headache, dizziness, and tingling of body parts.
    c. leg cramps, numbness of extremities, and edema.
    d. pain and cramping in the toes after walking.

54. A 21-year-old woman asks when she should perform a breast self-examination during the month. The nurse should inform the patient:
    a. "Any time you think of it."
    b. "At the same time each month."
    c. "About halfway through each month."
    d. "Two to three days after your menstrual period."

59

55. The nurse asks a patient to explain the meaning of the phrase, "Every cloud has a silver lining." This part of the examination is designed to assess:
    a. knowledge.
    b. judgment.
    c. association.
    d. abstract thinking.

56. Measurement of the patient's ability to sense the touch of a cotton ball on the forehead tests which cranial nerve?
    a. Optic
    b. Facial
    c. Trigeminal
    d. Oculomotor

57. The expected appearance of the oral mucosa in a light-skinned adult is:
    a. pinkish-red, smooth, and moist.
    b. light pink, rough, and dry.
    c. cyanotic, with rough nodules.
    d. deep red, with rough edges.

58. As part of the examination, the nurse will be assessing the patient's balance. The test that should be administered is the:
    a. Weber test.
    b. Romberg test.
    c. Allen test.
    d. Rinne test.

59. Part of the neurological examination is evaluating the response of the cranial nerves. To test cranial nerve VIII, the nurse should:
    a. ask the patient to read printed material.
    b. assess the directions of the gaze.
    c. assess the patient's ability to hear the spoken word.
    d. ask the patient to say "ah."

60. A student nurse is working with a patient who has asthma. The primary nurse tells the student that wheezes can be heard on auscultation. The student expects to hear:
    a. coarse crackles and bubbling.
    b. high-pitched whistling sounds.
    c. dry, grating noises.
    d. loud, low-pitched rumbling.

61. A physical examination is to be performed by the nurse on a patient who has cardiopulmonary disease. Knowing this information about the patient, the nurse is alert when checking the nails for the presence of:
    a. clubbing.
    b. paronychia.
    c. Beau lines.
    d. splinter hemorrhages.

62. During a physical examination, the patient tells the nurse that he has been told he has myopia. The nurse expects to find that the patient:
    a. is nearsighted.
    b. has decreased peripheral vision.
    c. has diminished night vision.
    d. experiences more glare, flashes, and floaters.

63. A nurse is evaluating a patient for conduction deafness in the right ear. In using the Weber test, the nurse appropriately places the tuning fork and confirms this type of deafness when:
    a. sound is not heard in either ear.
    b. sound is heard best by the patient in the left ear.
    c. sound is heard best by the patient in the right ear.
    d. sound is reduced and heard longer through air conduction.

64. An inspection of the lower extremities is being performed. The presence of arterial insufficiency is suspected when the nurse observes:
    a. increased hair growth.
    b. cooler skin temperatures.
    c. calf enlargement.
    d. brown pigmentation.

65. In the auscultation of the thorax, the nurse notes that the sounds heard over the trachea are expected to be:
    a. soft, low pitched, and breezy.
    b. harsh, loud, and high pitched.
    c. moist, crackling, and bubbling.
    d. medium pitched, intermittent, and grating.

66. During a physical examination, a nurse should assess the temperature of the patient's skin by using the:
    a. dorsal aspect of the hand.
    b. pads of the fingers.
    c. palmar surface of the hand.
    d. fingertips.

67. During the neurologic component of a physical examination, the nurse tests the function of the patient's cranial nerves. In testing cranial nerve III, the nurse determines the patient's ability to:
    a. smile and frown.
    b. move the tongue around.
    c. identify sweet and sour tastes.
    d. react to light with changes in pupil size.

68. The nurse is aware that which of the following are true regarding patients seeing their medical records?
    a. Patients are unable to see their records without a court order.
    b. Family members are able to view the patients' records.
    c. Copies of the patients' records can be provided to the patient with a provider's release.
    d. Patients should review the record in the presence of the primary care provider to ensure accuracy.

Practice Situation

For the case study in the chapter:

Mrs. Thatcher, an 85-year-old recent widow, comes to the health clinic for her annual physical examination. She reports feeling more tired than usual and has noticed that her feet are swelling. Mrs. Thatcher states that sometimes she feels short of breath after climbing the steps to her bedroom on the second floor. Her intake vital signs are T 98.2° F, P 100 and slightly irregular, BP 116/68, and R 24 and shallow. The nurse is acquainted with Mrs. Thatcher and notices that she is walking more slowly than usual to the examination room.

a. In the conceptual care map format, identify possible nursing diagnoses.

b. What treatments do you anticipate?

These are the patient's answers to the questions on a medical history form. What is the follow-up for these areas?

- Have you noticed any change in your vision? Yes
- Do you experience bleeding gums, cold sores, dry mouth, or cracked lips? Yes
- Do you smoke cigarettes? Yes
- Is there a burning sensation when you urinate? Yes

REVIEW QUESTIONS

- Which strategies are used to conduct a patient interview, health history, and review of systems?
- What are the environmental and patient care activities that should be completed before and during history taking and physical examination?
- How are the four physical assessment techniques used during the examination of each body system?
- Which factors are considered during the general survey?
- How are a focused and a head-to-toe physical assessment completed, including opportunities for patient education?
- What are the activities and specific documentation that are required at the completion of the physical assessment?

21 Ethnicity and Cultural Assessment

CHAPTER REVIEW

Match the description/definition in Column A with the correct term in Column B.

Column A

_____ 1. Focuses on the local, indigenous, and insider's culture

_____ 2. Process whereby a culture is passed from generation to generation

_____ 3. Arbitrarily assigning a race to a person on the basis of a societal dictate that associates social identity with ancestry

_____ 4. Process by which individuals from one cultural group merge with, or blend into, a second group

_____ 5. Process of being reared and nurtured within a culture and acquiring its characteristics

_____ 6. Mechanism of cultural change achieved through the exchange of cultural features resulting from firsthand contact between groups

_____ 7. Focuses on the outsider's world and especially on professional views

_____ 8. A statement, idea, or principle that has a broad application

_____ 9. A group of people having a common interest or identity

_____ 10. Belief that one's own culture is superior to that of another while using one's own cultural values as the criteria by which to judge other cultures

Column B

a. Acculturation

b. Assimilation

c. Generalization

d. Etic perspective

e. Enculturation

f. Rule of descent

g. Emic perspective

h. Ethnocentrism

i. Community

j. Socialization

Complete the following:

11. What is the difference between culture and ethnicity?

12. Explain culturally competent care.

13. People within a particular cultural group may differ in their beliefs and rituals.

    True _____   False _____

14. Briefly describe each of the following elements of culture:
    a. Learned

b. Symbolic

c. Shared

d. Integrated

15. How are stereotypes specifically detrimental in health care?

16. What are some examples of discrimination?

17. Identify examples of symbolic characteristics of a community.

18. How is the school system a part of cultural sharing?

19. Explain how nursing care may be influenced by patients' cultural rituals.

20. What is the goal of transcultural nursing?

21. What are the National Culturally and Linguistically Appropriate Standards (CLAS)?

22. What are the three cultures that the nurse brings into relationships with patients?

23. What cultural assessment tools are available?

24. How should a nurse assess a dark-skinned person for oxygenation?

25. An individual who is oriented to the present is more likely to exhibit which characteristics or behaviors? *Select all that apply.*
    a. Look to traditional approaches to health and healing. _____
    b. Delay personal gratification. _____
    c. Believe that time is flexible. _____
    d. Arrive late to scheduled appointments. _____
    e. Maintain a rigid time schedule. _____
    f. Be less likely to practice preventive health care. _____

26. How are the following influenced by culture?
    a. Hygienic care—

    b. Nutrition—

27. According to Purnell, what are the three levels of culture?

28. Patients from lower socioeconomic levels usually have poorer health and a shorter life expectancy.

    True _____   False _____

29. Impaired verbal communication is an accurate nursing diagnosis for a patient who speaks a language different from English.

    True _____   False _____

30. What are some interventions to use when working with a person who has come from a foreign country and speaks a different language?

31. Identify at least three of the areas, according to The Joint Commission, that should be assessed to ensure enhanced communication with culturally diverse individuals.

32. How can a patient's cultural background become a challenge for health care providers?

33. What are important aspects of nursing care that should be included when working with patients from other cultural backgrounds?

34. The nurse is assessing the patient's time orientation and space needs. Which of the following questions will elicit information in those areas? *Select all that apply.*
    a. How often do you have visitors to your home? _____
    b. Who or what helps you cope during difficult times? _____
    c. How do you define social activities? _____
    d. If a stranger touches you, how do you react or feel? _____
    e. Are you comfortable with the distance between us now? _____
    f. If the nurse tells you that you will receive a medication in "about half an hour," realistically, how much time will you allow before you call the nurses' station? _____

35. What are the four C's of culture?

36. Indicate which of the following statements are accurate, with consideration that not all individuals from a particular culture will always reflect the belief or practice. *Select all that apply.*
    a. Asians generally have a larger body stature than Anglo-Americans and Mexicans. _____
    b. Orthodox Jewish people require a kosher diet. _____

63

c. Self-care is valued among most American families. _____

d. Amish families tend to share health care costs. _____

e. Different-gender caregivers are acceptable for Muslim patients. _____

f. Nonverbal communication is important to Japanese individuals. _____

Select the best answer for each of the following questions:

37. Which of the following is the most important symbol of a culture?
    a. Tools
    b. Beliefs
    c. Clothing
    d. Language

38. Within transcultural nursing, sensitivity to social organization is the recognition of the patient's:
    a. use of language and gestures.
    b. definition of health and illness.
    c. status and expected role in the family.
    d. psychological characteristics and coping mechanisms.

39. Traditional Western medicine, in contrast to alternative therapy, uses which of the following?
    a. Prescribed medications
    b. Spiritual advising
    c. Acupuncture
    d. Music therapy

40. In working with patients from different cultural backgrounds, the nurse may find that the patient and family are not fluent in English. The nurse recognizes which of the following as an appropriate strategy for communicating with patients who are not fluent in English?
    a. Speaking in a louder tone of voice
    b. Responding to the patient by his or her first name
    c. Incorporating pictures and hand gestures
    d. Having a family member act as an interpreter for all communication

41. An older female who is Chinese is supposed to have chemotherapy. She is hesitant to agree to this treatment. The nurse who is culturally aware recognizes that this is most likely related to which of the following?
    a. Dependence on health care providers for information
    b. Reliance on family members for decision making
    c. Lack of motivation to participate in self-care
    d. Denial of traditional medical treatment

42. The nurse believes that a patient from another cultural background is using herbal remedies along with the prescribed medication to treat her arthritis. Which of the following should be the nurse's first action?
    a. Tell the patient that herbs will interfere with the prescribed medication.
    b. Ask the patient why additional remedies are being used.
    c. Determine which herbs are being used and their effectiveness.
    d. Contact the physician to alert him or her about the herbal remedies.

43. The patient is being prepared for surgery later in the afternoon. The nurse observes that the patient is wearing a religious charm on a chain around her neck. When asked, the patient says that she would like to keep it on. The nurse's best initial approach is to:
    a. remove the bracelet.
    b. tape the bracelet in place.
    c. ask the patient to remove the item and leave it with family members.
    d. determine if the item may remain in place during the procedure.

Practice Situation

Mr. R. is brought into the emergency department with chest pain and dyspnea. He speaks Spanish and does not appear to understand what you, the physician, and other nurses are trying to explain. No one in the immediate area speaks Spanish. Mr. R. appears frightened about what is happening.

a. How will you communicate with the patient while he is receiving emergency treatment?

b. After making sure that the patient is stabilized, what will you do next?

REVIEW QUESTIONS

- What are the characteristics of culture and ethnicity?
- How do cultural concepts affect a nurse's ability to provide culturally congruent care?
- Which factors contribute to cultural identity acquisition?
- What is transcultural nursing?
- What is cultural competence?

22 Spiritual Health

CHAPTER REVIEW

Complete the following:

1. What are the differences between spirituality and religion?

2. The three types of activities promoted by spiritual practices involve connecting with:

3. Identify examples of rituals associated with religion.

4. Although not all members of a religion will always practice in the same way, the nurse realizes that there are some commonalities. For patients who practice Hinduism, which of the following are anticipated health beliefs? *Select all that apply.*
   a. Health is viewed only physically. _____
   b. Illness is a buildup of toxins. _____
   c. Gua-sha therapy is used. _____
   d. Circumcision is regularly performed. _____
   e. Dietary restrictions exist. _____
   f. The soul is immortal. _____

5. How can the nurse provide spiritual care and assistance to a patient?

6. Briefly describe parish nursing and the role of the nurse in that system.

7. Identify how the nurse can be alert to signs of spiritual distress.

8. What nursing interventions are appropriate for a patient experiencing spiritual issues?

9. How can the nurse maintain spiritual health?

10. What does the acronym SPIRIT represent as a spiritual assessment framework?

11. Identify the following spiritual assessment cues that the patient may offer:
    a. Environmental—

    b. Situational—

Select the best answer for each of the following questions:

12. The process of moving beyond whom one is at the moment to whom one will become is known as:
    a. spirituality.
    b. transcendence.
    c. reflection.
    d. faith building.

13. In Fowler's Theory of Faith Development, Middle Adulthood (conjunctive faith) is characterized by which of the following behaviors?
    a. Spiritual growth happens as a result of finding meaning in social relationships.
    b. Concrete rules are rejected and personal meaning is found in one's own beliefs.
    c. There is a greater understanding of self and appreciation of different perspectives.
    d. An ability exists to accept multiple interpretations of reality.

14. When working with adolescent patients and discussing spirituality, the nurse is aware that patients in this age group often:
    a. have a good concept of a supreme being.
    b. question religious practices and values.
    c. give themselves over to spiritual tasks.
    d. fully accept the higher meaning of their faith.

65

15. The nurse's knowledge about spirituality begins with the nurse:
    a. looking at his or her own beliefs.
    b. researching all popular religions.
    c. sharing his or her faith with the patients.
    d. providing prayers and religious articles for patients.

16. A 76-year-old patient has just been admitted to the nursing unit with terminal cancer of the liver. The nurse is assessing the patient's spiritual needs and responds best by saying:
    a. "What do you believe happens to your spirit when you die?"
    b. "We would allow members of your church to visit you whenever you desire."
    c. "I notice you have a Bible—is that a source of spiritual strength to you?"
    d. "Has your terminal condition made you lose your faith or beliefs?"

17. While working with a patient to assess and support spirituality, the nurse should first:
    a. refer the patient to the agency chaplain.
    b. assist the patient to use faith to get well.
    c. provide a variety of religious literature.
    d. determine the patient's perceptions and belief system.

18. If a patient is identified as following traditional health care beliefs of Judaism, the nurse should prepare to incorporate which of the following into care?
    a. Faith healing
    b. Regular fasting
    c. Observance of the Sabbath
    d. Ongoing group meetings and prayer

19. The nurse has identified the following nursing diagnoses for his assigned patients. Of the following diagnoses, which one indicates the greatest potential need to plan for the patient's spiritual needs?
    a. Impaired health maintenance
    b. Ineffective individual coping
    c. Decreased adaptive capacity
    d. Impaired memory

20. The nurse anticipates the gender-related needs of the patients and tries to accommodate those needs whenever possible. A female nurse is arranged for the female patient who practices which of the following?
    a. Sikhism
    b. Judaism
    c. Catholicism
    d. Buddhism

Practice Situation

A patient is the adult daughter of parents who are Christian Scientists. She expresses that she tries to practice this faith but recently has accepted medical treatment to preserve her pregnancy. She tells you that she is conflicted about this and feels that she is "betraying her family and their beliefs" while still wanting to have a healthy baby.
a. Identify a nursing diagnosis, goal/outcome, and nursing interventions for this patient.

REVIEW QUESTIONS

- What is spirituality, and how is it practiced?
- What are the religious practices that promote spiritual health?
- How can nurses provide spiritual care?
- How can the spiritual assessment frameworks be used?
- Which nursing diagnoses are appropriate for the care of patients with spiritual concerns?
- What are the interdisciplinary aspects of planning when spiritual needs are identified?
- How are personalized spiritual care interventions and evaluation criteria incorporated into the patient's care plan?

23 Public Health, Community-Based, and Home Health Care

CHAPTER REVIEW

Match the description/definition in Column A with the correct term in Column B.

Column A

_____ 1. Occurrence

_____ 2. Consists of studies that are conducted once a disease is evident

_____ 3. Pervasiveness or extent

_____ 4. Generates a hypothesis of why the disease might be occurring in the community and then tests the hypothesis

_____ 5. Causes

Column B

a. Analytic epidemiology

b. Incidence

c. Etiological factors

d. Descriptive epidemiology

e. Prevalence

Complete the following:

6. What is the role of the public health nurse?

7. How are community health and public health different?

8. Identify examples of social determinants of health.

9. What is the role of the community-based nurse?

10. Home care nurses often need to be innovative when they are providing care in a patient's home. What possible items may be found in the home for safe disposal of used needles and syringes?

11. Which of the following are classified as skilled nursing services? *Select all that apply.*
    a. Meal preparation _____
    b. IV therapy _____
    c. Ostomy care _____
    d. Bathing _____
    e. Assistance with feeding _____
    f. Respiratory ventilation care _____

12. How are home health services funded?

13. What is end-of-life care for terminally ill patients called?

14. Provide an example for each of the following levels of health care prevention:
    a. Primary—

    b. Secondary—

    c. Tertiary—

15. Which of the following are examples of intrinsic or host factors? *Select all that apply.*
    a. Food sources _____
    b. Genetics _____
    c. Ethnic group _____
    d. Neighborhood safety _____
    e. Immunization status _____
    f. Place of employment _____

16. Provide at least three examples of vulnerable populations.

17. What online resources can the nurse use to answer the following questions?
    a. What is the recommended immunization schedule for children and adults?
    b. How many people live in a specific town, county, or state?

18. What is the nurse observing when performing a windshield survey?

19. Identify at least five items on the OASIS form.

20. For an issue with neighborhood safety, who are the stakeholders?

21. Identify a nursing diagnosis for a problem with the fresh water supply.

22. How are written materials assessed for their level of readability?

23. To achieve the QSEN competency of teamwork and collaboration in the community, whom may the nurse interact with to coordinate public health?

24. A patient has a history of a gastrointestinal (GI) disease with eight hospitalizations over the past 21 years. He eats a well-balanced diet that keeps his GI symptoms suppressed. Which level of prevention corresponds to his dietary management?

Select the best answer for each of the following questions:

25. It is important that critical aspects of *Healthy People 2020* be incorporated into health care delivery in the community. One of the overall goals of this plan is to:
    a. reduce funding for services.
    b. decrease health care costs.
    c. address health care disparity.
    d. establish the credentials of professionals providing services.

26. Health promotion is an important factor in cost reduction for health care delivery. The nurse assists the patient in a health promotion activity by:
    a. treating a foot ulcer.
    b. administering medication.
    c. obtaining an operative consent.
    d. discussing exercise and nutrition.

27. The student nurse is investigating different types of practice settings. In looking at community health nursing, the student recognizes that it:
    a. requires graduate-level educational preparation.
    b. includes direct care to individuals in specific areas.
    c. is the same as public health nursing.
    d. focuses on the incidence of disease.

28. In community health, the nurse works with patients from different populations who are extremely vulnerable. Which one of the following patients from a vulnerable population currently appears to be at the greatest risk?
    a. A substance abuser who shares needles and syringes
    b. An older adult taking medication for hypertension
    c. A physically abused patient in a shelter
    d. A schizophrenic patient in outpatient therapy

Practice Situation

You are visiting a patient in her home and observe the following during your assessment:

The patient is an 84-year-old female, with a history of heart disease, who lives alone in a second-floor apartment.

You notice that there is a wooden floor with a number of small rugs. There are papers and other items sitting in piles on the floor. When you wash your hands, you notice that the water temperature is quite hot and the lighting in the bathroom is dim. The patient's medications are sitting on the kitchen table, and the number in each bottle does not seem to match with how many should have been taken since her hospital discharge. In the refrigerator, you see that she has a large number of frozen meals and few fresh food items. The patient tells you that she does not feel like making meals because she cannot get to the grocery store by herself to purchase food.
a. What are your main concerns for this patient?

b. How can you assist the patient to meet her needs for health and safety?

REVIEW QUESTIONS

- What are the various types of community health nursing?
- How does the nurse address the three levels of prevention?
- Which factors have an impact on the health of a community?
- Who are some of the vulnerable individuals within a community, and what are the target populations for community-based care?
- How would you carry out a community or home health assessment using data collection tools such as the OASIS data set?
- What are possible nursing diagnoses for clients in the community or populations of interest?
- Which measurable goals can be used to develop community-based plans of care?
- Which collaborative interventions can be implemented to address the needs of the identified target population or client?

24 Human Sexuality

CHAPTER REVIEW

Match the description/definition in Column A with the correct term in Column B.

Column A

_____ 1. An individual who is sexually active with partners of either sex

_____ 2. The outward behavior of a person as a male or female and the perception of what constitutes gender-appropriate actions

_____ 3. A term most often associated with male homosexuality

_____ 4. A person's attraction to his or her own sex, the opposite sex, or both sexes when choosing a sexual partner

_____ 5. A person who has the desire to dress in the clothes of and be accepted as a member of the opposite sex

_____ 6. A person who has an overwhelming desire to be of the opposite sex

_____ 7. Having a gender identity or gender perception different from one's phenotypic gender

_____ 8. A person who has sexual interest in or sexual intercourse exclusively with partners of the opposite sex

_____ 9. Refers exclusively to female homosexuality

_____ 10. A person who has sexual interest in or sexual intercourse exclusively with members of his or her own sex

Column B

a. Transgendered

b. Gay

c. Bisexual

d. Gender role

e. Heterosexual

f. Homosexual

g. Lesbian

h. Transsexual

i. Sexual orientation

j. Transvestite

Complete the following:

11. The nurse is teaching patients about contraception. Identify which methods can be discussed for each of the following:
    a. Barrier methods _____

    b. Prescriptive _____

    c. Sterilization _____

12. How is infertility defined?

13. What are the areas of concern for sexual education?

14. What factors influence how a person identifies with gender?

15. For sexually transmitted diseases (STDs):
    a. Identify possible signs and symptoms of an STD.

    b. Risk of transmission can be reduced with:

    c. In addition to sexual transmission, HIV can be transmitted via:

69

16. How do the following affect sexual function?
    a. Chronic illness

    b. Work issues

    c. Poor body image

17. Which of the following are accurate statements regarding health characteristics of older adults? *Select all that apply.*
    a. There is continued interest in sex. _____
    b. Protection against STDs is not necessary. _____
    c. Modesty is increased. _____
    d. There are beginning role adjustments. _____
    e. Vaginal secretions are reduced. _____
    f. More time is necessary for erection. _____

18. A tool to assist nurses to become more comfortable with assessment of sexual health is the PLISSIT model. What is the meaning of this acronym?

    P ————
    L ————
    I ————
    S ————
    S ————
    I ————
    T ————

19. What areas should be included in the sexual history for a patient?

20. Specify how the following may influence sexuality and the nursing implications for each.
    a. Culture and religion

    b. Environment

21. Identify at least three types of medications that can influence sexual function.

22. For the Sexual Assault Nurse Examiner (SANE) and Sexual Assault Response Team (SART):
    a. To maintain a chain of evidence, the SANE/SART collects:

    b. The SANE and SART work with the patient to:

23. Which of the following are correct statements regarding domestic violence? *Select all that apply.*
    a. Domestic violence is always physical in nature. _____
    b. Leaving a domestic violence situation can be just as dangerous as staying. _____
    c. Total and complete privacy must be maintained during screening. _____
    d. Patient and family safety is the top priority. _____
    e. Nurses are not required to assess for indications of domestic violence. _____
    f. Victims may not accept written information from the nurse. _____

Select the best answer for each of the following questions:

24. The nurse is aware that sexuality is part of growth and development. The preschooler's interest in gender sexuality is characterized by which of the following?
    a. Asking questions associated with sex
    b. Learning how and why his or her anatomy differs from other children
    c. Playing and developing friendships with children of the opposite sex
    d. Spending most of his or her time with the parent of the opposite sex

25. A 58-year-old female asks the nurse what she can do to promote healthy sexual relations. On the basis of the patient's age, the nurse responds by saying:
    a. "Continue what you've been doing. Nothing should have changed."
    b. "I will refer you to a sexual therapist to better assist you."
    c. "Using a water-based lubricant may be helpful."
    d. "Reducing the frequency of intercourse may help you."

26. A patient states that she is afraid that she and her husband will not be able to maintain a healthy sexual relationship now that they have a baby in the house. To assist these patients, it would be most helpful for the nurse to first know:
    a. if they have similar parenting beliefs.
    b. how long they have been married.
    c. the level of knowledge they have regarding healthy sexual relationships.
    d. how comfortable they are in communicating their feelings to each other.

27. On completion of an assessment of a patient in the medical clinic, the nurse documents that the patient has dyspareunia on the basis of the patient's experience of:
    a. deficient or absent sexual desire.
    b. delay or absence of an orgasm.
    c. recurrent genital pain during intercourse.
    d. involuntary constriction of the vagina.

28. An adolescent female student who is sexually active visits the office of the school nurse. Which of the following statements best reflects her understanding of the effective use of contraception devices?
    a. "My boyfriend is able to withdraw before ejaculation, and that prevents me from getting pregnant."
    b. "I take my temperature every morning, and when it goes down for at least 2 days, we have unprotected sex."
    c. "We use 'foam' before each time that we have sex, and I haven't gotten pregnant yet."
    d. "I use a diaphragm and contraceptive cream."

29. A school nurse is responsible for teaching adolescents about STDs. When discussing chlamydia, the nurse instructs the students that it is:
    a. a viral infection that cannot be cured.
    b. treated with a full course of antibiotics.
    c. contracted via blood-borne exchange.
    d. prevented with the use of spermicidals.

30. The nurse is conducting a sexual history with a patient who is scheduled for cardiac surgery.
    The patient tells the nurse that he is nervous about resuming sexual activities. The nurse uses therapeutic communication with the patient when responding:
    a. "You are expressing a very normal concern—perhaps we could discuss your feelings further."
    b. "Don't worry. In about 2 months you will be able to return to your normal sexual patterns."
    c. "You can have sexual intercourse after your surgery, but there are serious risks."
    d. "Your partner will be nervous about resuming sexual activities, but that is normal."

31. A female nurse is working with a male patient. During the administration of medications, the male patient acts out sexually to the female nurse who is caring for him. The nurse should:
    a. ignore the behavior.
    b. get a male nurse to assume the care for this patient.
    c. immediately report the incident to the patient's physician.
    d. stop the action and tell the patient how you feel about the inappropriate behavior.

Practice Situations

You are working in the emergency department and have a female patient who appears to have been the victim of domestic violence.
a. What should you do for this patient?

b. What resources are available?

For the patient in the case study, Mr. Wells:
a. Fill in the following areas on the conceptual care map—admission and assessment information, laboratory tests, and medications.

b. Identify a potential nursing diagnosis and short-term goal for the patient.

REVIEW QUESTIONS

- How does sexual development occur throughout the life cycle?
- What are the structure and function of the male and female reproductive systems?
- What are the differences among sex, sexuality, and gender identity?
- How do the sexual response cycles work for men and women?
- What options are available for contraception?
- What are common sexually transmitted diseases, their causes, and treatments?
- Which factors can affect sexuality?
- Which factors can affect sexual function?
- What is the impact of family dynamics on sexuality?
- How is a sexual assessment conducted?
- Which nursing diagnoses are appropriate for patients with potential or identified sexuality concerns?
- How should a patient-centered care plan be designed to address sexuality needs?
- Which interventions will support enhanced patient sexuality?

25 Safety

CHAPTER REVIEW

Complete the following:

1. What are unintentional injuries?

2. The Joint Commission developed the National Patient Safety Goals, which are:

3. Identify how the following can affect individual safety.
   a. Musculoskeletal function

   b. Neurologic function

4. Which teaching should be included for an information session to new parents on infant safety?

5. How do the following environmental factors influence safety?
   a. Lighting

   b. Workplace hazards

6. Provide examples of safety hazards in the home environment.

7. Identify at least three substances that can lead to unintentional poisoning.

8. Which of the following can contribute to electrical shock? *Select all that apply.*
   a. Overloaded circuits _____
   b. Use of adhesives _____
   c. Use of appliances by sinks _____
   d. Use of kerosene heaters _____
   e. Uncovered electrical outlets _____
   f. Use of devices with frayed wires _____

9. Two of the commonly discussed forms of bioterrorism are:

10. Suffocation can occur as a result of:

11. Which of the following safety concerns are true for older adults? *Select all that apply.*
    a. Exposure to the Internet and TV should be reduced. _____
    b. Driving refresher courses may be indicated. _____
    c. Exercise should be discouraged. _____
    d. Caution should be taken with the water temperature. _____
    e. Medications should be taken in a well-lit area. _____
    f. Obstacles need to be removed from walking paths. _____

12. Adolescents are susceptible to which kinds of safety hazards?

13. The Centers for Medicare and Medicaid will not pay hospitals for the cost of additional care resulting from patient falls.

    True _____   False _____

14. Negative outcomes from the use of physical restraints include:

15. How can nurses avoid medication errors?

16. What are the sources of radiation exposure for nurses?

17. Which assessment questions can be used to determine a patient's susceptibility to injuries from fire and falls in the home?

18. Identify at least two possible safety-related nursing diagnoses and goals/outcomes.

19. The nurse needs to use a fire extinguisher and remembers the PASS acronym, which stands for:

20. Which interventions should the nurse use in the health care environment to reduce the possibility of patient falls?

21. Identify all of the accurate statements or actions involved in the use of physical restraints. *Select all that apply.*
    a. Never apply a restraint without first obtaining a medical order. _____
    b. Tie the restraints tightly in knots to prevent being dislodged. _____
    c. Application of restraints can be delegated to unlicensed assistive personnel. _____
    d. Use of the top two side rails on the bed is considered a restraint. _____
    e. Secure the restraints to the side rails of the beds. _____
    f. Assess the patient at least every hour while restraints are in use. _____

22. The most important way to prevent the spread of infection is for the nurse to:

23. Identify how the nurse can avoid the following procedure- and equipment-related events:
    a. Dislodging of a nasogastric tube—

    b. Inaccurate readings on glucose meters—

    c. Radiation exposure—

24. What is the purpose of this type of restraint?

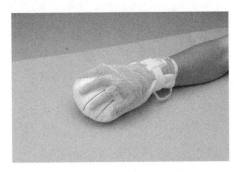

25. Assessment of a patient with a restraint in place should include:

26. The nurse collaborates with other members of the health care team. How does each of the following individuals promote patient safety?
    a. Occupational therapist

    b. Social worker

27. The use of restraints has been found to consistently reduce the number of patient injuries.

    True _____   False _____

28. Identify what should be in the teaching plan for individuals in their homes regarding:
    a. Fire safety—

    b. Carbon monoxide safety—

29. What are some of the common breaches in the safety standards of care that have led to litigation?

Select the best answer for each of the following questions:

30. The nurse has investigated safety hazards and recognizes that the leading cause of unintentional poisoning results from:
    a. carbon monoxide.
    b. contaminated food.
    c. decorative plants.
    d. lead.

31. An ambulatory patient is admitted to the extended care facility with a diagnosis of Alzheimer disease. In using a Fall Assessment tool, the nurse knows that the greatest indicator of risk is:
    a. confusion.
    b. impaired judgment.
    c. sensory deficits.
    d. history of falls.

32. The type of restraint used to prevent a patient from bending over in a wheelchair is a:
    a. wrist restraint.
    b. vest restraint.
    c. elbow restraint.
    d. mummy restraint.

33. A 79-year-old resident in a long-term care facility is known to "wander at night" and has fallen in the past. Which of the following is the most appropriate nursing intervention?
    a. The patient should be checked frequently during the night.
    b. An abdominal restraint should be placed on the patient during sleeping hours.
    c. A radio should be left playing at the bedside to assist in reality orientation.
    d. The patient should be placed in a room away from the activity of the nursing station.

34. The workmen cause an electrical fire when installing a new piece of equipment in the intensive care unit. A patient near the fire is on a ventilator. The first action the nurse should take is to:
    a. pull the fire alarm.
    b. attempt to extinguish the fire.
    c. use an Ambu bag and remove the patient from the area.
    d. call the physician to obtain orders to take the patient off the ventilator.

35. A visiting nurse completes an assessment of the ambulatory patient in the home and determines the nursing diagnosis *Risk for Injury Related to Decreased Vision*. On the basis of this assessment, the patient will benefit the most from:
    a. Installing fluorescent lighting throughout the house.
    b. Becoming oriented to the position of the furniture and stairways.
    c. Maintaining complete bed rest in a hospital bed with side rails.
    d. Applying physical restraints.

36. Which one of the following statements by the parent of a child indicates that further teaching by the nurse is required?
    a. "I make sure that my child wears a helmet when he rides his bicycle."
    b. "I have spoken to my teenager about safe sex practices."
    c. "My child is taking swimming classes at the community center."
    d. "Now that my child is 2 years old, I can let her sit in the front seat of the car with me."

37. The nurse assesses that the patient may need a restraint and recognizes that:
    a. an order for a restraint may be implemented indefinitely until it is no longer required by the patient.
    b. restraints should be ordered regularly for patient safety.
    c. no order or consent is necessary for restraints in long-term care facilities.
    d. restraints are to be periodically removed to have the patient re-evaluated.

38. Upon entering the patient's room, the nurse sees a fire burning in the trash can next to the bed. The nurse removes the patient and calls in the fire. The next action of the nurse is to:
    a. extinguish the fire.
    b. remove all of the other patients from the unit.
    c. close all the doors of patient rooms.
    d. move the trash can into the bathroom.

39. When applying a restraint, the nurse knows that:
    a. the padded side is away from the skin.
    b. it should be removed at least once each shift.
    c. the straps should be secured with a knot.
    d. two fingers' width should fit between the skin and the restraint.

40. A mother of a young child enters the kitchen and finds the child on the floor. There is a bottle of cleanser next to the child and particles of the substance around the child's mouth. The parent's first action should be to:
    a. provide ipecac syrup.
    b. call the Poison Control unit.
    c. check the child's airway and breathing.
    d. remove the particles of cleanser from the mouth.

Practice Situation

The patient is admitted to the hospital for evaluation after having fallen at home. The patient also appears to be disoriented.
    a. Based upon this patient's condition, what can you do to implement a restraint-free environment for this patient?

    b. How can falls be prevented in the patient's home environment?

REVIEW QUESTIONS

- What are common safety concerns in the home, community, and health care environments?
- What factors can affect safety?
- Which situations can alter safety in the home, community, and health care settings?
- Which safety factors can affect individuals at home, in the community, and in health care settings?
- Which nursing diagnoses are relevant for patient safety–related concerns and issues?
- How can nursing care plans that identify interventions to promote patient safety be prepared?
- Which safety measures should be implemented in the home, community, and health care settings?

26 Asepsis and Infection Control

CHAPTER REVIEW

Match the description/definition in Column A with the correct term in Column B.

Column A

_____ 1. Protein molecules on the surface of foreign invaders or nonliving substances such as toxins, chemicals, drugs, or particles

_____ 2. Involves a defense by the white blood cells (WBCs), T lymphocytes, in response to foreign microorganisms

_____ 3. Freedom from and prevention of the contamination that causes infection

_____ 4. Any disease-causing agent

_____ 5. A process used to destroy all microorganisms, including their spores

_____ 6. Specialized cells that recognize foreign invaders

_____ 7. Organisms that live on or in other organisms

_____ 8. Animals that carry the pathogens from one host to another

_____ 9. A defense system that involves antibodies and WBCs that are produced to fight antigens

_____ 10. Group of non-disease-causing microorganisms, such as bacteria, fungi, and protozoa, that live within or on the body

Column B

a. Antibodies

b. Pathogen

c. Vectors

d. Cellular immunity

e. Antigens

f. Normal flora

g. Humoral immunity

h. Asepsis

i. Sterilization

j. Parasites

Complete the following:

11. Identify what the nurse will assess for the following:
    a. Local inflammatory response—

    b. Systemic inflammatory response—

12. How do individuals acquire passive immunity?

13. Provide an example for each component in the chain of infection:
    a. Infectious agent—
    b. Source of infection—
    c. Portal of exit—
    d. Mode of transmission—
    e. Portal of entry—
    f. Susceptible host—

14. Health care–associated infections (HAIs):
    a. What are some of the causes of HAIs?

    b. How can nurses prevent HAIs?

15. Which of the following statements are accurate in relation to infectious control? *Select all that apply.*
    a. Females have a greater risk for urinary tract infection. _____

    b. Culture and ethnicity do not have an influence. _____
    c. Infants are less susceptible to infection. _____
    d. As people age, the immune system becomes more effective. _____
    e. Immobility increases the risk for infection. _____
    f. Older adults are at a greater risk for skin infection. _____

75

16. Which assessment questions should the nurse ask to determine if the patient may have an infection?

17. If an infection is present, what does the nurse expect to see with the patient's vital signs?

18. For the following, indicate which actions are performed under surgical asepsis. *Select all that apply.*
    a. Keep soiled items off of the floor. _____
    b. Avoid shaking linens. _____
    c. Teach patients the proper use of tissues. _____
    d. Avoid coughing or reaching across the sterile field. _____
    e. Keep all items above the waistline and in your sight. _____
    f. Pour liquids directly into the drain to avoid splashing. _____

19. Which nutrients need to be replaced to promote the body's defense mechanisms in the presence of an infection?

20. For drug-resistant microorganisms:
    a. Which factors have contributed to the development of resistant organisms?

    b. Provide at least two examples of resistant organisms in the hospital setting.

21. Why is the following nursing diagnosis a problem for infection control?
    Impaired skin integrity

22. Identify a web-based resource for evidence-based practice associated with infection control.

23. Contact precautions are used for: *Select all that apply.*
    a. Methicillin-resistant *Staphylococcus aureus* (MRSA). _____
    b. *Mycobacterium tuberculosis.* _____
    c. Hepatitis A. _____
    d. Pharyngeal diphtheria. _____
    e. Rubeola. _____
    f. Herpes simplex virus (HSV). _____

24. When is protective isolation used for a patient?

25. When putting on personal protective equipment (PPE), the correct order is:
    a. Gloves _____
    b. Mask _____
    c. Gown _____
    d. Goggles/eyewear _____

26. When there is a high risk of splashing or exposure to bodily fluids, the nurse should make sure to wear:

27. For proper hand washing, how should the nurse address the following:
    a. Cuts on the hands

    b. Visible dirt

    c. Artificial nails are in place

28. Identify the order in which the flaps of the sterile package should be opened.

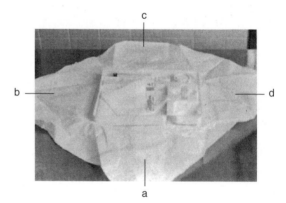

29. Identify the breaks in sterile technique in the two photos.

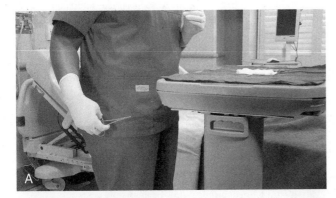

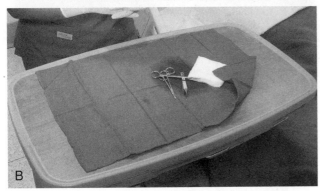

30. Which actions are considered part of Standard Precautions, rather than Transmission-Based Precautions? *Select all that apply.*
    a. Using a particulate respirator mask _____
    b. Discarding needles in a sharps container _____
    c. Keeping live flowers and plants away from the patient _____
    d. Cleaning equipment after use _____
    e. Performing hand hygiene _____
    f. Using gloves _____

31. What is the correct way to pour liquid into a sterile container on a sterile field?

Select the best answer for each of the following questions:

32. The patient has a 6-inch laceration on his right forearm. An infection develops at the site. Which of the following is a sign of a local inflammatory response observed by the nurse?
    a. Blanching of the skin
    b. Edema at the site
    c. Decrease in temperature
    d. Increase in the number of WBCs

33. A female patient has been undergoing diagnostic testing since admission to the medical unit in the hospital. The results of blood testing are sent back to the unit. Upon reviewing the results, the nurse will report the following abnormal finding to the physician:
    a. WBCs 14,000 cells/mm^3
    b. Lymphocytes 2000 cells/mm^3
    c. Neutrophils 65%
    d. Hemoglobin 14 g/dL

34. A nurse is observing a new staff member work with a patient. Of the following activities, which one has the greatest possibility of contributing to an HAI and requires correction?
    a. Washing hands before applying a dressing
    b. Taping a plastic bag to the bed rail for tissue disposal
    c. Placing a Foley catheter bag on the bed when transferring a patient
    d. Using an antiseptic to cleanse the skin before starting an intravenous line

35. The nurse works in a small rural hospital with a wide variety of patients. Of the patients admitted this afternoon, the nurse recognizes that the individual with the highest susceptibility to infection is the individual with which of the following?
    a. Burns
    b. Diabetes
    c. Pulmonary emphysema
    d. Peripheral vascular disease

36. The nurse employs surgical aseptic technique when:
    a. disposing of syringes in puncture-proof containers.
    b. placing soiled linens in moisture-resistant bags.
    c. washing hands before changing a dressing.
    d. inserting an intravenous catheter.

37. The patient has a large, deep abdominal incision that requires a dressing. The incision is packed with sterile half-inch packing and covered with a dry 4- x 4-inch gauze. When changing the dressing, the nurse accidentally drops the packing onto the patient's abdomen. The nurse should:
    a. throw the packing away, and prepare a new one.
    b. add alcohol to the packing and insert it into the incision.
    c. pick up the packing with sterile forceps, and gently place it into the incision.
    d. rinse the packing with sterile water, and put the packing into the incision with sterile gloves.

38. An adult patient has a viral infection. Which of the following vital signs is typical during the early stage of an infection?
    a. Increased blood pressure
    b. Normal temperature
    c. Decreased respiratory rate
    d. Increased oxygen saturation

39. The nurse recognizes that special care must be taken in the handling of which of the following in order to prevent the transmission of hepatitis C?
   a. Feces
   b. Blood
   c. Saliva
   d. Vaginal secretions

40. The parent of a preschool child asks the nurse how chickenpox (varicella zoster) is transmitted. The nurse identifies that the virus is transmitted:
   a. by a vector organism.
   b. through the air in droplets after sneezing or coughing.
   c. through person-to-person contact.
   d. by contact with contaminated objects.

41. The nurse is aware that it is important to break the chain of infection. An example of a nursing intervention that is implemented to control the portal of exit of infection for a patient is:
   a. using hand sanitizer.
   b. wearing disposable gloves.
   c. changing soiled dressings.
   d. administering vaccines.

42. The single most important technique to prevent and control the transmission of infections is:
   a. hand washing.
   b. the use of disposable gloves.
   c. the use of isolation precautions.
   d. sterilization of equipment.

43. A patient with active tuberculosis is admitted to the medical center. The nurse recognizes that admission of this patient to the unit will require the implementation by the staff of:
   a. droplet precautions.
   b. airborne precautions.
   c. contact precautions.
   d. protective isolation.

44. The nurse recognizes the appropriate procedures for sterile asepsis. Of the following, which action is consistent with surgical asepsis?
   a. Clean forceps may be used to move items on the sterile field.
   b. Sterile fields may be prepared well in advance of the procedures.
   c. Sterile items are kept well within a 1-inch outer border of the field.
   d. Wrapped sterile packages should be opened, starting with the flap closest to the nurse.

45. The nurse suspects that an older adult patient may be experiencing hypostatic pneumonia. Older adult patients may react differently to infectious processes, so the nurse is alert to an atypical sign, such as which of the following?
   a. Hypotension
   b. Confusion
   c. Erythema
   d. Chills

46. A patient requires a sterile dressing change for a midabdominal surgical incision. An appropriate intervention for the nurse to implement in maintaining sterile asepsis is to:
   a. put sterile gloves on before opening sterile packages.
   b. place the cap of the sterile solution well within the sterile field.
   c. place sterile items on the edge of the sterile drape.
   d. discard packages that may have been in contact with the area below waist level.

47. The nurse is preparing to assist with a dressing change. An appropriate technique that the nurse includes in performing correct hand hygiene is to:
   a. wash the wrists, then the hands.
   b. use a brush on the palms of the hands.
   c. maintain the scrub for at least 1 minute.
   d. wash well around watches and other jewelry.

48. A patient is found to have MRSA. An appropriate isolation procedure for the nurse to implement when working with this patient is to:
   a. leave all linen in the patient's room.
   b. use personal protective equipment for contact precaution.
   c. wipe the stethoscope off before removing it from the room.
   d. identify on the patient's door that droplet precautions are in place.

49. The nurse is observing the student put on sterile gloves. Which one of the following actions has contaminated the gloves?
   a. Keeping the package above waist level.
   b. Pulling the inner package edges apart with the thumbs and fingers.
   c. Grasping the second glove by the cuff.
   d. Adjusting the gloves by pinching and shifting with the other hand.

50. The unit manager observes the new staff nurse perform the following actions for a patient with isolation precautions. Which of the following actions should the unit manager address and correct with the new nurse?
   a. Keeping a thermometer, stethoscope, and blood pressure cuff in the patient's room.
   b. Documenting the precautions required in the patient's record.
   c. Using a particulate respirator mask for the patient who has tuberculosis.
   d. Coming out of the room in the PPE to quickly get another dressing.

Practice Situation

The patient had surgery this morning and has an incision on his right leg that is sutured and covered with a dry dressing. He will be in the medical center for 2 days.
   a. Identify a possible nursing diagnosis and goal/outcome for this patient related to infection control.

b. How can you help to prevent infection for this patient?

c. After the patient is discharged home, what can you teach the patient and family about infection control?

REVIEW QUESTIONS

- What are the body's defense mechanisms against infection?
- What are the components of the chain of infection?
- Which techniques should be used when assessing for infection or risk for infection?
- Which nursing diagnoses are possible for patients experiencing infection or at risk for infection?
- Which measurable goals are appropriate for patients experiencing complications from infection?
- Which interventions should be implemented in order to decrease the risk of infection and reverse the negative effects of infection?

27 Hygiene and Personal Care

CHAPTER REVIEW

Match the description/definition in Column A with the correct term in Column B.

Column A

_____ 1. A massage technique that employs long hand movements along the length of the back muscles

_____ 2. Unpleasant breath odor

_____ 3. Gums

_____ 4. Absence or loss of hair

_____ 5. Artificial part

_____ 6. Red, scaly areas with surface loss of skin tissue

_____ 7. Breakdown of the skin caused by fluid

_____ 8. Inflammation due to friction

_____ 9. Armpit

_____ 10. Surfaces that line the passages and cavities of the body, such as nasal, oral, vaginal, urethral, and anal areas

Column B

a. Alopecia

b. Excoriation

c. Maceration

d. Chafing

e. Mucous membranes

f. Axilla

g. Gingivae

h. Effleurage

i. Prosthetic

j. Halitosis

Complete the following:

11. How will the following alterations in the structure or function of the integument affect hygienic care?
    a. Ulcers—

    b. Decreased sensation—

    c. Pediculosis—

12. What are the purposes/benefits of the nurse bathing or helping to bathe the patient?

13. How do the following influence hygienic care?
    a. Age—

    b. Culture or ethnicity—

14. How can the nurse assess the patient's ability to perform hygienic self-care?

15. Which of the following are expected findings during a patient's bath? *Select all that apply.*
    a. Reddened gums _____
    b. Smooth, pliable skin _____
    c. Matted hair _____
    d. Ankle edema _____
    e. Rash on lower back _____
    f. Moist mucous membranes _____

16. Identify the ethical considerations associated with hygienic care.

17. For a massage:
    a. What are the benefits to the patient?

    b. What areas are able to be massaged by the nurse or unlicensed assistive personnel?

    c. Which techniques can be used for the massage?

18. When are the following bathing methods used?
    a. Complete bath—

    b. Partial bath—

    c. Shower—

19. What is the usual water temperature for a shower or bath?

20. For a patient with a cognitive impairment, how should hygienic care be adapted?

21. Guidelines for perineal care of a female patient include:

22. For a patient recovering from perineal surgery, what specific hygienic intervention may be used to cleanse the area?

23. What should be documented after hygienic care is provided?

24. Foot care includes:

25. For care of the patient's hair:
    a. The patient is unable to get out of bed and needs to have a shampoo. Which options are available for the nurse to use?

    b. What can be done for tangled and matted hair?

26. The patient has a very dry mouth and cracked lips. What should the nurse suggest?

27. When performing hygienic care, patients on anticoagulants should not use:

28. Which of the following are correct for care of the eyes, nose, and ears? *Select all that apply.*
    a. The eyes are cleaned from the inner to outer canthus. _____
    b. Hearing aids may be rinsed in warm water. _____
    c. Cerumen is removed by inserting a cotton-tipped applicator into the ear canal. _____
    d. Plastic eyeglasses are cleaned with bar soap, water, and a soft towel. _____
    e. Contact lenses are to be disinfected and stored in manufacturer-recommended solution. _____
    f. Crusting around a nasogastric tube in the nose can be removed with saline on a gauze pad. _____

29. Place the following steps for the bed bath in the correct order.
    a. Washing the legs _____
    b. Washing the arms and hands _____
    c. Perineal care _____
    d. Washing the back _____
    e. Cleaning the eyes _____
    f. Washing the chest and abdomen _____
    g. Washing the face, ears, and neck _____

30. Safety measures to implement upon finishing the bath include:

31. Indicate how the nurse can limit the spread of microorganisms for male and female perineal care.

32. Identify safety considerations for oral care of a comatose patient.

33. To prevent damage to a patient's dentures

34. Which of the following are correct in relation to shaving a patient? *Select all that apply.*
    a. Obtain consent from the patient to shave a beard or mustache. _____
    b. Apply cold water to the patient's face for 5 minutes before. _____
    c. Shave the patient in the direction away from the hair growth first. _____
    d. Keep the skin taut and use short strokes. _____
    e. Document any nicks or cuts during the procedure. _____

35. The nurse will be making the patient's bed. Which actions should be taken to prevent personal injury, promote patient comfort, and prevent the spread of microorganisms?

Select the best answer for each of the following questions:

36. A patient has a red, raised skin rash. During the bath, the priority action of the nurse is to:
    a. assess for additional inflammatory reactions.
    b. discuss the body image problems created by the presence of the rash.
    c. wash the skin thoroughly with hot water and soap.
    d. moisturize the skin to prevent drying.

37. The nurse is caring for a patient who has right-sided paralysis following a cerebrovascular accident (stroke). Which of the following factors would be most likely to result in decubitus ulcer formation for this patient?
    a. Poor nutrition
    b. Reduced mobility
    c. Excessive hydration
    d. Skin secretions

38. A nurse delegates the hygienic care of a male patient to the nursing assistant. In reviewing the patient assignment, the nurse instructs the assistant to make sure to use an electric razor to shave the patient with:
    a. thrombocytopenia.
    b. congestive heart failure.
    c. osteoarthritis.
    d. pneumonia.

39. The nurse delegates morning care to a new certified nursing assistant. Which of the following actions by the assistant would be evaluated as appropriate?
    a. Placing dentures in a tissue while not worn
    b. Cutting the patient's nails with scissors
    c. Using soap to cleanse around the eyes
    d. Washing the patient's legs from the ankle to the knee

40. A 61-year-old patient with diabetes mellitus has physician's orders for meticulous foot care. Which of the following is the best rationale for the order?
    a. The aging process causes increased skin breakdown.
    b. There is peripheral neuropathy with this pathology that places the patient at risk.
    c. The patient probably has a history of poor hygienic care.
    d. The lower extremities are difficult to see and therefore hard to maintain with good hygiene.

41. A nurse is instructing a patient with peripheral vascular disease about daily foot care.
    The nurse's instruction for the patient includes:
    a. soaking the feet 5-10 minutes each day.
    b. filing the nails into a curve shape.
    c. using commercial corn removers if needed.
    d. applying lotion to the feet and around the toes.

42. To administer oral care to a semi-comatose patient, the nurse should place the patient in which of the following positions?
    a. Reverse Trendelenburg
    b. High Fowler with the head to the side
    c. Side-lying with the head turned toward the nurse
    d. Supine with the neck slightly forward

43. A patient has recently experienced difficulty hearing out of both ears. Which of the following is the best nursing response to the patient?
    a. "Let's irrigate your ears with cool water."
    b. "Can you turn your head toward me when I am talking to you?"
    c. "Your hearing aid should not need a new battery for at least 3 months."
    d. "Try to avoid cleaning your ears with a Q-tip (cotton-tipped applicator)."

44. A patient has severe right-sided weakness and is unable to complete bathing independently. On the basis of this observation, the nurse identifies a nursing diagnosis of:
    a. powerlessness.
    b. hygiene self-care deficit.
    c. tissue integrity impairment.
    d. knowledge deficit of hygiene practices.

45. The nurse is preparing to assist the adult female patient with perineal care. The position of choice for this patient is:
    a. lithotomy.
    b. side-lying.
    c. supine.
    d. prone.

46. The nurse is completing a bed bath for a dependent adult male patient. During the perineal care, the patient has an erection. The nurse should:
    a. tell the patient just to relax.
    b. indicate that you cannot continue with the bath.
    c. ask the patient to do the care as well as he can.
    d. defer the care until a little later in the bath.

47. A patient on chemotherapy is experiencing stomatitis. The nurse advises the patient to use:
    a. normal saline rinses.
    b. a firm-bristle toothbrush.
    c. a commercial mouthwash.
    d. an alcohol and water mixture.

Practice Situations

Hygienic care is often delegated to unlicensed assistive personnel (UAP). When delegating this care:
a. What should you teach the UAP?

b. What should the UAP be told to report if observed during the care?

For Mr. Randall, the patient in the case study in the text, prepare a plan for his care for the 7 A.M.– to 3 P.M. shift.
    The medication schedule on the unit is follows:
    QID: 9 A.M. - 1 P.M. - 5 P.M. - 9 P.M.
    BID: 9 A.M. - 5 P.M.
    Q4H: 10 A.M. - 2 P.M. - 6 P.M. - 10 P.M. - 2 A.M. - 6 A.M.
    You can start the day by going in to visit the patient at 7:10 A.M. after receiving report.

REVIEW QUESTIONS

- What is the importance of hygiene in relation to skin, hair, nails, and mucous membranes?
- How do alterations in skin, hair, nails, and mucous membranes affect hygienic care?
- How does the nurse determine patients' hygiene status and need for assistance with care?
- What are the possible nursing diagnoses for patients who need assistance with hygiene or are experiencing alterations in self-care abilities?
- What measurable patient-centered goals are appropriate for patients with hygiene concerns and self-care alterations?
- How can nursing care plans be developed to include interventions to address the hygienic needs of patients?

28 Activity, Immobility, and Safe Movement

CHAPTER REVIEW

Match the description/definition in Column A with the correct term in Column B.

Column A

_____ 1. Increased muscle tone

_____ 2. Inability to move all four extremities

_____ 3. Death of cells, tissues, or organs

_____ 4. Manner of walking

_____ 5. Reduced blood flow

_____ 6. Lack of muscle tone

_____ 7. Wasting

_____ 8. Weakness on one side of the body

_____ 9. Awareness of posture and movement

_____ 10. Permanent fixation of a joint

Column B

a. Atrophy

b. Contracture

c. Ischemia

d. Hemiparesis

e. Quadriplegia

f. Necrosis

g. Proprioception

h. Gait

i. Flaccidity

j. Spasticity

Complete the following:

11. Provide examples of alterations in the following body systems that can lead to impaired mobility.
    a. Musculoskeletal—

    b. Neurologic—

    c. Cardiopulmonary—

12. Which assessment questions will help the nurse determine if a patient is experiencing difficulty with mobility?

13. Identify at least two of the complications associated with immobility in the following body systems and nursing interventions to eliminate or reduce their occurrence:
    a. Musculoskeletal—

    b. Cardiopulmonary—

    c. Gastrointestinal—

    d. Integumentary—

14. How does the nurse assess a patient's muscle strength?

15. While performing passive range of motion, the patient starts to grimace, moan, and become tense. The nurse should:

16. What is the purpose of "dangling?"

17. Provide three examples of special mattresses that may be used for immobile patients.

18. The nurse is teaching the aide about correct body mechanics. Which of the following principles are accurate and should be included in the teaching? *Select all that apply.*
    a. Elevate work surfaces to approximately neck height. _____
    b. Never lift more than 75 lb. independently. _____
    c. Push rather than pull patients or objects. _____
    d. Bend from the waist when lifting. _____
    e. Keep patients or objects close to the body to minimize reach. _____
    f. Keep the feet apart to provide a stable base. _____

19. What can the nurse do to prevent friction against the immobile patient's skin?

20. Range of motion:
    a. How many times daily is it usually performed?

    b. How many times should the joints be put through their motion?

21. When using a mechanical lift, which of the following techniques are appropriate? *Select all that apply.*
    a. Use the device only in life-threatening situations. _____
    b. At least two health care workers should carry out the procedure. _____
    c. Determine the operational status before using. _____
    d. Check the manufacturer's weight limit for the device before using. _____
    e. Use a transfer chair for confused or uncooperative patients. _____
    f. Instruct the patient in how the device will work. _____

22. A patient who is immobilized can suffer psychosocial effects. What can the nurse do to prevent or reduce this problem?

23. What are two recommendations and goals for logrolling a patient with a halo brace?

24. The nurse observes that the patient is extremely uncomfortable during position changes. What can the nurse do to avoid discomfort for the patient?

25. What criteria should be used to determine if the patient is strong enough to ambulate?

26. Identify some general safety measures to implement for a patient using an assistive device for ambulation.

27. Place the steps in the correct order for a patient rising from a chair with crutches.
    a. Move the crutches to a tripod position. _____
    b. Hands are holding the hand bar of the crutches and armrest of the chair.
    c. Move to front edge of the chair. _____
    d. Push off the chair and balance. _____

28. Select which of the following are correct for the use of antiembolism hose. *Select all that apply.*
    a. Knee-length hose should end 1 to 2 inches below the knee _____
    b. Application is after the patient is out of bed for at least 15 minutes _____
    c. DVT is checked with the Homan sign if there is calf redness or pain _____
    d. Draining wounds are covered with bandages _____
    e. Hose is applied over damp skin to facilitate application _____
    f. Hose should be washed at least every 3 days _____

Select the best answer for each of the following questions:

29. A patient has been on bed rest for a prolonged period of time. To specifically promote the use of isotonic exercise, the nurse will instruct the patient to:
    a. turn side to side in bed.
    b. perform pelvic floor exercises.
    c. repeatedly tighten the thigh muscle.
    d. use a trapeze to lift and hold the upper body off the bed.

30. An average-size male patient has right-sided hemiparesis, requiring minimal assistance with ambulation. The nurse helps this patient to walk by standing at his:
    a. left side and holding his arm.
    b. left side and holding one arm around his waist.
    c. right side and holding his arm.
    d. right side and holding the gait belt at the patient's back.

31. The nurse is working with a patient who has left-sided weakness. After instruction, the nurse observes the patient ambulate in order to evaluate the use of the cane. Which action indicates that the patient knows how to use the cane properly?
    a. The patient keeps the cane on the left side.
    b. Two points of support are kept on the floor at all times.
    c. There is a slight lean to the right when the patient is walking.
    d. After advancing the cane, the patient moves the right leg forward.

32. A patient with a fractured left femur has been using crutches for the past 4 weeks. The physician tells the patient to begin putting a little weight on the left foot when walking. Which of the following gaits should the patient be taught to use?
    a. Two-point
    b. Three-point
    c. Four-point
    d. Swing-through

33. While ambulating in the hallway of a hospital, the patient complains of extreme dizziness. The nurse, alert to a syncopal episode, should first:
    a. Support the patient and walk quickly back to the room.
    b. Lean the patient against the wall until the episode passes.
    c. Lower the patient gently to the floor.
    d. Go for help.

34. A patient is admitted to the medical unit following a cerebrovascular accident (stroke). There is evidence of left-sided hemiparesis, and the nurse will be following up on range-of-motion and other exercises performed in physical therapy. The nurse correctly teaches the patient and family members which one of the following principles of range-of-motion exercises?
    a. Move the joints quickly
    b. Work from the lower to upper body
    c. Flex the joint to the point of resistance
    d. Provide support above and below joints

35. Nurses need to implement appropriate body mechanics in order to prevent injury to themselves and patients. Which principle of body mechanics should the nurse incorporate into patient care?
    a. Flex the knees and keep the feet wide apart
    b. Assume a position far enough away from the patient
    c. Twist the body in the direction of movement
    d. Use the strong back muscles for lifting or moving

36. Following an assessment of a patient, the nurse identifies the nursing diagnosis *Activity Intolerance Related to Increased Weight Gain and Inactivity*. The physician wants the patient to improve her endurance and increase activity. Which of the following is an outcome identified by the nurse?
    a. Resting heart rate will be 90-100/minute.
    b. Blood pressure will be maintained between 140/80 and 160/90.
    c. Exercise will be performed 3 times per day over the next 2 weeks.
    d. Accommodation will be made for excess weight and fatigue.

37. A patient has been on prolonged bed rest, and the nurse is observing for signs associated with immobility. In assessment of the patient, the nurse is alert to a(n):
    a. increased blood pressure.
    b. decreased heart rate.
    c. increased urinary output.
    d. decreased peristalsis.

38. Two nurses are standing on opposite sides of the bed to move the patient up in bed with a draw sheet. Where should the nurses be standing in relation to the patient's body as they prepare for the move?
    a. Even with the thorax
    b. Even with the shoulders
    c. Even with the hips
    d. Even with the knees

39. A patient is leaving for surgery and, because of preoperative sedation, needs complete assistance to transfer from the bed to the stretcher. Which of the following should the nurse do first?
    a. Elevate the head of the bed.
    b. Explain the procedure to the patient.
    c. Place the patient in the prone position.
    d. Assess the situation for any potentially unsafe complications.

40. A patient has sequential compression stockings in place. Which of the following indicates that they are being implemented correctly?
    a. The ankle pressure is set at 40 mm Hg.
    b. Stockings are removed every hour during application.
    c. There is no space between the sleeve and the leg when the sleeve is not inflated.
    d. If there is an order for only one leg, the other sleeve is disconnected from the machine.

41. The nurse assesses that the patient has right-sided hemiparesis following a stroke. This individual most likely had ischemia to the:
    a. right side of the brain.
    b. left side of the brain.
    c. cerebellum.
    d. medulla oblongata.

42. An immobilized patient is suspected as having atelectasis. This is assessed by the nurse, upon auscultation, as:
    a. harsh crackles.
    b. wheezing on inspiration.
    c. diminished breath sounds.
    d. bronchovesicular whooshing.

43. The best approach for the nurse to use to assess the presence of deep vein thrombosis in an immobilized patient is to:
    a. measure the calf and thigh diameters.
    b. attempt to elicit the Homan sign.
    c. palpate the temperature of the feet.
    d. observe for a loss of hair and skin turgor in the lower legs.

44. A patient is getting up for the first time after a period of bed rest. The nurse should first:
    a. assess respiratory function.
    b. obtain a baseline blood pressure.
    c. assist the patient to sit at the edge of the bed.
    d. ask the patient if he or she feels lightheaded.

45. In order to promote respiratory function in the immobilized patient, the nurse should:
    a. encourage deep breathing and coughing every hour.
    b. use oxygen and nebulizer treatments regularly.
    c. change the patient's position q 4-8 hours.
    d. suction the patient every hour.

46. Antiembolism hose (stockings) are ordered for the patient on bed rest following surgery. The nurse explains to the patient that the primary purpose for the elastic stockings (TEDs) is to:
    a. keep the skin warm and dry.
    b. prevent abnormal joint flexion.
    c. apply external pressure.
    d. prevent bleeding.

47. To provide for the psychosocial needs of an immobilized patient, an appropriate statement by the nurse is:
    a. "The staff will limit your visitors so that you will not be bothered."
    b. "A roommate can be a real bother. You'd probably rather have a private room."
    c. "Let's discuss the routine to see if there are any changes we can make."
    d. "I think you should have your hair done and put on some make-up."

48. In order to reduce the chance of external hip rotation in a patient on prolonged bed rest, the nurse should implement the use of a:
    a. footboard.
    b. trapeze bar.
    c. bed board.
    d. trochanter roll.

49. In order to reduce the chance of plantar flexion (foot drop) in a patient on prolonged bed rest, the nurse should implement the use of:
    a. trapeze bars.
    b. high top sneakers.
    c. trochanter rolls.
    d. 30° lateral positioning.

50. Which of the following observations by the nurse indicates the correct use by the patient of a walker without wheels?
    a. Moving forward with both feet and then advancing the walker.
    b. Moving one foot forward, advancing the walker, and then moving the other foot.
    c. Sliding the walker while shuffling both feet forward.
    d. Lifting the walker forward one step, placing it on the ground, and then stepping forward into the walker.

51. Which one of the following is the best choice of protein for the immobile patient?
    a. Hot dog
    b. Grilled chicken
    c. Macaroni and cheese
    d. Grilled cheese sandwich

52. For the patient who is standing erect, which of the following indicates correct use of crutches?
    a. Axillary padding removed
    b. Crutches placed 10-12 inches to either side of each foot
    c. Elbow flexion of 60° for the handbar
    d. Three finger widths between the axilla and axillary piece of the crutch

53. Which of the following patients is expected to use a four-point crutch-walking technique? The patient who can bear weight:
    a. on both feet.
    b. partially on both feet.
    c. on both feet but has weak upper body strength and lower leg paralysis.
    d. on both feet but has strong upper body strength and lower body paralysis.

Practice Situation

The patient is admitted to the hospital after episodes of vertigo. The patient's family reports a history of two falls at home. The patient tells you that he is "steady on his feet."
a. How do you proceed with the assessment and care of this patient?

b. Identify a nursing diagnosis and patient goal/outcome for this patient.

c. Indicate the nursing interventions that you will implement to meet the QSEN competency for patient safety.

REVIEW QUESTIONS

- What are the functions of the musculoskeletal, neurologic, and cardiopulmonary systems in normal activity and movement?
- What are the changes in the musculoskeletal, neurologic, and cardiopulmonary systems that cause alterations in activity and movement throughout the life span?
- What are the effects of decreased activity and immobility on multiple body systems?
- What are the possible nursing diagnoses for patients experiencing immobility and impaired levels of activity?
- Which nursing care goals and outcome criteria are appropriate for patients experiencing complications from inactivity or immobility?
- Which interventions should be implemented to enhance patient activity, promote safety, and reverse the negative effects of immobility?

29 Skin Integrity and Wound Care

CHAPTER REVIEW

Match the description/definition in Column A with the correct term in Column B.

Column A

_____ 1. Brought together

_____ 2. Abnormal connection between two internal organs or between an internal organ and the outside of the body

_____ 3. Removal of necrotic tissue

_____ 4. Usually indicates bleeding and is bright red

_____ 5. Phenomenon that occurs through the relationship between friction and gravity

_____ 6. Partial or complete separation of the tissue layers during the healing process

_____ 7. Clear, watery fluid from plasma

_____ 8. Drainage is pink to pale red and contains a mix of clear fluid and red, bloody fluid

_____ 9. Necrotic tissue

_____ 10. Total separation of the tissue layers, allowing the protrusion of visceral organs through the incision

Column B

a. Dehiscence

b. Serous

c. Debridement

d. Eschar

e. Approximated

f. Serosanguineous

g. Evisceration

h. Fistula

i. Shear

j. Sanguineous

Complete the following:

11. How can the following affect skin integrity?
    a. Vascular disease—

    b. Malnutrition—

    c. Aging—

12. Provide an example of an open wound.

13. What type of wound heals by primary intention?

14. Identify how the following affect wound healing.

Decreased oxygenation	
Diabetes	
Infection	
Spinal injury	

15. How can the nurse prevent dehiscence and evisceration of a wound?

16. Fistulas can result in:

17. a. Full-thickness pressure ulcers are stages:
    b. Patients experiencing full-thickness wounds may have permanent loss of hair follicles, sweat glands, and skin color.

    True _____   False _____

18. What is included by the nurse in a focused wound assessment?

19. Using the Braden Scale, what is this patient's risk level?
    Responds to verbal commands, cannot always communicate discomfort _____
    Skin is occasionally moist _____
    Walks occasionally _____
    Makes slight position changes independently _____
    Posture steady in chair, slides down occasionally _____
    Eats more than 1/2 of meals and takes supplements _____

20. Identify what is pictured in the following photos:
    a.

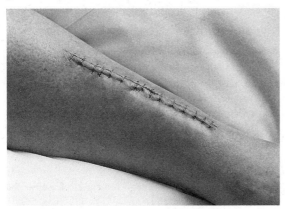

    b.

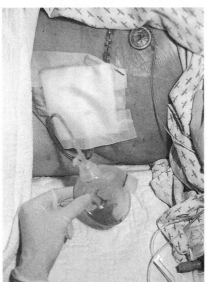

21. For pressure ulcers:
    a. What can lead to the development of ulcers?

b. Identify the areas on the body that are common sites for pressure ulcer development.

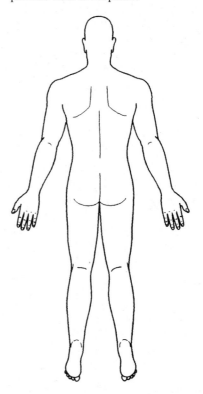

22. For documentation of the wound below:
    a. Measure the length and width of the wound.

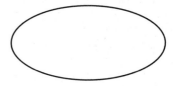

    b. Indicate the assessment in correct terminology for this wound that has blood-tinged exudate and an area of tissue loss under intact skin, forming a "lip" along the edges of the wound.

23. What does the nurse usually observe if the following are present at a wound?
    a. Maceration—

    b. Infection—

24. Identify the intervention(s) that should be implemented by the nurse to prevent pressure ulcer development. *Select all that apply.*
    a. Keep the head of the bed at 30 degrees or less. _____
    b. Use a moisture barrier ointment on the skin. _____
    c. Position the heels and elbows flat on the mattress. _____
    d. Turn the patient at least every 2 hours. _____
    e. Use hot water for bathing. _____
    f. Avoid use of antibacterial soaps. _____

25. Identify two methods for wound debridement.

26. For the following wounds, identify which type of dressing would be most effective:
    a. A simple, dry wound

    b. A wound with a moderate to heavy amount of exudate

27. What is the purpose of a drain in a wound?

28. For a T-tube or Penrose drain, what particular care must be provided by the nurse?

29. Identify the correct technique(s) for removal of staples and sutures. *Select all that apply.*
    a. The incision should be cleaned before removal. _____
    b. Cleansing occurs from the most to least contaminated. _____
    c. Sterile gloves are used. _____
    d. Staples should break when removed. _____
    e. Every other suture or staple should be removed first. _____
    f. Sutures are pulled out through the wound. _____

30. What are the five P's of circulation?

31. Which of the following is/are correct regarding the application of heat? *Select all that apply.*
    a. Vasoconstriction occurs with application. _____
    b. It promotes muscle relaxation. _____
    c. Aquathermia pads should be applied directly to the skin. _____
    d. It decreases edema. _____
    e. It is contraindicated for local abscesses. _____
    f. The patient should lie on the heat therapy device. _____

32. Wound irrigation:
    a. What is the purpose of irrigation?

    b. What solution can be used?

    c. What equipment provides the necessary pressure?

33. Place the steps in correct order for irrigation of a wound with a dressing.
    a. With the syringe about 1 inch above the wound, irrigate from least to most contaminated. _____
    b. Thoroughly dry the periwound area with sterile gauze. _____
    c. Fill the syringe with solution. _____
    d. Remove the old dressing. _____
    e. Continue until solution flow is clear. _____

34. When delegating simple, nonacute wound care to unlicensed assistive personnel (UAP), the nurse instructs the UAP to report:

35. Provide examples of general principles of asepsis that are used for wound care.

36. For wound cultures:
    a. What equipment is necessary for a wound culture?

    b. Can this skill be delegated to UAP?

    c. Where should the sample be taken in the wound?

37. As a general principle, when should the nurse discontinue a wound care procedure?

38. For applying bandages:
    a. Before wrapping a limb with a bandage, the nurse should:

    b. Limbs are bandaged in what direction?

c. What assessment is done after application?

d. How often is the bandage removed?

Select the best answer for each of the following questions:

39. The nurse determines that the patient's wound may be infected. In order to perform an aerobic wound culture, the nurse should:
    a. swab the necrotic tissue area.
    b. collect the culture before cleansing the wound.
    c. obtain a culturette tube and use sterile technique.
    d. place the used swab in a plastic bag and send it to the laboratory.

40. Pressure ulcers form primarily as a result of:
    a. nitrogen buildup in the underlying tissues.
    b. prolonged illness or disease.
    c. tissue ischemia.
    d. poor hygiene.

41. The nurse notes a patient's skin is reddened with a pink wound bed and serous fluid present. The nurse should classify this stage of ulcer formation as which of the following?
    a. Stage I
    b. Stage II
    c. Stage III
    d. Stage IV

42. The patient has rheumatoid arthritis, is prone to skin breakdown, and is also somewhat immobile because of arthritic discomfort. Which of the following is the best intervention for the patient's skin integrity?
    a. Having the patient sit up in a chair for 4-hour intervals.
    b. Keeping the head of the bed in a high Fowler position.
    c. Keeping a written schedule of turning and positioning.
    d. Encouraging the patient to perform pelvic muscle training exercises several times a day.

43. Upon changing the patient's dressing, the nurse notes that the wound appears to be granulating. An appropriate non-cytotoxic cleansing agent selected by the nurse is:
    a. sterile saline.
    b. hydrogen peroxide.
    c. povidone iodine (Betadine).
    d. sodium hypochlorite (Dakin solution).

44. A patient requires wound debridement. The nurse is aware that which one of the following statements is correct regarding this procedure?
    a. It allows the healthy tissue to regenerate.
    b. When performed by autolytic means, the wound is irrigated.
    c. Occlusive dressings provide the fastest debridement.
    d. Mechanical methods involve direct surgical removal of the eschar layer of the wound.

45. The nurse prepares to irrigate the patient's wound. The primary reason for this procedure is to:
    a. decrease scar formation.
    b. remove debris from the wound.
    c. improve circulation from the wound.
    d. decrease irritation from wound drainage.

46. When turning a patient, the nurse notices a reddened area on the coccyx. What skin care interventions should the nurse use on this area?
    a. Soak the area in normal saline solution.
    b. Apply a dilute hydrogen peroxide and water mixture and use a heat lamp to the area.
    c. Wash the area with an astringent and paint it with povidone-iodine (Betadine).
    d. Clean the area with mild soap, dry, and add a protective moisturizer.

47. A patient with a large abdominal wound requires a dressing change every 4 hours. The patient will be discharged to the home setting where the dressing care will be continued. Which of the following is true concerning this patient's care?
    a. Drinkable tap water should never be used for cleansing.
    b. A heat lamp should be used every 2 hours to rid the wound area of contaminants.
    c. Sterile technique should be emphasized to the patient and family.
    d. Sanitary pads or disposable diapers may be used as absorptive dressings.

48. Upon inspection of the patient's wound, the nurse notes that it appears infected and has a large amount of exudate. An appropriate dressing for the nurse to select on the basis of the wound assessment is:
    a. foam.
    b. hydrogel.
    c. hydrocolloid.
    d. transparent film.

49. A patient has a healing abdominal wound. The wound has granulation tissue and collagen formation. The wound is identified by the nurse as being in which phase of healing?
    a. Primary intention
    b. Inflammatory phase
    c. Proliferative phase
    d. Secondary intention

50. The nurse is concerned that the patient's midsternal wound is at risk for dehiscence. Which of the following is the best intervention to prevent this complication?
    a. Administering antibiotics to prevent infection
    b. Using appropriate sterile technique when changing the dressing
    c. Keeping sterile towels and extra dressing supplies near the patient's bed
    d. Having the patient splint the incision site when coughing

51. Following an injury, the patient has thick, yellow drainage coming from the wound. The nurse describes this drainage as:
    a. milky.
    b. serous.
    c. purulent.
    d. serosanguineous.

52. Which nursing entry is most complete in describing a patient's wound?
    a. Incision edges approximated without redness or drainage, two 4 x 4s applied.
    b. Wound appears to be healing well. Dressing dry and intact.
    c. Wound well approximated with minimal drainage.
    d. Small amount of drainage size of quarter, dressing applied.

53. The nurse recognizes that skin integrity can be compromised by being exposed to body fluids. The greatest risk exists for the patient who has exposure to:
    a. urine.
    b. purulent exudates.
    c. pancreatic fluids.
    d. serosanguineous drainage.

54. When cleaning a wound, the nurse should:
    a. go over the wound twice and discard that swab.
    b. move from the outer region of the wound toward the center.
    c. start at the drainage site and move outward with circular motions.
    d. use an enzymatic solution followed by a normal saline rinse.

55. The patient has a large, deep wound on the sacral region. The nurse correctly packs the wound by:
    a. filling ⅔ of the wound cavity.
    b. using dripping wet gauze.
    c. putting the dressing in tightly.
    d. extending only to the upper edge of the wound.

56. The nurse is aware that application of cold is indicated for the patient with which of the following?
    a. A fractured ankle
    b. Menstrual cramping
    c. An infected wound
    d. Degenerative joint disease

57. The nurse uses the Norton Scale in the extended care facility to determine the patient's risk for pressure ulcer development. Which one of the following scores, based on this scale, places the patient at the highest level of risk?
    a. 6
    b. 8
    c. 15
    d. 19

58. The patient requires bandaging to the lower extremity. The nurse correctly implements the use of a bandage by:
    a. using it as a replacement for underlying dressings.
    b. making sure the patient has distal pulses.
    c. keeping it loose for patient comfort.
    d. having the patient sit or stand when it is applied.

59. The patient is brought into the emergency department with a knife wound. The nurse correctly documents the patient's wound as a(n):
    a. acute wound.
    b. clean wound.
    c. chronic wound.
    d. contusion wound.

60. The nurse is planning a program on wound healing and includes information that smoking influences healing by:
    a. suppressing protein synthesis.
    b. creating increased tissue fragility.
    c. depressing systematic bone marrow function.
    d. reducing hemoglobin's ability to carry oxygen.

61. A patient on the medical unit is taking steroids and also has a wound from a minor injury. To promote wound healing for this patient, the nurse recommends that which of the following be specifically added?
    a. Iron
    b. Folic acid
    c. Vitamin C
    d. B-complex vitamins

62. A wound that results from surgery where the organ systems are likely to contain bacteria is known as a:
    a. clean wound.
    b. infected wound.
    c. contaminated wound.
    d. clean contaminated wound.

63. What happens during the inflammatory stage of wound healing?
    a. Collagen formation
    b. Scar tissue develops
    c. Coagulation cascade
    d. Wound contraction

64. Granulation tissue is assessed by the nurse as:
    a. "beefy" red and moist.
    b. pale gray and dry.
    c. dark black and hard.
    d. light pink and dry.

65. The nurse evaluates that the negative-pressure wound therapy is functioning properly by observing that:
    a. the negative-pressure setting is above 250 mm Hg.
    b. the suction tubing is directly on the wound.
    c. there is conformation of the dressing to the foam.
    d. painful stinging or burning is felt by the patient at the wound.

66. The patient is to have a dressing change with wound care. Last time, the patient was uncomfortable during the procedure. What should the nurse do to reduce discomfort for this care?
   a. Premedicate the patient 1/2 hour before the procedure.
   b. Swab the wound with a local anesthetic.
   c. Perform the wound care quickly.
   d. Continue with the procedure.

67. The unit manager is observing the new staff nurse perform a wet/damp-to-dry dressing change. Which of the following actions requires correction by the manager?
   a. Providing information on the procedure to the patient
   b. Applying clean, nonsterile gloves to remove the old dressing
   c. Holding the skin taut to remove the old tape
   d. Moistening the dressing to facilitate removal

68. Of these steps in the procedure, which of the following is done first in the wet/damp-to-dry dressing change?
   a. Preparing the packing gauze
   b. Irrigating the wound
   c. Moistening the packing
   d. Cleaning the wound with sterile saline

Practice Situation

- The patient has a 5-cm x 3-cm stage III pressure ulcer on his right heel. He identifies a pain level of 5 on a scale of 0 to 10. The patient appears fatigued and depressed. He tells you that the discomfort is wearing him down.

  When you inspect the wound, you notice that there is a small amount of serous drainage.

Using the conceptual care map:
a. Identify primary and secondary nursing diagnoses.

b. Identify relevant short-term goals for each nursing diagnosis and interventions.

c. Indicate how you will evaluate attainment of the goals.

- You are visiting a patient at home to teach her about wound care—cleansing and dressing. The patient tells you that she does not have a lot of money to buy supplies and asks if there is something she can do to save money.
  a. What are some money-saving ways to complete wound care?

REVIEW QUESTIONS

- What is the normal structure and function of skin?
- What are different factors that alter the skin's structure and function?
- How does the nurse complete a focused skin and wound assessment, including the use of risk assessment tools?
- Which nursing diagnoses may be appropriate for the patient with impaired skin integrity?
- What measurable patient-centered goals may be developed for patients with impaired skin integrity?
- Which interventions should be selected to prevent and treat impaired skin integrity?

30 Nutrition

CHAPTER REVIEW

Match the description/definition in Column A with the correct term in Column B.

	Column A	Column B
_____	1. Protein and caloric deficiency	a. Dysphagia
_____	2. Physical wasting	b. Marasmus
_____	3. Difficulty in swallowing	c. Aspiration
_____	4. Use of energy to change simple materials into complex body substances and tissue	d. Catabolism
_____	5. Inhalation of fluid or foreign matter into the lungs and bronchi	e. Cachexia
_____	6. Breaking down of substances from complex to simple, resulting in a release of energy	f. Anabolism
_____	7. Minimum amount of energy required to maintain bodily functions at rest while awake	g. Metabolism h. Basal metabolic rate
_____	8. Process of chemically changing nutrients, such as fats and proteins, into end products that are used to meet the energy needs of the body or stored for future use	

Complete the following:

9. What are the macronutrients and micronutrients?

10. For carbohydrates:
    a. What is the difference between simple and complex carbohydrates?

    b. Provide food examples for each type of carbohydrate.

    c. How much energy is provided by carbohydrates?

11. For fats:
    a. What types of fat are found in the body?

    b. What is the recommended daily fat intake?

c. Which are the fat-soluble vitamins?

d. The essential fatty acids are:

12. It is recommended that less than 7% of the total daily fat intake should be saturated fat. Which food(s) should the nurse advise the patient to avoid? *Select all that apply.*
    a. Corn oil _____
    b. Crackers _____
    c. Cheese _____
    d. Trout _____
    e. Cashews _____
    f. Ice cream _____

13. What role do proteins play in the body?

14. An individual with a decrease of water in the body is anticipated to have what problems?

15. Food(s) high in vitamin A include: *Select all that apply.*
    a. Carrots _____
    b. Bread _____
    c. Pumpkin _____
    d. Canola oil _____
    e. Green, leafy vegetables _____
    f. Nuts _____

16. How can the nurse help the patient to eat healthier foods?

17. The nurse instructs the patient that vitamin C is important in the body for:

18. What is the general role of the B-complex vitamins?

19. Coffee contains a significant amount of which B vitamin?

20. The patient is on a diuretic and losing potassium. The nurse instructs the patient to increase the dietary intake of which of the following? *Select all that apply.*
    a. Bread _____
    b. Bananas _____
    c. Tomatoes _____
    d. Orange juice _____
    e. Smoked meat _____
    f. Cheese _____

21. For antioxidants:
    a. Antioxidants are thought to prevent the development of what problems?

    b. Vitamin E can act as an antioxidant. Identify at least two food sources of this vitamin.

22. For the child with a milk allergy or other digestive difficulty, what type of formulas will be recommended?

23. How can an individual's culture influence nutritional intake?

24. What effects occur in the following systems from a nutritional deficiency?
    a. Musculoskeletal—

    b. Cardiopulmonary—

25. The patient who is lactose intolerant should avoid:

26. Obesity is a major health problem throughout the world. Which of the following is/are true regarding obesity? *Select all that apply.*
    a. One out of every three adults is overweight. _____
    b. The prevalence of obesity in the United States more than tripled among children and adolescents from 1980–2008. _____
    c. Obese teenagers are less likely to become obese adults. _____
    d. A person with a body mass index (BMI) greater than 40 is classified as morbidly obese. _____
    e. Obesity is more common in white teenagers. _____
    f. High BMI levels increase the risk for hypertension. _____

27. Identify the primary treatment option for individuals with eating disorders.

28. Two common ways to obtain information about a patient's food intake are:

29. A focused physical assessment for nutritional status should include:

30. The nurse is weighing the patient daily. What principles are applied?

31. For the following patients, calculate the BMI and provide an interpretation:
    a. 61 kg–1.65 m
    b. 72 kg–1.8 m
    c. 95 kg–1.7 m

32. What indicators are associated with metabolic syndrome?

33. Identify which of the following signs and symptoms is/are associated with a nutritional deficit. *Select all that apply.*
    a. Dry, stiff hair _____
    b. Pink, moist oral membranes _____
    c. Constipation _____
    d. Decreased albumin level _____
    e. Petechiae _____
    f. White, evenly colored teeth _____

95

34. How can the nurse prevent aspiration?

35. The patient has an iron deficiency. What foods should the nurse recommend?

36. For the Quality and Safety Education for Nurses QSEN competency of teamwork and collaboration, who should be included in the planning of care for a patient with an identified nutritional concern?

37. For the patient who is a vegetarian, what foods should the nurse recommend in the diet in order for the patient to obtain essential amino acids?

38. The nurse is assessing the patient for dysphagia.
    a. What are the signs and symptoms?

    b. How can the nurse assist an adult with feeding?

39. The patient's percutaneous endogastric (PEG) tube becomes occluded. What actions should the nurse take to try to remove the occlusion?

40. For total parenteral nutrition (TPN):
    a. Which patients may benefit from this option?

    b. What monitoring is done regularly?

    c. What complications can occur?

41. For insertion of a nasogastric tube:
    a. What position should the patient be in for the insertion?

    b. What should the nurse do if resistance is felt?

    c. How should the tube be anchored after insertion?

42. For nasogastric tube feedings:
    a. The nurse can proceed with the next feeding if the residual is less than _____ mL.

    b. Continuous feedings are usually administered with the use of a:

    c. What equipment is required specifically for gravity feedings?

Select the best answer for each of the following questions:

43. While doing a nutritional assessment of a low-income family, the community health nurse determines the family's diet is inadequate in protein content. The nurse suggests which of the following lower-cost foods to increase protein content?
    a. Rice
    b. Beans
    c. Potatoes
    d. Citrus fruits

44. The school nurse suspects that the junior high student may have anorexia nervosa. This eating disorder is characterized by:
    a. a lack of control over eating patterns.
    b. self-imposed starvation.
    c. binge-purge cycles.
    d. excessive exercise.

45. A patient is pregnant for the first time. In regards to her nutritional status, she should:
    a. limit her weight gain to a maximum of about 25 lb.
    b. increase her vitamin A and milk product consumption.
    c. approximately double her protein intake.
    d. increase her intake of folic acid.

46. The patient has had throat surgery and is able to have clear liquid oral intake. The nurse should offer the patient:
    a. fresh squeezed orange juice.
    b. chicken noodle soup.
    c. apple juice.
    d. oatmeal.

47. The nurse is discussing dietary intake with a patient who is on a renal diet. The nurse informs the patient that the diet will specifically include a(n):
    a. restriction of potassium, Phosphorous, protein, and sodium.
    b. increase in complex carbohydrates.
    c. increase in folic acid intake.
    d. reduction in caffeine intake.

48. When introducing a feeding to a patient with an indwelling tube for enteral nutrition, the nurse should first:
    a. irrigate the tube with normal saline solution.
    b. verify measured placement tape markings.
    c. place the patient in a supine position.
    d. determine residual volume.

49. A patient is having a nasogastric tube removed. The nurse should:
    a. apply wall suction during the removal.
    b. insert 50 to 100 mL of water to clear the tube.
    c. ask the patient to take a deep breath and hold it.
    d. remove the tube slowly in small increments.

50. A patient is seen in the outpatient clinic for follow-up of a nutritional deficiency. In planning for the patient's dietary intake, the nurse includes a complete protein, such as:
    a. eggs.
    b. oats.
    c. lentils.
    d. peanuts.

51. While assisting the patient with meal selection, the nurse realizes that patients who practice Islam or Judaism share an avoidance of:
    a. alcohol.
    b. shellfish.
    c. caffeine.
    d. pork products.

52. Following a surgical procedure, the patient is advanced to a full liquid diet. The nurse is able to recommend which one of the following foods for this patient?
    a. Yogurt
    b. Pureed meats
    c. Soft fresh fruit
    d. Canned soup

53. The nurse is speaking with parents of a child at a day care center. The parents ask the nurse about the nutritional needs of their toddler. An appropriate finger food that is identified by the nurse is:
    a. nuts.
    b. popcorn.
    c. Cheerios.
    d. hot dogs.

54. A nasogastric tube is inserted in order for the patient to receive intermittent tube feedings. After radiologic verification, the next most reliable method of checking for tube placement is for the nurse to:
    a. place the end of the tube in water and observe for bubbling.
    b. auscultate while introducing air into the tube.
    c. measure the pH of aspirated secretions.
    d. ask the patient to speak.

55. The nurse recognizes that the individual with an inborn error of metabolism with a failure to properly metabolize amino acids has:
    a. diabetes.
    b. kwashiorkor.
    c. Crohn disease.
    d. phenylketonuria.

56. The nurse recommends that the patient include which of the following foods as a good source of omega-3?
    a. Salmon
    b. Chicken
    c. Lamb
    d. Liver

57. Which of the following techniques used by the new staff nurse for administering medications via an enteral tube requires correction by the charge nurse?
    a. Giving the medications in their liquid form
    b. Adding the medications to the tube feeding
    c. Dissolving powdered medications in sterile water
    d. Flushing with 15 to 30 mL of sterile water after administration

58. The nurse is inserting a nasogastric tube. During the insertion, the patient starts to gag and becomes dyspneic. Which action should the nurse take?
    a. Withdraw the tube and start again.
    b. Provide water for swallowing.
    c. Check the back of the throat for coiling.
    d. Use an anesthetic or analgesic spray.

59. On the basis of information for North America, which waist circumference size puts a man in the high-risk category for heart disease?
    a. 35 inches
    b. 40 inches
    c. 45 inches
    d. 50 inches

Practice Situation

You are working with an older adult patient with a history of cardiac disease who lives at home alone. While visiting with the patient, you notice that there are many frozen meals and canned foods, while there are no fresh fruits or vegetables in the kitchen. The patient tells you that she does not feel like making her meals all of the time and falls back on ready-made foods. You recognize that there may be a nutritional deficiency.
a. What focused assessment will you perform to determine if a deficiency exists?

b. Identify a nursing diagnosis and goal for this patient.

c. How will you assist the patient to avoid foods that will adversely affect her condition and include those that will be more nutrient dense?

REVIEW QUESTIONS

- What is the role of nutrition and food metabolism in normal body structure and function?

- Which nutritional imbalances can result in physical alterations, psychological disturbances, and the development of disease?
- What are the critical aspects of a thorough nutritional assessment?
- Which nursing diagnoses are possible for patients experiencing an alteration in nutrition?
- What nursing care goals and outcome criteria may be developed for patients experiencing complications from an alteration in nutrition?
- How does the nurse implement and evaluate the interventions designed to address nutritional needs?

31 Cognitive and Sensory Alterations

CHAPTER REVIEW

Match the description/definition in Column A with the correct term in Column B.

	Column A	Column B
C	1. A change in the environment sufficient to evoke a response	a. Cognition
i	2. Age-related hearing loss	b. Myopia
j	3. Crossing over of sensory pathways	c. Stimulus
h	4. Speech or language impairment	d. Gustation
f	5. Sense of smell	e. Anosmia
B	6. Nearsightedness	f. Olfaction
A	7. Knowing influenced by awareness and judgment	g. Presbyopia
e	8. Complete loss of the sense of smell	h. Aphasia
D	9. Sense of taste	i. Presbycusis
G	10. Age-related farsightedness	j. Decussate

Complete the following:

11. For the following lobes of the brain, identify a problem that the patient may experience if that area is damaged.
    a. Frontal lobe—

    b. Occipital lobe—

12. Identify sensory changes that occur with aging.

13. What are some of the causes of delirium?

14. a. What is the difference between exogenous and endogenous depression?

    b. How is depression usually treated?

15. Children are more prone to otitis media because:

16. Which of the following are commonly associated with Meniere disease? *Select all that apply.*
    a. Hypertension. _____
    b. Hearing loss. _____
    c. Vertigo. _____
    d. Dyspnea. _____
    e. Tinnitus. _____
    f. Persistent cough. _____

17. Identify what changes occur with the following visual alterations:
    a. Presbyopia—

    b. Cataracts—

    c. Glaucoma—

d. Diabetic retinopathy—

e. Macular degeneration—

18. Identify if the findings indicate that this female patient has metabolic syndrome.
    - BP 140/90
    - Fasting blood sugar 90 mg/dL
    - Waist circumference 30 inches
    - Low high-density lipoprotein cholesterol 60 mg/dL
    - Triglycerides 120 mg/dL

19. What does the nurse expect to find for a patient who has had a right-sided cerebrovascular accident (CVA)?

20. Describe what happens to the person with dementia.

21. Provide examples of situations that can lead to sensory overload and sensory deprivation for patients.

22. What lifestyle choices place the patient at risk for cognitive and sensory problems?

23. The Mini-Mental State Examination (MMSE) can be used to determine:

24. Which laboratory tests can be performed to determine if there is a reason for a cognitive or sensory alteration?

25. How can a loss or decline in the sense of taste create problems for patients?

26. For the patient with dementia, identify interventions to ensure safety and achievement of basic activities of daily living.

27. What should the nurse do for patients with tactile deficits?

28. Identify a home safety concern for a patient with an olfactory deficit.

29. What nursing interventions should be instituted in the acute care setting for patients with the following alterations?
    a. Visual

    b. Auditory

30. For the patient with a cognitive alteration who is being discharged, what are some home care considerations?

Select the best answer for each of the following questions:

31. With advancing age, which of the following normal physiological changes in sensory function occurs?
    a. Decreased sensitivity to glare
    b. Increased number of taste buds
    c. Decreased sensitivity to pain
    d. Difficulty discriminating vowel sounds

32. Which of the following occupations poses the least risk for sensory alterations?
    a. Librarian
    b. Welder
    c. Computer programmer
    d. Construction worker

33. The nurse is working with a patient with a moderate hearing impairment. To promote communication with this patient, the nurse should:
    a. use a louder tone of voice than normal.
    b. select a public area to have a conversation.
    c. approach a patient quietly from behind before speaking.
    d. use visual aids such as the hands and eyes when speaking.

34. The patient has experienced a CVA (stroke) with resultant expressive aphasia. The nurse promotes communication with this patient by:
    a. speaking loudly and slowly.
    b. speaking to the patient on the unaffected side.
    c. using a picture chart for the patient's responses.
    d. using hand gestures to convey information to the patient.

35. The patient was working in the kitchen and was splashed in the face with a caustic cleaning agent. His eyes were affected and he was brought to the hospital for treatment. After cleansing and evaluation, his eyes were bandaged. When assisting this patient to eat, the nurse should:
    a. feed the patient the entire meal.
    b. allow the patient to experiment with foods.
    c. encourage the family to feed the patient.
    d. orient the patient to the location of the foods on the plate.

36. An older adult patient in a nursing home has visual and hearing losses. The nurse is alert to which of the following signs that represents the effects of sensory deprivation?
    a. Depression
    b. Diminished anxiety
    c. Improved task completion
    d. Decreased need for physical stimulation

37. During a home safety assessment, the nurse identifies that there are a number of hazards present. Of the following hazards that are noted by the nurse, which one represents the greatest risk for this patient with diabetic peripheral neuropathy?
    a. Cluttered walkways
    b. Absence of smoke detectors
    c. Improper water heater settings
    d. Lack of bathroom grab bars

38. The nurse in the pediatric clinic is checking the basic visual acuity of a 3½ year old child. The nurse should have the child:
    a. identify crayon colors.
    b. read the standard Snellen chart.
    c. read a few lines from a children's book.
    d. follow the peripheral movement of an object.

39. For a patient with receptive aphasia (Wernicke aphasia), which one of the following nursing interventions is the most effective?
    a. Providing the patient with a letter chart to use to answer complex questions
    b. Using a system of simple gestures to communicate
    c. Speaking louder and slower.
    d. Obtaining a referral for a speech therapist

40. The nurse recommends follow-up auditory testing for a child who was exposed in utero to:
    a. rubella.
    b. excessive oxygen.
    c. alcohol ingestion.
    d. respiratory infection.

41. The nurse is working with older adult patients in an extended care facility. In order to enhance the patients' gustatory sense, the nurse should:
    a. mix foods together.
    b. assist with oral hygiene.
    c. make sure foods are extremely spicy.
    d. provide foods of similar texture and consistency.

42. A home safety measure specific for a patient with diminished olfaction is the use of:
    a. extra lighting in hallways.
    b. amplified telephone receivers.
    c. smoke detectors on all levels.
    d. mild water heater temperatures.

43. The nurse has completed the admission assessment for a patient admitted to the hospital's subacute care unit. Of the following nursing diagnoses identified by the nurse, which takes the highest priority?
    a. Social isolation
    b. Risk for injury
    c. Adjustment, impaired
    d. Communication, impaired verbal

44. The patient is being discharged to home after being evaluated for Meniere disease and episodes of dizziness. Which one of the following statements alerts the nurse that further reinforcement is necessary for safety?
    a. "I'll be careful in the morning when I first get out of bed."
    b. "It will be good to get back to my job on the train."
    c. "I have a small bench that I can use when I'm taking a shower."
    d. "I'm going to be changing to brighter light bulbs in the hallways."

Practice Situations

• The patient had a left CVA that resulted in right-sided weakness in the upper and lower extremities. There is some expressive aphasia noted, although the patient is improving in being able to communicate.
    a. Identify a possible nursing diagnosis for this patient, along with a goal/outcome and appropriate nursing interventions.

• Using the case study example in the text, fill in the assessment data on the conceptual care map with the information noted on Mrs. Matson.

REVIEW QUESTIONS

• What is the normal structure and function of cognition and sensation?
• How do alterations in the structure and function of cognition and sensation impact patients' abilities?
• How does the nurse assess patients' cognitive and sensory function?
• What are some nursing diagnoses for patients who need assistance or modifications in care due to cognitive or sensory deficits?
• What are goals for patients with cognitive or sensory alterations?
• How does the nurse use nursing care plans that include interventions to enhance patients' cognitive and sensory function?

32 Stress and Coping

CHAPTER REVIEW

Complete the following:

1. How is stress defined?

2. Identify the three types of stress.

3. Provide examples of different stressors that may be encountered by individuals.

4. For the fight-or-flight response, which is/are the physiological response(s)? *Select all that apply.*
   a. Bradycardia. _____
   b. Pupil constriction. _____
   c. Increased blood pressure. X_____
   d. Palpitations. _____
   e. Decreased gastric motility. X_____
   f. Bradypnea. X_____

5. Briefly explain what happens in each stage of the general adaptation syndrome (GAS).

   a. Alarm reaction—

   b. Resistance—

   c. Exhaustion—

6. a. Negative stress is termed—

   b. Positive stress is termed—

7. How is the local adaptation syndrome (LAS) different from GAS?

8. Determine whether the following individual appears to have a strong or low sense of coherence.

   Mr. B. has had a lot of extra responsibilities at work that have kept him late in his office. On his way home, he stops at a nearby park and walks around to gather his thoughts. When he gets home, he takes time to speak with his wife and two children. During his free time, Mr. B. enjoys working outside and reading.

9. Stress-induced hyperglycemia may result from:

10. What is a stress appraisal?

11. Which personality factors reduce the negative consequences of stress?

12. How do fear and anxiety differ?

13. Describe the following levels of anxiety.
    a. Mild—

    b. Moderate—

    c. Severe—

    d. Panic—

14. Unresolved and chronically suppressed anger can lead to:

15. Identify what problem is manifested with the following patient: The patient is sitting alone, displaying a flat affect. She has expressed an inability to fall asleep, malaise, and lack of energy. Her outward appearance is untidy.

16. Provide at least two examples of how prolonged stress can affect an individual.

17. Which of the following are accurate statements regarding stress? *Select all that apply.*
    a. Most stressors for older adults involve loss and grieving. _____
    b. Young adults experience more interpersonal stressors. _____
    c. Children are able to deal with multiple stressors for a long time. _____
    d. Culture has little impact upon the response to stress. _____
    e. The arrival of a sibling can become a stressor for a child. _____
    f. Cognitive changes can influence an individual's ability to cope. _____

18. For a patient with a different cultural background, the nurse should be alert to which signs or behaviors that may indicate stress?

19. Which of the following questions by the nurse will specifically assess information on stress-related physical symptoms? *Select all that apply.*
    a. How have you dealt with stressful situations in the past? _____
    b. Have you experienced any changes in your life recently? _____
    c. Whom do you talk to about your feelings and problems? _____
    d. Have you experienced episodes of hyperventilating? _____
    e. Does your cultural or spiritual background provide you with certain beliefs that are helpful in times of stress? _____
    f. Do you experience any muscle tension in your neck, back, and head? _____

20. The patient was recently told that he has a serious renal disorder and may need a transplant. He is experiencing a lack of sleep, anxiety, and a poor outlook.
    a. Identify a possible nursing diagnosis for this patient and a goal/outcome.

    b. Indicate what nursing interventions are appropriate.

21. Identify at least five examples of stress management strategies.

22. What are some of the principles of effective time management?

23. What foods should the nurse encourage the patient to include in the diet to facilitate stress reduction and improve well-being?

24. What progressive relaxation therapy has been used to treat stressed patients?

Select the best answer for each of the following questions:

25. A recommended intervention for a lifestyle stress indicator and reduction in the incidence of heart disease is:
    a. regular physical exercise.
    b. attendance at a support group.
    c. self-awareness skill development.
    d. time management.

26. The nurse is involved in crisis intervention with a family where the father has just loss his job and is experiencing periods of depression. The mother has a chronic debilitating illness that has put added responsibilities on the adolescent child who is having behavioral problems. The nurse intervenes to specifically focus the family on their feelings by:
    a. discussing past experiences.
    b. working on time management skills.
    c. encouraging the use of the family's current coping skills.
    d. pointing out the connection between the situation and their responses.

27. A child and his mother have gone to the playroom on the pediatric unit. His mother tells him he cannot have a toy another child is playing with. The child cries, throws a block, and runs over to kick the door. This child is using a mechanism known as:
    a. denial.
    b. conversion.
    c. displacement.
    d. compensation.

28. Patients undergoing stress may undergo periods of regression. The nurse assesses this regressive behavior in the situation where an:
    a. adult patient exercises to the point of fatigue.
    b. 8-year-old child sucks his thumb and wets the bed.
    c. adult patient avoids speaking about health concerns.
    d. 11-year-old child experiences stomach cramps and headaches.

103

Chapter **32** **Stress and Coping**

29. During the end-of-shift report, the nurse notes that a postoperative patient had been nervous and preoccupied during the evening and that no family visited. To determine the amount of anxiety that the patient is experiencing, the nurse should ask:
    a. "How serious do you think your illness is?"
    b. "You seem worried about something. Would it help to talk about it?"
    c. "Would you like for me to call a family member to come support you?"
    d. "Would you like to go down the hall and talk with another patient who had the same surgery?"

30. Nurses in the medical center are working with patients experiencing posttraumatic stress disorder (PTSD) following a natural disaster. An approach that is appropriate and should be incorporated into the plan of care is:
    a. suppression of anxiety-producing memories.
    b. reinforcement that the PTSD is short term.
    c. promotion of relaxation strategies.
    d. focus on physical needs.

31. A 72-year-old patient is in a long-term care facility after having had a CVA (stroke). The patient is noncommunicative, the enteral feedings are not being absorbed, and respirations are becoming labored. Which stage of GAS is the patient experiencing?
    a. Alarm reaction
    b. Resistance stage
    c. Exhaustion stage
    d. Reflex pain response

32. A corporate executive works 60 to 80 hours/week. The patient is experiencing some physical signs of stress. The practitioner teaches the patient to direct her attention to positive images, such as a favorite vacation spot. This is an example of which of the following health promotion interventions?
    a. Guided imagery
    b. Time management
    c. Regular exercise
    d. Progressive relaxation

33. The patient is assessed by the nurse as experiencing a crisis. The nurse plans to:
    a. complete an in-depth evaluation of stressors and responses to the situation.
    b. allow the patient to work through independent problem solving.
    c. focus on immediate stress reduction.
    d. recommend ongoing therapy.

34. While working with patients who are experiencing a significant degree of stress, the nurse is aware that a priority assessment area is:
    a. the patient's primary activities of daily living needs.
    b. what else is happening in the patient's life.
    c. how the stress has influenced the patient's activities of daily living.
    d. whether the patient is thinking about harming himself, herself, or others.

35. The patient demonstrates unrealistic levels of worry and tension without an identifiable cause. This is termed a(n):
    a. social anxiety disorder.
    b. generalized anxiety disorder.
    c. obsessive-compulsive disorder.
    d. posttraumatic stress disorder.

36. An individual who is overwhelmed with and distraught over the new diagnosis of heart disease will most likely use which strategy to relieve stress?
    a. Direct action
    b. Problem-focused
    c. Emotion-focused
    d. Physiological

37. Which of the following interventions requires a referral to a therapist with specialized training?
    a. Guided imagery
    b. Biofeedback
    c. Time management
    d. Progressive relaxation

Practice Situations

One of your friends is a nurse on the oncology unit, where there have been a number of difficult patient situations and deaths. He has worked there for 4 years, but you notice that he has recently become more irritable, taken frequent sick days, and is now complaining about headaches and fatigue.
a. What do you suspect is happening to your colleague?

b. What can you do to assist your colleague?

The patient is assessed with the Holmes-Rahe Life Stress Inventory (refer to the text) and found to have the following life events occurring:
Divorce, death of a close friend, a son going off to college, and a change in her responsibilities at work
a. What is the score of this patient, and what is its meaning?

REVIEW QUESTIONS

- What are the key concepts associated with the body's physiological and psychological responses to stress?
- What are the normal nervous, endocrine, immune, and psychological responses to stress?
- How is health affected by stress?
- Which assessment techniques are used for recognizing signs and symptoms of stress?
- What are possible stress-related nursing diagnosis statements?
- Which stress-reduction goals and patient outcomes may be developed?
- How are patient-centered care plans developed and interventions designed to address stress-related conditions?
- What is the potential impact of stress on nurses?

33 Sleep

CHAPTER REVIEW

Match the description/definition in Column A with the correct term in Column B.

Column A

e   1. An uncontrollable desire to sleep that can occur at any time

d   2. Clenching or the grinding of teeth from side to side

a   3. The recording of brain waves and other physiological variables, such as muscle activity and eye movements, during sleep

B   4. Bedwetting at night

C   5. Excessive daytime sleepiness lasting at least 1 month

Column B

a. Polysomnography

b. Nocturnal enuresis

c. Hypersomnia

d. Bruxism

e. Narcolepsy

Complete the following:

6. What physiological and psychological changes occur during sleep?

7. According to a normal non-rapid eye movement (NREM)/ rapid eye movement (REM) sequence, when does a patient experience dreams and become difficult to arouse?

8. What is the recommended amount of uninterrupted time that nurses should provide patients for sleep?

9. The nurse is working with a patient who is totally blind. How can this affect the individual's sleep patterns?

10. Which of the following statements is/are accurate regarding sleep? *Select all that apply.*
    a. Humans spend one-half of their lives sleeping. _____
    b. Adults normally fall asleep within 10 minutes. _____
    c. There are usually three sleep stages. _____
    d. NREM sleep alternates with REM sleep in about 5-minute intervals. _____
    e. Pain can adversely affect the quality of sleep. _____
    f. Individuals who are awakened from sleep will begin their cycle again with the first stage of NREM sleep. _____

11. What physical problems may occur for individuals who sleep less than average?

12. What are two sleep-related safety concerns for infants and toddlers?

13. Which of the following sleep-related behaviors are associated with toddlers and preschoolers? *Select all that apply.*
    a. They usually sleep 10 to 12 hours per night. _____
    b. Bedtime rituals are important. _____
    c. They awaken more and take longer to go back to sleep. _____
    d. Sleeping in the parents' room is recommended. _____
    e. Naps are no longer necessary. _____
    f. Nightmares may occur. _____

14. What are causes of dyssomnias?

15. The nurse is working with a patient who is experiencing insomnia. What interventions should be included in the teaching plan for this patient?

16. Identify a potential safety hazard for a patient who is experiencing narcolepsy.

17. The nurse is alert to patients who may be predisposed to obstructive sleep apnea, including those individuals with which of the following risk factor(s) of? *Select all that apply.*
    a. Heart disease _____
    b. Renal disease _____
    c. Nasal polyps _____
    d. Obesity _____
    e. Arthritis _____
    f. Alcohol use _____

18. What problems can occur with prolonged sleep apnea?

19. Which of the following is/are associated with sleep deprivation? *Select all that apply.*
    a. Excitability _____
    b. Nausea _____
    c. Extreme weight loss _____
    d. Increased focus _____
    e. Hallucinations _____
    f. Increased sensitivity to pain _____

20. For the nursing diagnosis *Disturbed Sleep Pattern related to the schedule and noise on the unit and manifested by frequent awakenings,* what nursing interventions should be implemented?

21. For an individual with somnambulism, what is the biggest safety factor?

22. Identify the effects of the following factors on sleep:
    a. Exercise—

    b. Stress—

    c. Family relationships—

23. The nurse asks a male patient who is having difficulty sleeping if he drinks beverages with caffeine. He responds that he often has tea around 9 P.M. What should the nurse recommend that may assist the patient to sleep?

24. The patient tells the nurse that she has been scheduled for a polysomnography evaluation. She does not understand what this test will tell her provider. How will you explain the purpose of this test?

25. Identify what the equipment in the photo is and what sleeping disorder it is used to treat.

26. Provide an example of a common bedtime ritual for an adult and/or child.

Select the best answer for each of the following questions:

27. The nurse recognizes the stages of sleep and knows that a patient is most easily aroused in which stage?
    a. NREM 1
    b. NREM 2
    c. NREM 3
    d. NREM 4

28. Which of the following is an antidepressant medication that may be prescribed to promote sleep?
    a. Elavil
    b. Haldol
    c. Versed
    d. Benadryl

29. Which of the following is associated with a patient who has hypersomnia?
    a. Sleeping less than 6 hours a night
    b. Having trouble waking up in the morning
    c. Falling asleep during a conversation
    d. Having difficulty falling asleep

30. The patient has expressed difficulty in sleeping. Upon further investigation by the nurse, the patient identifies the following behaviors. Which one should the nurse focus on that may be interfering with the patient's sleep?
    a. Exercising after work
    b. Taking a warm bath before bedtime
    c. Having one or two glasses of wine after dinner
    d. Eating a bedtime snack of crackers and juice

31. The mother of a 2-year-old tells the nurse that the child has started crying and resisting going to sleep at the scheduled bedtime. The nurse should advise the parent to:
    a. offer the child a bedtime snack.
    b. eliminate one of the naps during the day.
    c. allow the child to sleep longer in the mornings.
    d. maintain consistency in the same bedtime ritual.

32. An 11-year-old child in middle school is currently experiencing sleep-related fatigue during classes. Which of the following should the nurse ask the parents first?
    a. "What are the child's usual sleep patterns?"
    b. "Is there anything else going on at home or school?"
    c. "Do you think that there is a medical reason for the problem?"
    d. "Are you allowing the child stay up late."

33. In describing the sleep patterns of older adults, the nurse recognizes that they:
    a. require more sleep than middle-aged adults.
    b. are more difficult to arouse.
    c. take less time to fall asleep.
    d. have a decline in stage 4 sleep.

34. For a patient who is currently taking a diuretic, the nurse should inform the patient that he or she may experience:
    a. nocturia.
    b. nightmares.
    c. reduced REM sleep.
    d. increased daytime sleepiness.

35. As a result of recent studies regarding sudden infant death syndrome and infant safety during sleep, the nurse instructs the parents to:
    a. cover the infant loosely with a blanket.
    b. provide a stuffed toy for comfort.
    c. place the infant on its back.
    d. use small pillows in the crib.

36. A 74-year-old patient has been having sleeping difficulties. In order to have a better idea of the patient's problem, the nurse should respond with which of the following?
    a. "What do you do just before going to bed?"
    b. "Why don't you try napping more during the daytime?"
    c. "You should always eat something just before bedtime."
    d. "Let's make sure that your bedroom is completely darkened at night."

37. Which of the following information provided by the patient's bed partner is most associated with sleep apnea?
    a. Restlessness
    b. Talking during sleep
    c. Somnambulism
    d. Excessive snoring

38. In teaching methods to promote positive sleep habits at home, the nurse instructs the patient to:
    a. use the bedroom only for sleep or sexual activity.
    b. eat a large meal 1 to 2 hours before bedtime.
    c. exercise vigorously before bedtime.
    d. stay in bed if sleep does not come after ½ hour.

39. The nurse is discussing sleep habits with the patient in the sleep assessment clinic. Of the following activities performed before sleeping, the nurse is alert to the one that may be interfering with the patient's sleep, which is:
    a. listening to classical music.
    b. finishing office work.
    c. drinking warm milk.
    d. reading novels.

40. Older adults at the community center are having a discussion on health issues that is being led by a nurse volunteer. One of the participants asks the nurse what to do about not being able to sleep well at night. The nurse informs the participants that sleep in the evening may be enhanced by:
    a. drinking an alcoholic beverage before bedtime.
    b. using an over-the-counter sleeping agent.
    c. wearing loose, comfortable clothing.
    d. eating a large meal before bedtime.

Practice Situation

You are working on a medical unit in an acute care hospital. Having worked on the day shift (8 A.M. to 4 P.M.) for 6 months, you are now asked to rotate every 5 days to the night shift (12 A.M.– to 8 A.M.) while one of the staff members is away on family leave.

a. What strategies should you use to minimize the effect of this change in your circadian rhythm?

b. What signs and symptoms should you be alert for that may indicate an inadequate amount of sleep?

REVIEW QUESTIONS

- What is the physiology and function of sleep?
- What are the characteristics of common sleep disorders?
- Which assessment techniques should be used for determining sleep patterns?
- Which nursing diagnoses are appropriate for patients with sleep disturbances?
- How are patient goals determined for individual sleep problems?
- Which interventions should be implemented to promote sleep?

34 Diagnostic Testing

CHAPTER REVIEW

Match the description/definition in Column A with the correct term in Column B.

Column A

_____ 1. Insertion of a needle directly into the vein

_____ 2. Involves removing fluid from the peritoneal cavity

_____ 3. Soft tissue radiographs that allow visualization of the underlying breast tissue

_____ 4. Radiologic procedure in which the use of a special scanner allows cross-sectional images of an organ to be visualized

_____ 5. Involves removing a larger collection of cells, as in a tumor or mass, and may be used to detect cancer in the skin, breast, or liver

_____ 6. Involves the use of a superconducting magnet and radiofrequency waves that cause hydrogen nuclei to emit signals

_____ 7. A procedure that provides visualization of soft tissue organs by recording and measuring the reflection of sonic waves

_____ 8. Removes fluid from the pleural space

_____ 9. Contains chemically altered filter paper that changes color when stool containing blood is placed on it

_____ 10. A recording of the electrical current generated by the heart during depolarization and repolarization of the cardiac muscle

Column B

a. Magnetic resonance imaging (MRI)

b. Thoracentesis

c. Biopsy

d. Electrocardiogram

e. Hemoccult

f. Ultrasound

g. Mammogram

h. Paracentesis

i. Venipuncture

j. Computed tomography (CT)

Complete the following:

11. What are the components of a complete blood count?

12. The nurse anticipates that testing will be done for the patient who is taking an anticoagulant. Identify at least two specific tests that may be ordered to assess this patient's status.

13. Glucose testing is done to determine the presence of which pathologic condition?

14. The patient asks about "good cholesterol." Which one of these should the nurse identify to the patient?
Low-density lipoprotein (LDL) _____
High-density lipoprotein (HDL) _____

15. Which of the following is/are normal values for a urinalysis? *Select all that apply.*
a. Clear to slightly hazy _____
b. Specific gravity 1.050 _____
c. Very pale yellow color _____
d. Positive ketones _____
e. Negative protein _____
f. Positive bilirubin _____

16. C-reactive protein (CRP) is used as a marker for which disorders?

17. The nurse anticipates that which of the following cardiac markers may be ordered for the patient to determine possible tissue damage? *Select all that apply.*
    a. Triglycerides _____
    b. Myoglobin _____
    c. Serum creatinine _____
    d. Troponin T _____
    e. Aspartate aminotransferase _____
    f. Total creatine kinase _____

18. The patient has stools that are black and tarry in appearance. The nurse recognizes that this finding is associated with:

19. Which test is performed for the patient with a suspected tapeworm and how must the sample be sent to the laboratory?

20. The patient is to have a culture and sensitivity done. How do you explain this test to the patient?

21. What disorders can be diagnosed with a chest radiograph?

22. The patient had a diagnostic test with contrast media. Following the test, the nurse notices that the patient has developed a rash and does not feel well. What does the nurse suspect that the patient may be experiencing?

23. Which of the following requires that the patient be fasting? *Select all that apply.*
    a. Glucose _____
    b. Cholesterol _____
    c. Low-density lipoprotein _____
    d. Blood urea nitrogen (BUN) _____
    e. Complete blood count _____
    f. Albumin _____

24. The patient is to have an MRI. What instruction should the nurse provide to the patient for this test?

25. What should screening for colorectal cancer for individuals older than age 50 include?

26. What is ultrasound commonly used to determine?

27. What is a critical question to ask young and middle adult female patients who are having diagnostic tests?

28. What is the most critical area to monitor during a bronchoscopy?

29. What are the procedures being done in the following two photos, and what patient care should the nurse provide after each one?
    a.

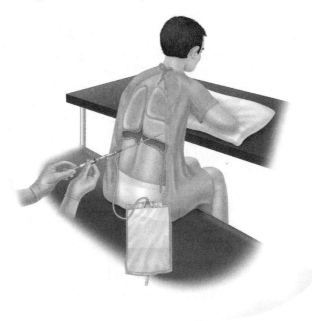

    b.

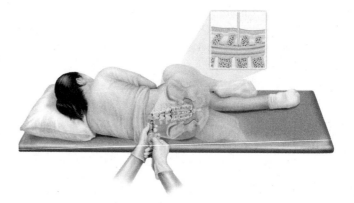

30. The patient is extremely anxious about the diagnostic tests to be performed. Identify a potential nursing diagnosis and goal for this individual.

31. The nurse is going to perform a venipuncture and asks the unlicensed assistive personnel (UAP) to get collection tubes for a blood chemistry and blood culture. The UAP is told to get tubes with what color stoppers?

32. Identify at least two National Patient Safety Goals for patients having diagnostic tests.

33. Indicate the standard precautions that are used for:
    a. Venipuncture—

    b. Urine collection—

34. While a patient is going through a procedure, what can the nurse do to provide support and comfort?

35. How does the nurse carefully manage collection and transfer of specimens?

36. The nurse instructs the female patient to do a clean-catch urine specimen collection. Place the steps the patient should take in the correct order.
    a. Urinate a small amount into the toilet. _____
    b. Finish urinating, close and wipe off the container. _____
    c. Cleanse the perineum from front to back, repeating with new wipes. _____
    d. Prepare the sterile specimen cup. _____
    e. Place the cup into the urine stream and collect 30 mL of urine. _____
    f. Separate the labia. _____

37. For a timed urine collection:
    a. What should be done with the initial voiding?

    b. What should be done if a voiding is not collected during the time period?

38. Sputum collection is usually ordered when what disease processes are suspected?

39. Identify all of the following that are correct for sputum collection:
    a. Samples should be collected first thing in the morning. _____
    b. Clean containers are used. _____
    c. Oral care is provided before and after. _____
    d. A specimen of 2 to 10 mL is needed. _____
    e. The patient expectorates directly into the container. _____
    f. Suctioning for specimen collection can be delegated to the UAP. _____

40. The patient starts to gag during the throat culture. The nurse should:

41. After most procedures, the nurse should monitor the patient's:

42. Identify what the following laboratory results indicate:
    a. Female patient, red blood cells (RBCs) 3.7 cells/mm^3

    b. 8-year-old child, white blood cells (WBCs) 8000 cells/ mm^3

    c. Platelets 75,000 cells/mm^3

    d. BUN 30 mg/dL

43. CT scan can be used on the brain to diagnose:

44. To verify the presence of Crohn disease, the nurse anticipates that there will be an order for which test(s)?

45. For collection of a stool specimen, identify the action required for the following:
    a. Multiple specimens are required.

    b. The sample has toilet paper mixed in.

Select the best answer for each of the following questions:

46. The nurse is checking the laboratory reports for the patient who has diabetes mellitus. Which finding indicates that the patient has the diabetes under control?
    a. hgb A_{1c} below 3%
    b. hgb A_{1c} 3% to 6%
    c. hgb A_{1c} 7% to 11%
    d. hgb A_{1c} over 11%

47. Which of the following is found in higher amounts when jaundice is present?
    a. Albumin
    b. Bilirubin
    c. Alkaline phosphatase
    d. Gamma-glutamyltransferase

48. The nurse is teaching the UAP how to collect a specimen for blood glucose monitoring. The patient demonstrates correct technique when:
    a. calibrating the meter to the strip.
    b. using the center of the tip of a finger for the puncture.
    c. holding the finger upright after puncture.
    d. vigorously squeezing the fingertip after puncture.

49. When obtaining a urine specimen for urinalysis from a patient with an indwelling catheter, the nurse should:
    a. apply sterile gloves for the procedure.
    b. clamp the drainage tubing for 30 to 60 minutes before specimen collection begins.
    c. disconnect the catheter from the drainage tubing and collect the urine in a specimen cup.
    d. insert a small-gauge needle directly into the catheter tubing to draw up the urine.

50. Instruction to the patient for collection of a midstream sample includes:
    a. use of a clean specimen cup.
    b. collection of 200 mL of urine for testing.
    c. voiding some urine first and then collecting the sample.
    d. washing the perineal area back and forth with Betadine.

51. Although care is taken with all patients having a venipuncture, the nurse is especially alert to the potential for continued bleeding for the patient who regularly takes:
    a. aspirin.
    b. insulin.
    c. calcium.
    d. Lasix.

52. Which of the following statements is accurate for Hemoccult testing?
    a. A large sample is required.
    b. Surgical asepsis is used.
    c. Ova and parasites can be identified.
    d. The strip changes color when blood is found.

53. A lumbar puncture is ordered for the patient suspected of having:
    a. peritonitis.
    b. meningitis.
    c. sinusitis.
    d. glomerulonephritis.

54. The patient is going to have a cystoscopy tomorrow. The nurse is aware that a possible complication of this procedure is:
    a. hematuria.
    b. pneumonia.
    c. thrombophlebitis.
    d. compartment syndrome.

Practice Situation

The patient is going to have an arthroscopy of his left knee in the morning. The patient is aware of what will be done during the procedure and does not appear to be anxious, having had this done before on the right knee. You will focus on making sure that the preparation of the patient is completed.

a. What will you do to make sure that patient safety and comfort are maintained?

b. What is your plan of care for the patient after the procedure?

c. What do you anticipate to be a primary need for the patient after the arthroscopy?

REVIEW QUESTIONS

- What are the types of cells found in blood and their functions?
- What are the common blood tests, their purposes, and their normal values?
- What are some other laboratory tests, such as urine and stool studies, and their purposes and normal values?
- What is the purpose of common diagnostic tests?
- Which assessment procedures should be implemented for patients undergoing diagnostic tests?
- Which nursing diagnoses are appropriate for patients having diagnostic testing?
- Which goals are appropriate for patients having diagnostic tests?
- What is the nurse's role before, during, and after diagnostic tests and procedures?

35 Medication Administration

CHAPTER REVIEW

Match the description/definition in Column A with the correct term in Column B.

Column A	Column B
____ 1. Severe allergic reaction	a. Adverse effects
____ 2. Unpredictable patient response to medication	b. Medication interaction
____ 3. Predictable but unwanted and sometimes unavoidable reactions to medications	c. Allergic reaction
____ 4. Occurs when the combined effect is greater than the effect of either substance if taken alone	d. Side effects
____ 5. Severe, unintended, unwanted, and often unpredictable drug reactions	e. Antagonism
____ 6. The desired result or action of a medication	f. Synergistic effect
____ 7. Unpredictable immune responses to medications	g. Idiosyncratic reaction
____ 8. Occurs when the drug action is modified by the presence of a certain food or herb or another medication	h. Therapeutic effect
____ 9. Result from a medication overdose or the buildup of medication in the blood due to impaired metabolism and excretion	i. Anaphylactic reaction
____ 10. Occurs when the drug effect is decreased by taking the drug with another substance	j. Toxic effects

Complete the following:

11. What is the difference between the terms *drug* and *medication*?

12. For the following, identify whether it is a chemical, generic, or trade (brand) name:
    a. Lasix
    b. acetaminophen
    c. fentanyl
    d. acetylsalicylic acid
    e. Prozac

13. Which of the following is the most effective way in the acute care environment to determine the patient's identity before administering medications? *Select all that apply.*
    a. Check the patient's medical record number on the ID band. _____
    b. Use the patient's room number. _____
    c. Compare an ID photo with the patient. _____
    d. Check the patient's date of birth. _____
    e. Use the bar code system, if available. _____
    f. Call the patient by name. _____

14. For the following individuals, identify special considerations to be taken when administering medications:
    a. A woman who is pregnant—

    b. An infant—

    c. An older adult—

15. Which organs are affected by the following?
    a. Metabolism of drugs—

    b. Excretion of drugs—

16. If a medication is administered that has an onset of action of 1/2 hour and the medication is given at 8:00 A.M., when should the nurse return to evaluate the patient's response?

17. The patient has come to the clinic for treatment of an infection and is given a new antibiotic. What should the nurse do to promote patient safety?

18. Provide examples of synergistic and antagonist drugs.

19. What are examples of common over-the-counter medications that patients may purchase?

20. For the following, identify what is missing in the medication orders:
    Patient—J. Smith
    August 20, 2014 10:00 A.M. B.Careful, MD
    a. Digoxin 0.125 mg PO
    b. Lasix 40 mg daily

21. When is special documentation required on the computerized or paper medication admission record (MAR) for medication administration?

22. a. What route is being used in the photo?

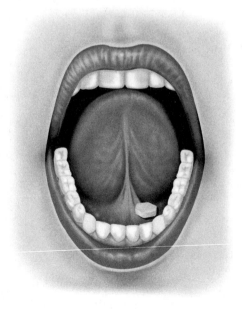

    b. Provide an example of a medication given by this route.

23. What general types of medications cannot be crushed for administration through an enteric tube?

24. Although unlicensed assistive personnel do not normally administer medications in the acute care area, what can the nurse delegate to this caregiver regarding the patient's medications?

25. Identify the topical medication route(s). *Select all that apply.*
    a. Cough suppressant _____
    b. Vaginal suppository _____
    c. Transdermal patch _____
    d. Patient-controlled analgesia drip _____
    e. Ear irrigation _____
    f. Antiseptic throat spray _____

26. From the following supplies, select those needed for an injection to an average-size adult:
    Available syringes—tuberculin (1 mL), 50 U insulin, 3 mL
    Available needles—5/8 inch, 1 inch, 1 1/2 inch
    a. Intramuscular (IM) injection—

    b. Subcutaneous injection—

27. Which specific assessments should be done by the nurse before administration of the following types of medications?
    a. Antihypertensive—

    b. Bronchodilator—

    c. Narcotic analgesic—

    d. Anticoagulant—

    e. Antipyretic—

28. Identify at least three ways that nurses can reduce medication errors.

29. For the following abbreviations and dose designations, which one(s) are appropriate to use? *Select all that apply.*
    a. PO _____
    b. OD _____
    c. .5 mg _____
    d. prn _____
    e. mL _____
    f. bid _____

30. Calculate the following dosages:
    a. Prescriber's order: 20 mg IM q4h
       Available: 40 mg/mL
       How much should be given? Identify the amount on the syringe.

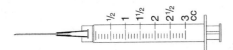

    b. Prescriber's order: 250 mcg PO tid
       Available: 0.5 mg scored tablets
       How many tablets should be given?

    c. Prescriber's order: 750 mg IM
       Available: 500 mg/mL
       How much should be given?

    d. Prescriber's order: 100 mg PO bid
       Available: 50 mg capsules
       How many capsules should be given?

    e. Prescriber's order: 10,000 U subcutaneous
       Available: 20,000 U/mL
       How much should be given?

    f. Prescriber's order: 30 U regular insulin
       Available: regular insulin U-100
       Identify the amount prepared on the syringe.

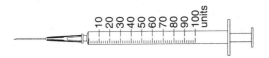

31. Identify the angle of insertion and the type of injection that is being administered.
    a.
    b.
    c.

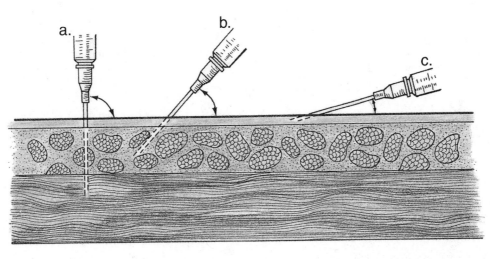

32. Identify the "Six Rights" of medication administration:
    Right _____
    Right _____
    Right _____
    Right _____
    Right _____
    Right _____

33. When does the nurse perform the three checks of the medications to be given?

34. Identify at least three assessment questions that the nurse should ask a patient about his or her medication history.

35. The patient has been newly diagnosed with a heart-related condition and is prescribed a number of different medications. The patient is unsure about the medications and would like to know what they are and how they work.
    a. Identify a nursing diagnosis for this individual.

    b. Identify a relevant goal for the patient.

36. Identify special considerations for administration of medications to children.

37. When is oral medication administration contraindicated?

38. Which type of oral medications should be given last?

39. The nurse is to administer medications through the patient's nasogastric tube. Which of the following techniques is/are correct? *Select all that apply.*
    a. Check the placement of the tube before giving medications. _____
    b. Crush all of the patient's tablets and capsules. _____
    c. Flush the tube before and after with 5 mL of water. _____
    d. Have the patient sit upright for the medication administration. _____
    e. Keep the patient's head elevated after the administration for at least 30 minutes. _____
    f. Replace gastric suction, if used, right after giving the medications. _____

40. What do the following abbreviations mean?
    a. pc—

    b. bid—

    c. prn—

    d. IV—

    e. qid—

41. The nurse is to apply transdermal patches to his patients. Which of the following techniques is/are correct? *Select all that apply.*
    a. Use the same location for the new transdermal patch. _____
    b. Place transdermal patches over bony areas. _____
    c. Write initials, date, and time on patches before applied. _____
    d. Massage the patch when it is in place. _____
    e. Remove patches if the patient requires defibrillation. _____
    f. Clean the skin site where the patch will be placed. _____

42. For administration of ear drops:
    a. To prevent nausea, pain, and dizziness during the administration, the nurse should:

    b. The ear canal is straightened in an adult patient by:

43. What does the nurse ask the patient to do first before administering nasal medications?

44. For inhaled medications:
    a. What assessment does the nurse do before administration?

    b. The patient is taking a steroid via an inhaler. What should be done after administration?

    c. How does the patient/nurse determine the amount of doses in a container?

45. The patient is placed in what position for the following:
    a. Vaginal suppository insertion—

b. Rectal suppository insertion—

46. What type of asepsis is used for administration of parenteral medications?

47. The nurse prepares the injection in the medication room and needs to bring it to the patient down the hall. What is the correct technique for covering the needle for transport?

48. The nurse is preparing an injection from an ampule. What special safety techniques are used?

49. Two medications are to be given, one from an ampule and one from a vial. Identify the correct order of the procedure for putting the medications into the same syringe. The ampule and vial have both been prepared.
    a. Draw an amount of air into the syringe equal to the vial's medication dose. _____
    b. Draw up the amount of medication ordered from the ampule. _____
    c. Verify the total dose in the syringe. _____
    d. Attach a filter needle to the syringe. _____
    e. Insert the needle into the vial and instill the air into the space above the medication. _____
    f. Draw the medication from the vial. _____

50. Identify the sites for subcutaneous injections on the figures below.

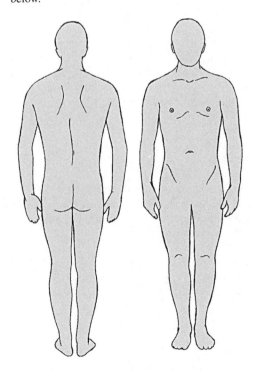

51. For intradermal injections:
    a. When is this type of injection route used?

    b. Where can the injection be given?

52. An IM injection is to be given into the ventrogluteal muscle. The nurse should aspirate before administering the medication.

    True _____   False _____

53. Indicate the maximum amount of medication that should be given for each of the following injections:
    a. Subcutaneous—

    b. Deltoid injection—

54. Describe how a Z-track injection is given.

55. EpiPen injections can be done through the patient's clothes.

    True _____   False _____

56. How can intravenous (IV) medications be administered to the patient?

57. Special considerations for administration of IV medications include:

58. The older adult patient has several medications at home and tends to forget whether the daily doses have been taken. What can the nurse do to assist this patient with the medications?

59. What is the "Ask Me 3" program?

60. How can the patient and nurse evaluate the effectiveness of insulin?

61. A patient is nauseated, has been vomiting for several hours, and needs to receive an antiemetic medication. The nurse recognizes that administration of the medication, considering the patient's status and the medication, is best via which route(s)? *Select all that apply.*
    a. Oral _____
    b. Enteral _____
    c. Parenteral _____
    d. Inhalation _____
    e. Topical—rectal suppository _____
    f. Topical—nasal application _____

62. Bar-code scanning is used to verify what?

63. What instructions does the nurse give the patient specifically for buccal and sublingual medications?

64. The patient is to use a traditional metered-dose inhaler (MDI). Place the steps of the procedure in the correct order.
    a. Patient places the mouthpiece of the inhaler in the mouth. _____
    b. Patient removes inhaler and exhales through pursed lips. _____
    c. Patient takes a deep breath and blows out completely. _____
    d. Patient inhales slowly and pushes the canister. _____
    e. Patient shakes the MDI. _____
    f. Patient continues to inhale for 3 to 5 seconds and hold the breath to 5 to 10 seconds. _____

65. How are medications that are reconstituted in vials mixed?

66. The nurse assesses the area where an injection will be given. What assessment findings will require the need to use a different site?

67. Identify the anatomic landmarks for the following injections:
    a. Deltoid—

    b. Vastus lateralis—

68. Identify the steps in the procedure of a direct IV push of a medication through a saline lock (intermittent access port).

Select the best answer for each of the following questions:

69. The Kefauver-Harris Drug Amendments were passed in 1962 in order to:
    a. classify habit-forming medications as narcotics.
    b. mandate accuracy in drug labeling.
    c. require proof of drug safety and efficacy before marketing.
    d. categorize drugs on their abuse and addiction potential.

70. Which of the following is a correct technique for use of an insulin pen?
    a. Clean the pen tip with household soap.
    b. Prime the pen with 2 units before use.
    c. Cover the needle until the next dose.
    d. Empty the pen and complete the dosage with a new pen, if necessary.

71. A medication order that is to be administered immediately is:
    a. diazepam 10 mg IV stat.
    b. Lanoxin 0.125 mg PO daily.
    c. ibuprofen 300 mg q4h prn.
    d. Ativan 1 mg IV on call for surgery.

72. Which one of the following actions performed by the new staff nurse and observed by the nurse manager requires additional instruction?
    a. Giving medications 20 minutes before the scheduled time.
    b. Applying a topical medicated cream without gloves.
    c. Alternating the sides of the cheeks for buccal medications.
    d. Documenting on the MAR that the patient refused the medication.

73. The patient tells the nurse that he is experiencing nausea, vomiting, clumsiness, and blurred vision. He says that he has been taking a lot of vitamins. On the basis of the patient's symptoms, which vitamin does the nurse suspect is creating the adverse effects?
    a. Vitamin B_3
    b. Vitamin C
    c. Folic acid
    d. Vitamin A

74. The patient asks the nurse about different herbal therapies that may promote physical stamina and mental concentration. On the basis of the patient's request, the nurse provides information on:
    1. ginseng.
    2. ginger.
    3. echinacea.
    4. chamomile.

75. The patient is taking an herbal remedy for mild anxiety and difficulty sleeping. It also has the potential to interact with antidepressant medications. The nurse expects that this patient is taking:
    a. chamomile.
    b. St. John's wort.
    c. echinacea.
    d. Gingko biloba.

76. The patient is to be given the medication that is enclosed in a cylindrical gelatin coating. The nurse knows that this medication comes in the form of a:
    a. tablet.
    b. powder.
    c. capsule.
    d. suppository.

77. The patient receiving an IV infusion of morphine sulfate begins to experience respiratory depression and decreased urine output. This effect is described as:
    a. toxic.
    b. allergic.
    c. therapeutic.
    d. idiosyncratic.

78. The patient is to receive a medication via the buccal route. The nurse plans to implement which of the following actions?
    a. Place the medication inside the cheek.
    b. Crush the medication before administration.
    c. Utilize sterile technique to administer the medication.
    d. Offer the patient a glass of orange juice after administration.

79. The physician orders 100 mg of a hypnotic medication to help the patient sleep. The label on the medication bottle reads Seconal 50 mg. How many tablets should the nurse give the patient?
    a. 1/2
    b. 1
    c. 1 1/2
    d. 2

80. The physician has ordered 6 mg morphine sulfate every 3 to 4 hours prn for a patient's postoperative pain. The unit dose in the medication dispenser has 15 mg in 1 mL. How much solution should the nurse give?
    a. 1/5 mL
    b. 1/3 mL
    c. 2/5 mL
    d. 1/4 mL

81. The nurse is documenting administration of a medication that is given at 10 A.M., 2 P.M., and 6:00 P.M.. The medication that the nurse is documenting is:
    a. morphine sulfate 10 mg q4h prn.
    b. Inderal 10 mg PO bid.
    c. diazepam 5 mg PO tid.
    d. Keflex 500 mg PO q8h.

82. The nurse is working on the pediatric unit. In preparing to give medications to a preschool-age child, an appropriate interaction by the nurse is:
    a. "Do you want to take your medication now?"
    b. "Would you like the medication with water or juice?"
    c. "Let me explain about the injection that you will be getting."
    d. "If you don't take the medication now you will not get better."

83. A patient has a prescription for a medication that is administered via an inhaler. In order to determine if the patient requires a spacer for the inhaler, the nurse will determine the:
    a. dosage of medication required.
    b. ability of the patient to control the rate of inhalation.
    c. schedule of administration.
    d. use of a dry powder inhaler (DPI).

84. The student nurse reads the order to give a 10-month-old patient an intramuscular injection. The appropriate and preferred muscle to select for a child is the:
    a. deltoid.
    b. dorsogluteal.
    c. ventrogluteal.
    d. vastus lateralis.

85. The nurse administers the IM medication of iron by the Z-track method. The medication was administered by this method to:
    a. provide faster absorption of the medication.
    b. reduce discomfort from the needle.
    c. provide more even absorption of the drug.
    d. prevent the drug from irritating sensitive tissue.

86. The patient is ordered to have eyedrops administered daily to both eyes. Eyedrops should be instilled on the:
    a. cornea.
    b. outer canthus.
    c. lower conjunctival sac.
    d. opening of the lacrimal duct.

87. Following the administration of eardrops to the left ear, the patient should be positioned:
    a. prone.
    b. upright.
    c. right lateral.
    d. dorsal recumbent with hyperextension of the neck.

88. An order is written by the prescriber for Demerol 500 mg IM q3-4h prn for pain. The nurse recognizes that this is significantly more than the usual therapeutic dose. The nurse should:
    a. call the prescriber to clarify the order.
    b. give 50 mg IM as it was probably intended to be written.
    c. refuse to give the medication and notify the nurse manager.
    d. administer the medication and watch the patient carefully.

89. An order is written for 80 mg of a medication in elixir form. The medication is available in 80 mg/tsp strength. The nurse prepares to administer how much?
   a. 2 mL
   b. 5 mL
   c. 10 mL
   d. 15 mL

90. The nurse prepares to administer an intradermal injection for the administration of medication for:
   a. pain.
   b. allergy sensitivity.
   c. anticoagulant therapy.
   d. low-dose insulin requirements.

91. The nurse is evaluating the integrity of the ventrogluteal injection site. The nurse finds the site by locating the:
   a. middle third of the lateral thigh.
   b. anterior aspect of the upper thigh.
   c. acromion process and axilla.
   d. greater trochanter, anterior iliac spine, and iliac crest.

92. The patient is to receive heparin by injection. The nurse prepares to inject this medication in the patient's:
   a. scapular region.
   b. vastus lateralis.
   c. posterior gluteal.
   d. abdomen.

93. A medication is prescribed for the patient and is to be administered by IV bolus injection. A priority for the nurse before the administration of medication via this route is to:
   a. set the rate of the IV infusion.
   b. check the patient's mental alertness.
   c. confirm placement of the IV line.
   d. determine the amount of IV fluid to be administered.

94. The nurse recognizes that an example of a Schedule II medication is:
   a. heroin.
   b. diazepam.
   c. morphine.
   d. acetaminophen.

95. A priority for the nurse in the administration of oral medications and prevention of aspiration is:
   a. checking for a gag reflex.
   b. assessing the ability to cough.
   c. allowing the patient to self-administer.
   d. using straws and extra water for administration.

Practice Situation

You are the new staff nurse on the unit and the following situations occur during your first week. Identify what you should do in each case.

   a. Your colleague has prepared the medications for one of her assigned patients but gets called away and asks you to administer the medications to her patient.

   b. The medication dosage needs to be carefully calculated on the basis of the patient's body weight. Your calculation leads to a result that you are pretty sure about, but it is a medication that you have never given before.

   c. The patient is to receive two IV medications that are incompatible with each other.

   d. The liquid medication is ordered in a dose that is less than 10 mL.

   e. The patient tells you that the pill "doesn't look like the one I usually take."

   f. You give one of the medications to the wrong patient.

   g. The patient does not have a hospital ID wristband in place.

   h. You see your fellow staff nurse documenting all of the patients' medications before they are given.

   i. The liquid medication has spilled on the label, making it difficult to read clearly.

   j. The dosage requires 1/2 of a pill, which is scored.

   k. You have taken out a medication from the drawer system for the patient that is a controlled substance. While placing the pills in the cup, you drop them on the floor.

   l. The patient needs the medications crushed and one is enteric coated.

   m. One of the medications in the patient's drawer is expired, and the other one is not the correct generic equivalent.

REVIEW QUESTIONS

- How do government, facility, and professional regulations affect medication administration by nurses?
- What are the physiological outcomes of medication actions?
- How are prescription and nonprescription medications different?
- What are the common medication forms and routes?
- Which measures are planned by the nurse in order to administer medications safely?
- Which assessments are necessary for safe medication administration?
- What nursing diagnoses are related to safe medication administration?
- How are individual patient goals determined for medication administration?
- What are the guidelines and essential nursing actions for safely administering medications?

36 Pain Management

CHAPTER REVIEW

Match the description/definition in Column A with the correct term in Column B.

Column A

h   1. Results from nerve injury

i   2. Physiological pain

j   3. Excessive sensitivity

f   4. Occurs after an amputation when the brain continues to receive messages from the area of the amputation

b   5. Pain that extends to other areas

d   6. Pain that is perceived by an individual but has no physical cause

e   7. Pain from noninjury stimuli

c   8. Greatly exaggerated pain reaction to stimuli

A   9. The administration of medications before a painful event

g   10. Unpleasant, abnormal sensation

Column B

a. Preemptive analgesia

b. Radiating pain

c. Hyperalgesia

d. Psychogenic pain

e. Allodynia

f. Phantom pain

g. Dysesthesia

h. Neuropathic pain

i. Somatic pain

j. Hyperpathia

Complete the following:

11. Identify at least two causes of unrelieved pain.

12. When should nurses assess pain?

13. A patient is having severe, acute pain from kidney stones. On the basis of the patient's experience, the nurse anticipates which of the following in the patient's assessment? *Select all that apply.*
    a. Tachycardia _____
    b. Diaphoresis _____
    c. Pupil dilation _____
    d. Muscle relaxation _____
    e. Hypertension _____
    f. Bradypnea _____

14. What area of the body is most sensitive to pain?

15. Identify and briefly describe the four steps in the pain conduction process.

16. What is the difference between the pain threshold and pain tolerance?

17. Identify the three major types of pain.

18. What are the specific sensations associated with neuropathic pain?

19. Which pathologies can alter the pain experience?

122

20. Identify physiological changes that can occur when an individual is experiencing pain.

21. How can the following factors influence the pain experience?
    a. Gender

    b. Disability

    c. Morphology

22. The infant is assessed as follows:
    Facial expression—grimace
    Cry—whimper
    Breathing pattern—change in breathing
    Arms—flexed
    Legs—flexed
    State of arousal—fussy

According to the Neonatal Infant Pain Scale, what would the score be for this infant and would you identify that the infant was in pain?

23. What strategies can be implemented to help a child with pain relief/management?

24. How is medication administration adapted for older adults with pain?

25. The patient is unable to speak. Identify how the nurse can assess this individual's level of pain.

26. Indicate the meaning of the following acronym:
    S—
    O—
    C—
    R—
    A—
    T—
    E—
    S—

27. What behaviors and/or psychological responses can be observed for a patient in pain?

28. The new staff nurse is working with unlicensed assistive personnel. The nurse is aware that which pain relief actions can be delegated to this person?

29. Identify at least three nursing actions that should be implemented to reduce legal risks associated with pain management.

30. Herbal remedies may be used by patients to help with pain relief. What is a consideration for the nurse in regard to this treatment?

31. How can the nurse use distraction to help the patient manage his or her pain?

32. The patient is given a fentanyl transdermal patch. He asks why he does not have an intravenous (IV) medication. The nurse explains that there are advantages to this method, including:

33. Which of the following are opioid analgesic medications that may be used for pain management? *Select all that apply.*
    a. Acetaminophen _____
    b. Morphine _____
    c. Hydromorphone _____
    d. Ibuprofen _____
    e. Pentazocine _____
    f. Oxycodone _____

34. What is the major side effect associated with narcotic analgesics?

35. For the patient who has patient-controlled analgesia (PCA), identify the following:
    a. Medications usually administered—
    b. Frequency of assessment—
    c. Precautions—

36. What is a nerve block is used for?

37. A large percentage of patients become addicted to analgesic medications.

    True _____   False _____

38. Indicate at least two Joint Commission standards for pain management.

Select the best answer for each of the following questions:

39. Which one of the following nursing interventions for a patient in pain is based on the gate control theory?
    a. Giving the patient a back massage.
    b. Changing the patient's position in bed.
    c. Giving the patient a pain medication.
    d. Limiting the number of visitors.

40. The patient tells the nurse about a burning sensation in the epigastric area. The nurse should describe this type of pain as:
    a. referred.
    b. radiating.
    c. visceral.
    d. superficial.

41. The nurse must frequently assess a patient experiencing pain. When assessing the intensity of the pain, the nurse should:
    a. ask about what precipitates the pain.
    b. question the patient about the location of the pain.
    c. offer the patient a pain scale to objectify the information.
    d. use open-ended questions to find out about the sensation.

42. The nurse on a postoperative care unit is assessing the quality of the patient's pain. In order to obtain this specific information about the pain experience from the patient, the nurse should ask:
    a. "What does your discomfort feel like?"
    b. "What activities make the pain worse?"
    c. "How much does it hurt on a scale of 0 to 10?"
    d. "How much discomfort are you able to tolerate?"

43. The patient will be going home on medication administered through a PCA system. To assist the family members with an understanding of how this therapy works, the nurse explains that the patient:
    a. has control over the frequency of the IV analgesia.
    b. can choose the dosage of the drug received.
    c. may request the type of medication received.
    d. controls the route for administering the medication.

44. An older patient with mild musculoskeletal pain is being seen by the primary care provider. The nurse anticipates that treatment of this patient's level of discomfort will include:
    a. fentanyl.
    b. diazepam.
    c. acetaminophen.
    d. meperidine.

45. The nurse tells the patient in advance that the urinary catheter insertion may feel uncomfortable. This is most accurately an example of:
    a. distraction.
    b. reducing pain perception.
    c. anticipating a response.
    d. self-care maintenance.

46. A patient with chronic back pain has an order for a transcutaneous electrical nerve stimulation unit for pain control. The nurse is aware that this therapy is contraindicated for the patient with:
    a. a pacemaker.
    b. muscle pain.
    c. diabetes.
    d. arthritis.

47. A terminally ill patient with liver cancer is experiencing great discomfort. A realistic goal in caring for the patient is to:
    a. increasingly administer narcotics to oversedate the patient and thereby decrease the pain.
    b. continue to change the analgesics until the right narcotic is found that completely alleviates the pain.
    c. adapt the analgesics as the nursing assessment reveals the need for specific medications.
    d. withhold analgesics as they are not being effective in relieving discomfort.

48. Nurses working with patients in pain need to recognize and avoid common misconceptions and myths about pain. In regards to the pain experience, which of the following is correct?
    a. Chronic pain is mostly psychological in nature.
    b. Regular use of analgesics leads to drug addiction.
    c. The patient is the best authority on the pain experience.
    d. The amount of tissue damage is accurately reflected in the degree of pain perceived.

49. A nonpharmacologic approach that the nurse may implement for patients experiencing pain that focuses on creating a calm state with controlled breathing and relaxation is:
    a. acupressure.
    b. meditation.
    c. biofeedback.
    d. hypnosis.

50. The nurse consults with the primary care provider of a patient who is experiencing continuous, severe pain. In planning for the patient's treatment, the nurse is aware of the principles of pain management and that it is appropriate to expect treatment to include:
    a. focusing on intramuscular administration of analgesics.
    b. waiting for pain to become more intense before administering opioids.
    c. administering opioid with nonopioid analgesics for severe pain experiences.
    d. administering large doses of opioids initially to patients who have not taken the medications before.

51. Upon entering the room, the nurse discovers that the patient is experiencing acute pain. An expected assessment finding for this patient is:
    a. bradycardia.
    b. diaphoresis.
    c. bradypnea.
    d. decreased muscle tension.

52. Which of the following is an example of multimodal analgesia?
    a. Ginseng
    b. Massage
    c. IV morphine
    d. Tylenol with codeine

53. Knowing the major side effect of nonsteroidal antiinflammatory drug medications, the nurse instructs the patient to:
    a. apply sunscreen before going outdoors.
    b. take the medication with food.
    c. avoid taking it with other drugs.
    d. take the medication in the morning.

54. The nurse expects to administer which of the following medications for a narcotic overdose?
    a. Naloxone
    b. Meperidine
    c. Butorphanol
    d. Dezocine

Practice Situation

A 72-year-old female patient visits the primary care provider's office for assessment of ongoing joint discomfort, stiffness, and more difficulty getting around. The discomfort is described by the patient as a 2 to 3 on a pain scale of 0 to 10. The patient is diagnosed with osteoarthritis and given medication.

Use the conceptual care map to input the information.

a. What signs, symptoms, or behaviors do you expect this patient to demonstrate?

b. Identify a potential nursing diagnosis, a goal, and nonpharmacologic interventions for this patient.

c. What medications do you anticipate will be prescribed or recommended?

REVIEW QUESTIONS

- How is pain defined?
- What is the role of the nurse in pain management?
- How are the physiology of pain and its perception connected?
- Which factors influence pain perception and response?
- How can the individual physiological, behavioral, and psychosocial responses to pain be assessed?
- What nursing diagnoses are appropriate for patients experiencing pain?
- What are the nursing care goals and outcome criteria for patients experiencing pain?
- How can pain management care, including prescribed medications and alternative and complementary pain relief interventions, be planned, implemented, and evaluated?

CHAPTER REVIEW

Match the description/definition in Column A with the correct term in Column B.

Column A

_____ 1. Improves comfort, decreases pain or symptoms

_____ 2. Replaces dysfunctional body part

_____ 3. Restores function or appearance to traumatized or malnourished tissues

_____ 4. Establishes or confirms a condition

_____ 5. Removes a part of the body that is diseased

_____ 6. Improves personal appearance

Column B

a. Diagnostic

b. Ablative

c. Cosmetic

d. Palliative

e. Reconstructive

f. Transplant

Complete the following:

7. Briefly describe what happens in each of the perioperative phases:
   a. Preoperative

   b. Intraoperative

   c. Postoperative

8. What is meant by a "time-out" during surgery?

9. Identify the positions in which the patient should be placed for the following surgical procedures:
   a. Gynecologic—

   b. Cardiac—

   c. Renal—

   d. Rectal—

10. What are the roles of the scrub nurse and the circulating nurse?

11. The patient is extremely overweight and has difficulty lying in the supine position. What can the nurse do to position the patient more comfortably?

12. Identify what is included in skin preparation for surgery.

13. What information is commonly included in the hand-off communication between the intraoperative and the postoperative/postanesthesia care recovery unit (PACU) nurse?

14. The patient has been moved to the PACU. What are the priority assessments that the nurse should make for this patient?

15. Provide examples for each of the following types of surgery:
    a. Elective—

    b. Urgent—

    c. Emergency—

    d. Minor—

    e. Major—

16. What factors make the following patients a greater risk for surgery?
    a. Infants—

    b. Older adults—

    c. Obese individuals—

    d. Patient with schizophrenia—

    e. Patient with a cardiac disease—

    f. Patient with diabetes—

17. The nurse is observing the patient who is receiving an inhaled general anesthetic for malignant hyperthermia. Which of the following is/are signs of this serious disorder? *Select all that apply.*
    a. High fever _____
    b. Muscle relaxation _____
    c. Hypotension _____
    d. Tachycardia _____
    e. Erythema _____
    f. Bradypnea _____

18. What is the immediate treatment for malignant hyperthermia?

19. For spinal anesthesia:
    a. What is the major postoperative problem related to the anesthesia?

    b. What can be done to alleviate the problem?

20. Identify at least three critical questions to ask a patient in the preoperative phase.

21. Baseline information to obtain before surgery should include:

22. The nurse is normally the first one to change the surgical dressing.

    True _____   False _____

23. a. What is the patient using in the photo?

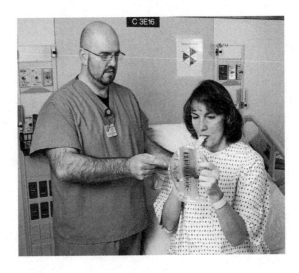

    b. What is this device used to prevent?

24. For the following nursing diagnosis, identify a goal/outcome and nursing intervention.
    Anxiety related to concern over the surgery as evidenced by pacing, tachycardia, diaphoresis, and verbalization of anxiousness.

25. What are the key nursing interventions in the preoperative phase?

26. When teaching a patient deep-breathing technique, what is the order for instruction?
    a. Inhale as deeply as possible. _____
    b. Take slow deep breaths, inhaling through the nose, and feeling the abdomen push against the hands. _____
    c. Exhale slowly through pursed lips, stopping when the hands touch.
    d. Hold the breath for 3 to 5 seconds. _____
    e. Rest the palms of the hands on the rib cage, with middle fingers touching.
    f. Assume an upright position. _____

27. Along with deep-breathing techniques, identify at least four topics that are included in preoperative patient teaching.

28. For informed consent:
    a. What is included in the consent?

    b. What is the nurse's role?

29. Why are surgical patients kept NPO?

30. For postoperative pain:
    a. The nurse assesses the patient's pain level at least every _____ hours.
    b. How is the pain level assessed?

    c. What is the benefit of providing pain relief to the post-operative patient?

31. For each of the following postoperative complications, indicate the nursing intervention(s) to prevent or treat the problem.
    a. Airway obstruction—

    b. Thrombophlebitis—

32. Atelectasis is specifically characterized by what signs and symptoms?

33. The care for an evisceration includes:

34. What factors can create a delay in surgical wound healing?

35. For patient safety, when the nurse leaves the room of a patient in the postoperative phase, he or she should:

36. What postoperative complications are seen in the photo?

37. The patient in the PACU in an ambulatory surgery center is scheduled to be discharged, but he has not been able to urinate. What should the nurse do?

38. Which of the following are appropriate actions for a surgical scrub and gowning? *Select all that apply.*
    a. Leaving on nail polish and short artificial nails. _____
    b. Removing all rings. _____
    c. Keeping the back turned toward the sterile area. _____
    d. Having the work area above waist level. _____
    e. Keeping the hands above the elbows. _____
    f. Wet and lather the hands to the wrists. _____

39. Indicate the order in which the surgical attire is removed.
    a. Eyewear _____
    b. Mask _____
    c. Gloves _____
    d. Gown _____

40. Documentation of the surgical wound needs to include what assessments?

41. During the surgical procedure, the circulating nurse notices that the surgeon has broken sterile technique. The nurse should:

Select the best answer for each of the following questions:

42. A 43-year-old patient is scheduled to have a gastrectomy. Which of the following is a major preoperative concern?
    a. An IV infusion is present.
    b. The patient's brother had a tonsillectomy at age 11.
    c. The patient smokes a pack of cigarettes a day.
    d. The patient has worked as a computer programmer.

43. An appendectomy is appropriately documented by the nurse as:
    a. diagnostic surgery.
    b. palliative surgery.
    c. ablative surgery.
    d. reconstructive surgery.

44. An obese patient is admitted for abdominal surgery. The nurse recognizes that this patient is more susceptible to the postoperative complication of:
    a. anemia.
    b. seizures.
    c. protein loss.
    d. dehiscence.

45. The nurse is working in a postoperative care unit in an ambulatory surgery center. Of the following patients that have come to have surgery, the patient at the greatest risk during surgery is a:
    a. 43-year-old taking an antihypertensive agent.
    b. 27-year-old taking an anticoagulant agent.
    c. 78-year-old taking an analgesic agent.
    d. 10-year-old taking an antibiotic agent.

46. A 92-year-old patient is scheduled for a colectomy. Which normal physiological change that accompanies the aging process increases this patient's risk for surgery?
    a. An increased tactile sensation
    b. An increased metabolic rate
    c. A relaxation of arterial walls
    d. Reduced glomerular filtration

47. The nurse is completing the preoperative checklist for an adult female patient who is scheduled for an operative procedure later in the morning. To evaluate renal function, the nurse reviews the results of the:
    a. fasting blood sugar.
    b. serum glutamate pyruvic transaminase.
    c. blood urea nitrogen (BUN).
    d. human chorionic gonadotropin.

48. The nurse is evaluating the following for the informed consent: *"Patient describes surgical procedures and post-operative treatment"* and determines that the patient has not achieved this outcome. The nurse should:
    a. teach the patient all about the procedure.
    b. inform the surgeon so that information can be provided.
    c. ask the unit manager to assist with a teaching plan.
    d. obtain the consent, as this is expected with preoperative anxiety.

49. Which of the following statements most accurately reflects nursing accountability in the intraoperative phase?
    a. "I would like to see the patient have a regional anesthetic rather than a general anesthetic."
    b. "There seems to be a missing sponge, so a recount should be done of all the sponges that have been removed."
    c. "Did the patient receive the medications and sign the consent?"
    d. "The patient looks to be reactive and stable."

50. The patient will have an incision in the lower left abdomen. Which of the following measures by the nurse will help decrease discomfort in the incisional area when the patient coughs postoperatively?
    a. Applying a splint directly over the lower abdomen
    b. Keeping the patient flat with her feet flexed
    c. Turning the patient onto the right side
    d. Applying pressure above and below the incision

51. A patient is in the PACU recovering from a vagotomy and pyloroplasty. Which of the following is a normal expectation of the patient in this stage of recovery?
    a. A subdued level of consciousness and neurologic function
    b. Pain that is relieved with nonpharmacologic measures
    c. Returned normal bowel sounds on auscultation
    d. Voluntary bladder control and function

52. The patient is scheduled for abdominal surgery and has just received the preoperative medications. The nurse should:
    a. keep the patient quiet.
    b. obtain the consent.
    c. prepare the skin at the surgical site.
    d. place the side rails up on the bed or stretcher.

53. The nurse is completing the preoperative checklist for an adult patient who is scheduled for an operative procedure later in the morning. Which of the following preoperative assessment findings for this patient indicates a need to contact the anesthesiologist?
    a. Temperature = 101° F
    b. Pulse = 84
    c. Respirations = 20
    d. Blood pressure = 130/74

54. The patient tells the nurse that "blowing into this tube thing (incentive spirometer) is a ridiculous waste of time." The nurse explains that the specific purpose of the therapy is to:
   a. directly remove excess secretions from the lungs.
   b. increase pulmonary circulation.
   c. promote lung expansion.
   d. stimulate the cough reflex.

55. The patient asks the nurse the purpose of having medications (sedatives) given before surgery. The nurse should inform the patient that these particular medications:
   a. decrease body secretions.
   b. reduce preoperative fear.
   c. promote emptying of the stomach.
   d. ease the introduction of the anesthesia.

56. A patient in the PACU who has received general anesthesia in an ambulatory surgery center:
   a. has to meet identified criteria in order to be discharged home.
   b. will remain in the recovery area longer than a hospitalized patient.
   c. is allowed to ambulate as soon as being admitted to the recovery area.
   d. is immediately given liberal amounts of fluid to promote the excretion of the anesthesia.

57. Following abdominal surgery, the nurse suspects that the patient may be having internal bleeding. Which of the following findings is indicative of this complication?
   a. Restlessness
   b. Increased blood pressure
   c. Slow, shallow respirations
   d. Increased urinary output

58. The patient is transferred to the PACU at 10 A.M. It is now 11:30 A.M., and the patient is not experiencing any complications or difficulties. The nurse will plan to measure the patient's vital signs every:
   a. 15 minutes.
   b. 30 minutes.
   c. 1 hour.
   d. 4 hours.

59. The patient had surgery in the morning that involved the right femoral artery. To assess the patient's circulation status to the right leg, the nurse will make sure to check the pulse at which arterial site?
   a. Radial
   b. Ulnar
   c. Brachial
   d. Dorsalis pedis

60. Upon admission to the PACU, the patient who has no orthopedic or neurologic restrictions is positioned with the:
   a. bed flat and the patient's arms to the sides.
   b. patient's neck flexed and body positioned laterally.
   c. head of the bed slightly elevated with the patient's head to the side.
   d. patient's arms crossed over the chest and the bed in high Fowler position.

61. A patient who is scheduled for surgery is found to have thrombocytopenia. A specific postoperative concern for the nurse for this patient is:
   a. hemorrhage.
   b. wound infection.
   c. fluid imbalance.
   d. respiratory depression.

62. During stage III of general anesthesia, the nurse expects that the patient will:
   a. become drowsy.
   b. lose respiratory function.
   c. experience muscle tension.
   d. have regular breathing.

63. For which of the following types of anesthesia will the patient lose consciousness?
   a. General anesthesia
   b. Regional anesthesia
   c. Epidural anesthesia
   d. Spinal anesthesia

64. Patient assessment reveals restlessness, chest pain, dyspnea, cyanosis, leg pain, and a dysrhythmia. The nurse suspects that the patient may have a(n):
   a. airway obstruction.
   b. anxiety reaction.
   c. pulmonary embolism.
   d. hypovolemic shock.

65. The nurse is assessing the patient in the postoperative period and finds that there is a possible pneumonia. This is based on the finding of which specific sign or symptom?
   a. Fever
   b. Chills
   c. Adventitious sounds
   d. Rust-colored sputum

Practice Situations

The patient has had a repair of an abdominal hernia in the outpatient surgery center. He has a small dressing over the surgical site. His recovery has been as expected, with no difficulties. His wife has been allowed into the recovery area to help him get his things together to go home. She asks you what she should expect and just wants to confirm what to do in case there are problems.
a. What do you tell the patient's wife to help her at home?

Put the following information from the case study in the text, Ms. Logan, into the conceptual care map format.
a. Assessment data

b. Treatment and medication orders

REVIEW QUESTIONS

- How are the perioperative phases different?
- What are the different types of surgery?
- Which safety measures are critical to employ during the perioperative period?
- What alterations can occur during the perioperative period?
- What vital perioperative assessment data needs to be obtained?
- Which nursing diagnoses are appropriate for each perioperative stage?
- What are the nursing care goals and outcome criteria for surgical patients?
- How does the nurse evaluate the effectiveness of the perioperative nursing interventions?

Chapter **37** **Perioperative Nursing Care**

38 Oxygenation and Tissue Perfusion

CHAPTER REVIEW

Match the description/definition in Column A with the correct term in Column B.

Column A

_____ 1. Collapse of lung tissue in the distal part of the lung

_____ 2. An inflammation of the larger airways, increased production of mucus, and chronic cough

_____ 3. An enlargement of small air sacs on the distal end of terminal bronchioles

_____ 4. A reaction of airways to stimulation by irritants, allergens, pollutants, or cold air through constriction and spasms

_____ 5. An infection in the lungs

Column B

a. Asthma

b. Emphysema

c. Pneumonia

d. Chronic bronchitis

e. Atelectasis

Complete the following:

6. The normal heart rate is _____ beats per minute.

7. Identify cardiovascular alterations that can influence oxygenation.

8. What are the causes of the following disorders?
   a. Emphysema—

   b. Pneumonia—

   c. Atelectasis—

9. How do scoliosis and kyphosis affect respiration?

10. Identify at least five assessment questions that the nurse should ask the patient in regards to cardiopulmonary function?

11. For the physical assessment, which areas will the nurse focus on to determine the patient's oxygenation status?

12. Define the following terms:
    a. Cyanosis—

    b. Hemoptysis—

    c. Hypercapnia—

    d. Arrhythmia—

    e. Necrosis—

    f. Hypoxemia—

13. For the patient with emphysema:
    a. The results of the *forced vital capacity* (FVC), *forced expiratory volume* (FEV1), and *forced expiratory flow* (FEF) are expected to be _____ than normal.

b. The results of the *residual volume* (RV) and *functional residual capacity* (FRC) are expected to be _____ than normal.

14. For the patient with heart failure:

   a. Hemoglobin levels may be _____.

   b. Potassium levels may be _____.

15. What abnormalities can be found with a chest radiograph?

16. What concerns does the nurse have for the patient undergoing a cardiac catheterization?

17. Identify at least three nursing diagnoses related to oxygenation.

18. Identify at least two related goal/outcome statements for patient oxygenation.

19. What measures can the nurse implement to promote a patient's oxygenation?

20. Oxygen saturation should be at a minimum of _____%.

21. What is required when oxygen is going to be used by a patient at home?

22. For the Quality and Safety Education for Nurses competency of Teamwork and Collaboration, what other health team members will most likely be involved in the care of a patient with an oxygenation deficit?

23. The patient is admitted to the hospital with an exacerbation of his emphysema. The patient's wife asks why the oxygen level is "not turned up high" to help her husband breathe better. The nurse responds by explaining to the patient's spouse:

24. Indicate safety considerations associated with the oxygen delivery methods pictured:

   a.

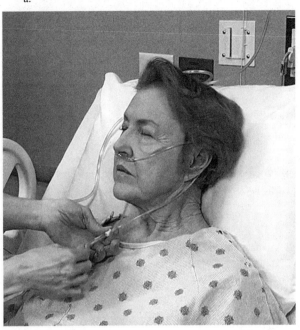

   b.

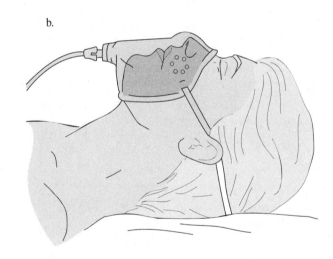

25. a. Continuous positive airway pressure (CPAP) is used for:

   b. Barriers to CPAP compliance include:

   c. What is the difference between CPAP and biphasic positive airway pressure (BIPAP)?

26. When would a bag-valve-mask (BVM) or Ambu bag be used?

27. Identify the following for airway insertion and care:

	Oropharyngeal Airway	Nasopharyngeal Airway
Size		
Insertion		
Nursing Care		

28. What emergency equipment should be in the room of a patient with a tracheostomy?

29. Indicate interventions that can be used to promote cardio-pulmonary function.

30. Identify at least three classifications of medications that are expected to be part of the treatment for:
   a. Pulmonary disease—

   b. Cardiovascular disease—

31. An unlicensed assistive personnel (UAP) is checking on the patient with a nasopharyngeal airway who has oxygen in place and requires frequent suctioning. What do you tell the UAP to report to you regarding this patient's status?

32. The patient who needs nasotracheal suctioning has an excessive amount of secretions. How does the nurse ventilate this patient before suctioning?

33. The nurse recognizes that suctioning through the patient's nares is contraindicated for the patient who has which of the following? *Select all that apply.*
   a. Epistaxis _____
   b. Chronic obstructive pulmonary disease _____
   c. Coagulation disorder _____
   d. Reactive airway disease _____
   e. An upper neck injury _____
   f. Hypertension _____

34. To clear the suction catheter and check that the suction is functioning, the nurse uses:

35. Identify the pressures to be set for suction of the following:
   a. Tracheostomy:

   b. Oropharyngeal:

36. Identify the correct sequence for cleaning the tracheostomy once the sterile field and solutions are prepared.
   a. Gently clean the outer area of the tracheostomy from the stoma outward. _____
   b. Clean the inner cannula, if nondisposable. _____
   c. Apply sterile gloves. _____
   d. Pat the outer area of the tracheostomy dry with sterile gauze. _____
   e. Dip the cotton swab into the sterile normal saline solution. _____

37. For a patient with a chest tube, indicate what the nurse should do for the following:
   a. Positioning for a patient with a pneumothorax—

   b. Bubbling in the water-seal chamber—

   c. Drainage is collecting in the coiled tube—

   d. Assessment of the drainage system should be done at least every _____ hours or per agency policy.

Select the best answer for each of the following questions:

38. The nurse is working on a respiratory care unit in the hospital. Upon entering the room of a patient with emphysema, it is noted that the patient is experiencing respiratory distress. The nurse should:
   a. instruct the patient to breathe rapidly.
   b. place the patient in the supine position.
   c. go to contact the physician.
   d. provide oxygen at 2 L/minute via nasal cannula.

39. An older patient has developed kyphosis and is at a greater risk for developing pneumonia primarily because the:
   a. resulting paralysis immobilizes him, and secretions will increase in his lungs.
   b. innervation to the phrenic nerve is absent, preventing chest expansion.
   c. abnormal chest shape prevents efficient ventilatory movement.
   d. trauma decreases the ability of his red blood cells to carry oxygen.

40. The patient has experienced a myocardial infarction resulting in damage to the left ventricle. A possible complication the patient may experience that the nurse is alert to is:
   a. jugular neck vein distention.
   b. pulmonary congestion.
   c. peripheral edema.
   d. liver enlargement.

41. A patient has recently had a mitral valve replacement. To prevent excess serosanguinous fluid accumulating, the nurse anticipates that care will include:
   a. increased oxygen therapy.
   b. frequent chest physiotherapy.
   c. incentive spirometry on a regular basis.
   d. chest tube placement in the thoracic cavity.

42. All of the following patients are experiencing increased respiratory secretions and require intervention to assist in their removal. Chest percussion is indicated and appropriate for the patient experiencing which of the following?
   a. Thrombocytopenia
   b. Cystic fibrosis
   c. Osteoporosis
   d. Spinal fracture

43. The nurse is working on a pulmonary unit at the local hospital. The nurse is alert to one of the early signs of hypoxia in the patients, which is:
   a. cyanosis.
   b. restlessness.
   c. a decreased respiratory rate.
   d. a decreased blood pressure.

44. In teaching a patient about an upcoming diagnostic test, the nurse identifies that which one of the following uses an injection of contrast material?
   a. Cardiac catheterization
   b. Pulmonary function test
   c. Echocardiography
   d. Electrocardiogram.

45. At a community health fair, the nurse informs the residents that the pneumococcal vaccine is recommended for patients:
   a. only older than age 65.
   b. aged 40 to 60 years of age.
   c. of any age who have a chronic lung disease.
   d. in any age group who are currently experiencing flu-like symptoms.

46. The unit manager is orienting a new staff nurse and evaluates which of the following as an appropriate technique for nasotracheal suctioning?
   a. Placing the patient in a supine position
   b. Preparing for a clean or nonsterile technique
   c. Suctioning the oropharyngeal area first, then the nasotracheal area
   d. Applying intermittent suction for 10 to 15 seconds during catheter removal

47. The patient has chest tubes in place following thoracic surgery. In working with a patient who has a chest tube, the nurse should:
   a. keep the drainage collection device upright.
   b. clamp off the tubes except during patient assessments.
   c. milk or strip the tubes every 15 to 30 minutes to maintain drainage.
   d. remove the tubing from the connection to check for adequate suction power.

48. The patient has supplemental oxygen in place and requires suctioning to remove excess secretions from the airway. In order to promote maximum oxygenation, an appropriate action by the nurse is to:
   a. suction continuously for 30-second intervals.
   b. increase the amount of suction pressure to 200 mm Hg.
   c. replace the oxygen and allow rest in between suctioning passes.
   d. complete a number of suctioning passes until the catheter comes back clear.

49. A patient with a chest tube in place is being transported via stretcher to another room closer to the nurse's station. During the transport, the chest tube pulls out from the pleural space. The nurse immediately:
   a. clamps the tube.
   b. tells the patient to hyperventilate.
   c. covers the site with an occlusive dressing.
   d. pushes the tube back into the chest opening.

50. The patient is admitted to the medical center with a diagnosis of right-sided heart failure. In assessment of this patient, the nurse expects to find:
   a. dyspnea.
   b. confusion.
   c. dizziness.
   d. peripheral edema.

51. A flow rate of oxygen of 2 L per minute is providing what percent of oxygenation?
   a. 24%
   b. 28%
   c. 32%
   d. 36%

Practice Situation

You are working with a 72-year-old patient who has had left-sided congestive heart failure for several years. She is admitted to the hospital with dyspnea and 2+ peripheral edema.

a. What medical treatment do you anticipate for this patient?

b. Which independent nursing actions can you implement to assist the patient to achieve necessary oxygenation?

REVIEW QUESTIONS

- How do the anatomy and physiology of the cardiovascular and respiratory systems function in relation to ventilation and perfusion?
- What are common alterations in structure and function of the cardiovascular and respiratory systems?
- How does the nurse assess the cardiac and respiratory systems?
- Which nursing diagnoses are appropriate for patients with problems of decreased oxygenation?
- What goals are indicated for patients experiencing complications from decreased oxygenation?
- How does the nurse evaluate interventions used to enhance patient oxygenation, promote safety, and reverse negative effects of decreased oxygenation?

39 Fluid, Electrolyte, and Acid-Base Balance

CHAPTER REVIEW

Match the description/definition in Column A with the correct term in Column B.

Column A

_____ 1. Decreased serum calcium level

_____ 2. Increases intravascular volume but does not cause fluid shifts in or out of the cell

_____ 3. An abnormal collection of fluid within the peritoneal cavity

_____ 4. Decreased serum sodium level

_____ 5. Fluid overload

_____ 6. Decreased oxygen concentration of arterial blood

_____ 7. Increased blood glucose level

_____ 8. Increased serum potassium level

_____ 9. Pulls water from the cell to the extracellular fluid compartment, leading to cell shrinkage

_____ 10. The abnormal accumulation of fluid in the interstitial spaces

Column B

a. Hyperglycemia

b. Hyperkalemia

c. Hypertonic

d. Isotonic

e. Hyponatremia

f. Hypocalcemia

g. Hypoxemia

h. Edema

i. Ascites

j. Hypervolemia

Complete the following:

11. Identify whether the following solutions are hypertonic, isotonic, or hypotonic.
    a. 0.9% NaCl
    b. 5% Dextrose/Water (D_5W)
    c. 0.33% NaCL
    d. Lactated Ringer (LR)
    e. Dextrose 5% in Lactated Ringer (D_5LR)

12. What are two of the body's compensatory mechanisms for acid-base balance?

13. For the following individuals, indicate what blood type(s) are compatible:
    a. A person with type A blood—

    b. A person with type O blood—

14. What are the criteria for blood donation?

15. The nurse is observing the patient who is receiving blood/blood products. In the first 15 minutes, the nurse stops the transfusion for an acute hemolytic reaction, which is characterized by: *Select all that apply.*
    a. Chills _____
    b. Wheezing _____
    c. Chest pain _____
    d. Itching _____
    e. Lumbar pain _____
    f. Vomiting _____

16. The nurse is evaluating the severity of the patient's dehydration. A _____% loss of total body weight (TBW) indicates a mild dehydration.

17. For the following electrolyte imbalances, indicate at least two underlying causes and two nursing interventions:

Electrolyte Imbalance	Underlying Causes	Nursing Interventions
Hypokalemia		
Hyperkalemia		
Hypocalcemia		
Hypercalcemia		

18. Alterations in sodium levels can be caused by:

19. Which age groups are most susceptible to fluid and electrolyte imbalances?

20. How can the use of diuretics alter fluid and electrolyte balance?

21. Which of the following should be recommended for a patient requiring potassium supplementation? *Select all that apply.*
    a. Bacon _____
    b. Cheese _____
    c. Broccoli _____
    d. Oranges _____
    e. Tomatoes _____
    f. Wheat germ _____

22. Identify the underlying causes of the following acid-base imbalances:

Acid-Base Imbalance	Underlying Causes	Nursing Interventions
Respiratory acidosis		
Metabolic alkalosis		
Metabolic acidosis		

23. The nurse anticipates finding which of the following clinical manifestations for the patient who is dehydrated? *Select all that apply.*
    a. Dry skin _____
    b. Oliguria _____
    c. Weight gain _____
    d. Hypertension _____
    e. Bounding pulses _____
    f. Urine specific gravity > 1.030 _____

24. When an isotonic fluid volume excess occurs:
    a. What clinical manifestations are expected?

    b. Which nursing interventions are appropriate?

25. The nurse is assessing a patient's level of hydration. Which assessments should be made specific to the following body systems?
    a. Neurologic—

    b. Cardiovascular—

26. Identify at least three medical conditions that can create fluid and electrolyte imbalances.

27. What happens to the patient's blood pressure if the blood volume is reduced?

28. For calculation of the patient's intake and output, the nurse recognizes that fluids include:

29. How does the nurse calculate the urinary output of a baby?

30. Where should the nurse assess a patient's skin turgor?

31. Which specific fluids are recommended when there is a loss of fluid and electrolytes from strenuous exercise (adults) or severe diarrhea (adults and children)?

32. Identify the Six Rights for IV fluids:
    a. Right _____
    b. Right _____
    c. Right _____
    d. Right _____
    e. Right _____
    f. Right _____

33. What are the guidelines for IV administration of potassium?

34. Identify three of the veins in the photo that are used for peripheral IV therapy.

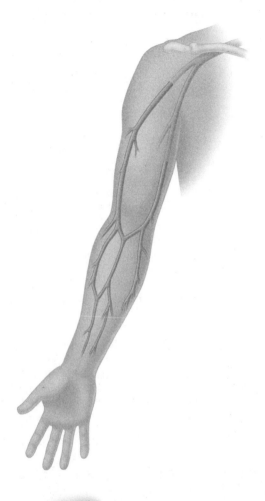

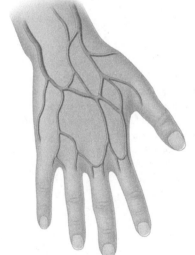

35. What veins are used for newborns, infants, and children?

36. What criteria are used for selection of a vein for IV therapy?

37. Regarding central venous catheters:
    a. What are they used for?

    b. How is placement confirmed?

    c. What type of asepsis is necessary?

38. An advantage of a peripherally inserted central catheter (PICC) is:

39. Identify the correct sequence for care of a Mediport central venous access device.
    a. Flush all lumens per agency policy. _____
    b. Hold a Huber needle at a 90° angle to the port. _____
    c. Fully insert the needle until it meets resistance. _____
    d. Cleanse the site 2 inches around the port with chlorhexidine prep. _____
    e. Hold the port between the thumb and index finger. _____
    f. Cover the Huber needle with a nontransparent dressing. _____

40. The nurse is going to prepare an IV for the patient. What assessments of the solution should be made before administration?

41. The primary care provider has ordered IV infusions for the patient at 3000 mL/24 hours. The nurse will be using an IV infusion device for the administration. What rate will the nurse set on the infusion device?

42. In order to infuse a continuous IV through an intermittent access, the nurse must first:

43. The nurse is measuring intake and output for the patient. This is what has been observed during the first 4 hours of the 8-hour shift:
    The patient ate/drank 1 cup of tea, 1/2 pint of milk, a bowl of cold cereal, an 8-oz glass of orange juice, a sandwich, a banana, and 2 cups of water. Cups are 8 oz.

139

The patient voided 850 mL of urine and had 75 mL of drainage in the Hemovac.
a. What is the intake and output in milliters for this 4-hour time period?

b. Is there a positive or negative fluid balance noted?

44. For the following, identify the IV complication and nursing considerations:
a. IV flow is sluggish, and the catheter cannot be flushed.

b. Chest pain, shoulder pain, dyspnea, and tachycardia

45. What should be included in the documentation for the patient with an IV?

46. For the patient with a central venous catheter, identify the correct action(s). *Select all that apply.*
a. A signed consent is required before insertion. _____
b. Cleansing the site with soap and water before insertion is recommended. _____
c. Gauze dressings are changed every 48 hours. _____
d. The central venous catheter is sutured to the vein used. _____
e. Needle-free connectors are used.
f. Have the patient wear a mask and turn the head away for dressing changes. _____

47. For administration of blood products:
a. What is checked with another nurse before administration?

b. What is the rate of the infusion?

c. How long can the blood be infused?

d. What is the most common cause of a transfusion reaction?

48. The patient is receiving total parenteral nutrition (TPN). Identify at least three responsibilities of the nurse for safe administration of this fluid.

49. Identify the correct sequence for this stage of insertion of a peripheral IV.
a. Cleanse the site with 2% chlorhexidine and allow the site to air dry. _____
b. Apply clean gloves. _____
c. Repalpate the selected vein. _____
d. Insert the IV catheter at a 10- to 30-degree angle. _____
e. Apply the tourniquet with a quick-release knot. _____
f. Advance the catheter. _____

50. When maintaining a peripheral IV, indicate what the nurse should do for the following:
a. The IV solution is discolored.

b. The IV solution will not infuse.

51. For peripheral and central venous sites, what should the nurse write on the dressing or dressing label?

Select the best answer for each of the following questions:

52. A patient is brought into the emergency department after having had severe diarrhea. Arterial blood gases are assessed, and the nurse anticipates that this patient will demonstrate the following results:
a. pH—7.3, $PaCO_2$—38 mm Hg, HCO_3—19 mEq/L
b. pH—7.5, $PaCO_2$—34 mm Hg, HCO_3—20 mEq/L
c. pH—7.35, $PaCO_2$—35 mm Hg, HCO_3—24 mEq/L
d. pH—7.52, $PaCO_2$—48 mm Hg, HCO_3—28 mEq/L

53. When a patient's serum sodium level is 120 mEq/L, the priority nursing assessment is to monitor the status of which body system?
a. Neurologic
b. Gastrointestinal
c. Pulmonary
d. Hepatic

54. An 8-year-old is admitted to the pediatric unit with pneumonia. On assessment, the nurse notes that the child is warm and flushed, is lethargic, has difficulty breathing, and has crackles on auscultation. The nurse determines that the child is suffering from:
a. metabolic acidosis.
b. metabolic alkalosis.
c. respiratory acidosis.
d. respiratory alkalosis.

55. Arterial blood gases are obtained for the patient. The patient's results space = 7.48, CO_2 = 42, HCO_3 = 32. These are consistent with which one of the following acid-base imbalances?
    a. Metabolic acidosis
    b. Metabolic alkalosis
    c. Respiratory acidosis
    d. Respiratory alkalosis

56. The nurse is aware that the compensating mechanism most likely to occur in the presence of respiratory acidosis is:
    a. hyperventilation to decrease the CO^2 levels.
    b. hypoventilation to increase the CO^2 levels.
    c. retention of HCO_3 by the kidneys to increase the pH level.
    d. excretion of HCO_3 by the kidneys to decrease the pH level.

57. Of all of the following patients, the nurse recognizes that the individual who is most at risk for a fluid volume deficit is a:
    a. 6-month-old learning to drink from a cup.
    b. 42-year-old with severe vomiting.
    c. 90-year-old with frequent headaches.
    d. 12-year-old who is moderately active in 80° F weather.

58. A patient experiences a loss of intracellular fluid. The nurse anticipates that the IV therapy that will be used to replace this type of loss is:
    a. 0.33% normal saline.
    b. 10% dextrose.
    c. 5% dextrose in lactated Ringer.
    d. dextrose 5% in ½ NS.

59. The patient has been experienced an extensive burn and now has bradycardia, muscle weakness, and abdominal cramping. Which of the following laboratory values would be most desirable for the nurse to obtain on the basis of the patient's assessment?
    a. Serum potassium
    b. Serum magnesium
    c. Serum sodium
    d. Serum calcium

60. The physician orders 1000 mL of D5RL with 20 mEq KCl to run for 8 hours. Using an infusion set with a drop factor of 15 gtt/mL, the nurse calculates the flow rate to be:
    a. 12 drops/minute.
    b. 22 drops/minute.
    c. 32 drops/minute.
    d. 42 drops/minute.

61. The nurse will be starting a new IV infusion and needs to select the site for the insertion. In selection of a site, the nurse should:
    a. use sites on an extremity away from a dialysis graft.
    b. start with the most proximal site.
    c. look for hard, cordlike veins.
    d. use the patient's dominant arm.

62. A patient has IV therapy for the administration of antibiotics and is stating that the "IV site hurts and is swollen." Which of the following information assessed on the patient indicates the presence of phlebitis, as opposed to infiltration?
    a. Intensity of the pain
    b. Amount of subcutaneous edema
    c. Skin discoloration of a bruised nature
    d. Warmth of the skin surrounding the IV site

63. For a child who has ingested the remaining contents of an aspirin bottle, the nurse suspects signs and symptoms consistent with:
    a. metabolic alkalosis.
    b. metabolic acidosis.
    c. respiratory alkalosis.
    d. respiratory acidosis.

64. A patient complains of a headache and nausea and vomiting during a blood transfusion. Which one of the following actions should the nurse take immediately?
    a. Check the vital signs.
    b. Stop the blood transfusion.
    c. Slow down the rate of blood flow.
    d. Notify the physician and blood bank personnel.

65. For a patient with a nursing diagnosis of *fluid volume excess,* the nurse is alert to which one of the following signs and symptoms?
    a. Dry mucous membranes
    b. Weak, thready pulse
    c. Hypertension
    d. Flushed skin

66. A patient is currently taking Lasix and Digoxin. As a result of the medication regimen, the nurse is alert to the presence of:
    a. cardiac dysrhythmias.
    b. severe diarrhea.
    c. hyperactive reflexes.
    d. peripheral cyanosis.

67. For the patient with a vitamin D deficiency and inadequate calcium intake, the nurse observes for:
    a. anxiety.
    b. diaphoresis.
    c. Chvostek sign.
    d. nausea and vomiting.

68. The single best indicator of fluid status is the nurse's assessment of the patient's:
    a. skin turgor.
    b. daily body weight.
    c. intake and output.
    d. serum electrolyte levels.

Chapter **39** **Fluid, Electrolyte, and Acid-Base Balance**

69. An IV of 50 mL is to be infused over 30 minutes. A microdrip infusion set will be used. The nurse calculates the infusion rate as:
    a. 30 gtt/min.
    b. 50 gtt/min.
    c. 100 gtt/min.
    d. 200 gtt/min.

70. A patient is admitted to the hospital with a diagnosis of adrenal insufficiency. In preparing to complete the admission history, the nurse anticipates that the patient will have experienced increased serum levels of:
    a. magnesium.
    b. sodium.
    c. chloride.
    d. potassium.

71. In reviewing the results of the patient's blood work, the nurse recognizes that the unexpected value that should be reported to the physician is:
    a. calcium 9 mg/dL.
    b. sodium 140 mEq/L.
    c. potassium 3.1 mEq/L.
    d. magnesium 1.9 mEq/L.

72. The nurse anticipates that the patient with a *fluid volume deficit* will manifest a(n):
    a. decreased urine specific gravity.
    b. decreased body weight.
    c. increased blood pressure.
    d. increased pulse strength.

73. The nurse recognizes that the patient, on the basis of the imbalance that is present, will require fluid replacement with isotonic solution. One of the isotonic solutions that may be ordered by the physician is:
    a. 0.45% saline.
    b. lactated Ringer solution.
    c. 5% dextrose in normal saline.
    d. 5% dextrose in lactated Ringer solution.

74. A patient has severe anemia and will be receiving blood transfusions. The nurse prepares and begins the infusion. Ten minutes after the infusion has begun, the patient develops tachycardia, chills, and low back pain. After stopping the transfusion, the nurse should:
    a. administer an antipyretic.
    b. begin an infusion of epinephrine.
    c. run normal saline through the blood tubing.
    d. obtain and send urine and blood specimens to the laboratory.

75. Mild hypoxemia is present with which of the following PaO_2 concentrations?
    a. 90 mm Hg
    b. 70 mm Hg
    c. 50 mm Hg
    d. 30 mm Hg

76. The patient has a continuous IV infusion of 0.9% NS. For this infusion, the tubing should be changed every:
    a. 24 hours.
    b. 48 hours.
    c. 72 hours.
    d. time the bag is changed.

77. For the patient who needs fluid replacement, which of the following should be avoided?
    a. Juice
    b. Water
    c. Coffee
    d. Lemon-lime soda

78. The nurse anticipates that the blood product that will be used for the patient with acute renal failure should be:
    a. albumin.
    b. platelets.
    c. whole blood.
    d. cryoprecipitate.

79. The nurse requires additional instruction if he/she selects which of the following IV catheter sizes for a patient who will be receiving a blood transfusion?
    a. 26 gauge
    b. 22 gauge
    c. 20 gauge
    d. 18 gauge

80. The patient has heart failure and is on a restricted sodium diet. Which of the following foods in the patient's diet is the nurse most concerned about?
    a. Celery
    b. Baked fish
    c. Canned soup
    d. Dried fruit

81. The mucous membranes of a normally hydrated individual are:
    a. dry.
    b. red.
    c. moist.
    d. sticky.

82. The patient has a PICC line in place. Which of the following actions indicates that additional instruction is necessary for the new staff nurse?
    a. The PICC site is kept dry and protected.
    b. The lumen is flushed with 10 mL of preservative-free saline.
    c. The catheter is measured from the site to the hub outside the body.
    d. The blood pressure is measured on the arm with the PICC line.

83. A critical measure for patients with hypocalcemia and hypomagnesemia is:
    a. encouraging increased fluid intake.
    b. implementing seizure precautions.
    c. checking for digitalis toxicity.
    d. administering analgesics.

84. The nurse is assessing the patient's average daily intake and recognizes that it should be a total for fluids and food of:
    a. 1500 mL.
    b. 2000 mL.
    c. 2500 mL.
    d. 3000 mL.

85. The nurse anticipates that which of the following diagnostic tests will be done to determine the patient's renal function?
    a. Creatinine
    b. Calcium level
    c. Hemoglobin
    d. Serum albumin

86. The nurse is assessing a patient's peripheral edema. An obvious indentation that lasts several seconds is classified as:
    a. 1+.
    b. 2+.
    c. 3+.
    d. 4+.

Practice Situation

The patient comes to the outpatient emergency center with a high fever. He tells you that he has had the fever for several days, along with periods of diaphoresis and vomiting.
a. What other signs and symptoms do you anticipate?

b. What results do you expect for the following laboratory tests?
   • Urine specific gravity
   • Hematocrit
   • BUN

c. Identify a possible nursing diagnosis, patient goal/outcome, and nursing interventions.

REVIEW QUESTIONS

• What is the normal structure and function of fluids, electrolytes, acids, and bases in the body?
• What are the differences between the common fluid, electrolyte, and acid-base imbalances and their underlying causes?
• What are the assessment priorities for patients with fluid, electrolyte, and acid-base imbalances?
• Which are the most common nursing diagnoses related to fluid, electrolyte, and acid-base imbalances?
• How can nursing goals and outcomes be integrated into the plan of care for patients with fluid and electrolyte imbalances?
• Which nursing interventions are implemented to maintain normal fluid, electrolyte, and acid-base balance or to correct imbalances?

40 Bowel Elimination

CHAPTER REVIEW

Complete the following:

1. What factors can influence bowel elimination?

2. What are hemorrhoids?

3. What signs and symptoms are associated with diarrhea?

4. Indicate the possible cause(s) of diarrhea. *Select all that apply.*
   a. Reduced fluid intake _____
   b. Food-borne pathogens _____
   c. Hypothyroidism _____
   d. Low-fiber diet _____
   e. Psychological stress _____
   f. Administration of narcotic analgesics _____

5. Straining during defecation can stimulate the _____

   _____, which could cause _____.

6. For *Clostridium difficile* (C. Diff):
   a. Cause/etiology

   b. Common symptoms

7. What is a primary concern for the patient who is incontinent?

8. A patient is to have a stool test for occult blood. The nurse is instructing the patient about the preparation for the test and tells the patient to avoid which foods?

9. What is a cardinal sign of a fecal impaction?

10. The patient tells the nurse that he has a "lot of gas." The nurse notes that he has some abdominal distention as well. What interventions may help the patient?

11. For the ostomy that is pictured, which stoma will produce fecal material?

12. Which of the following is/are accurate statements regarding bowel elimination? *Select all that apply.*
    a. The meconium passed by newborns is brown and liquid. _____
    b. Breast-fed infants have feces that are yellow, soft, and liquid. _____
    c. Control of defecation starts at about 3 years of age. _____
    d. Constipation can be a problem for school-age children. _____
    e. Bowel elimination problems are prevalent in long-term care facilities. _____
    f. Older adults suffer more from diarrhea. _____

13. Identify two possible causes of constipation.

14. Indicate how the following foods may influence bowel elimination:
   a. Pasta and cheese

   b. Spicy foods

   c. Figs

   d. Chocolate

15. Identify the factor(s) that will promote bowel elimination. *Select all that apply.*
   a. Lack of privacy _____
   b. Immobility _____
   c. Squatting _____
   d. Calcium supplements _____
   e. Anesthesia _____
   f. Emotional stress _____

16. The patient who is taking iron supplements is told to expect the stool to appear:

17. During the physical assessment of the gastrointestinal (GI) system, what is included in the inspection of the patient?

18. Which diagnostic test does the nurse anticipate will be ordered for the patient with prolonged diarrhea?

19. The nurse recognizes that the major side effect from an upper or lower GI series is:

20. For an endoscopy:
   a. What instructions are provided to the patient to prepare for the test?

   b. What should the patient expect during the procedure?

   c. After the procedure, what safety measures should be taken?

21. For a colonoscopy:
   a. What preparation is required before the examination?

   b. What are the similarities to an endoscopy?

   c. Colonoscopies are recommended to be done:

22. What can overuse of laxatives lead to?

23. How does the nurse promote bowel elimination for the patient who is immobile or cognitively impaired?

24. Which type(s) of enteral tube is/are used for gastric lavage?

25. Identify the principles that the nurse should incorporate into the teaching of an unlicensed assistive personnel (UAP) for proper bedpan use.

26. The use of laxatives and cathartics is contraindicated for patients with:

27. Enemas are used to:

28. Identify the correct procedures for administration of a rectal suppository to stimulate bowel evacuation. *Select all that apply.*
   a. Apply sterile gloves for the procedure. _____
   b. Place the patient in a right, side-lying position. _____
   c. Insert the suppository with the rounded end inserted first.
   d. Insert the suppository above the internal anal sphincter. _____
   e. Embed the suppository into the feces. _____
   f. Return to evaluate the response in about 30 to 45 minutes. _____

145

29. In accordance with the Quality and Safety Education for Nurses competency for patient-centered care, what specific concerns will the nurse have for the patient who has just had an ileostomy?

30. To assist the patient with a colostomy to reduce odor and gas, the nurse suggests avoidance or reduction of which foods?

31. For enema administration:
   a. When is it contraindicated?

   b. Can it be delegated to an UAP?

   c. If the patient cannot assume the usual position, what can be done?

   d. What should the nurse do if the patient experiences abdominal distention or rigidity?

   e. How far is the tube inserted for an adult patient?

   f. If a noncommercial solution in a bag is given, how high should the bag be for gravity drainage?

32. Identify the correct sequence for replacing an ostomy pouch, one-piece system.
   a. Center opening over stoma and secure in place. _____

   b. Perform hand hygiene and apply new clean gloves. _____

   c. Fill in leaks with barrier paste and allow to dry. _____

   d. Remove the backing or apply stoma adhesive, allow to dry. _____
   e. Gently tug on pouch to ensure it is secure. _____
   f. Assess the seal. _____

33. For ostomy care, identify the following:
   a. How long can the pouching system stay in place if there are no complications?

   b. What do you do if skin barrier fragments remain on the patient's skin?

   c. When should the ostomy bag be emptied?

34. Identify at least three strategies to include in the teaching for a patient who struggles with episodes of constipation.

35. Identify the expected appearance of an ostomy stoma. *Select all that apply.*
   a. Dry _____
   b. Dark red with whiter areas _____
   c. Moist _____
   d. Reddish-pink _____
   e. Purplish-blue _____
   f. Budding slightly above the skin _____

Select the best answer for each of the following questions:

36. The nurse recognizes that changes in elimination occur with the aging process. An expected change in bowel elimination is that:
   a. chewing processes are less efficient.
   b. esophageal emptying time is increased.
   c. changes in nerve innervation and sensation cause diarrhea.
   d. absorptive processes are increased in the intestinal mucosa.

37. A 6-month-old infant has severe diarrhea. The major problem associated with severe diarrhea is:
   a. pain in the abdominal area.
   b. electrolyte and fluid loss.
   c. presence of excessive flatus.
   d. irritation of the perineal and rectal area.

38. The patient is seen in the gastroenterology clinic after having experienced changes in his bowel elimination. A colonoscopy is ordered, and the patient has questions about the examination. Before the colonoscopy, the nurse teaches the patient that:
   a. light sedation is normally used.
   b. no metallic objects are allowed.
   c. no special preparation is required.
   d. swallowing of an opaque liquid is required.

39. The patient has been admitted to an acute care unit with a diagnosis of upper GI bleeding. The nurse suspects that the feces will appear:
   a. bright red.
   b. pus filled.
   c. black and tarry.
   d. white or clay colored.

40. The patient asks the nurse to recommend bulk-forming foods that may be included in the diet. Which of the following should be recommended by the nurse?
    a. Whole grain cereals
    b. Fruit juice
    c. Rare meats
    d. Milk products

41. For the patient with diarrhea, the nurse recommends:
    a. fresh vegetables.
    b. milk products.
    c. cold sodas.
    d. mashed potatoes.

42. While undergoing a soapsuds enema, the patient complains of mild abdominal cramping. The nurse should:
    a. clamp the tubing.
    b. immediately stop the infusion.
    c. lower the container to slow the infusion.
    d. advance the enema tubing 2 to 3 inches.

43. The nurse is caring for patients on a postoperative unit in the medical center. The nurse is alert to the possibility that for 24 to 48 hours of the postoperative period, patients may experience the following as a result of the anesthetic used during the surgery:
    a. colitis.
    b. stomatitis.
    c. paralytic ileus.
    d. gastrocolic reflex.

44. The patient receiving a tube feeding develops diarrhea. The nurse should:
    a. adjust the rate of the infusion.
    b. change the container every 8 hours.
    c. request that psyllium be added to the feeding.
    d. monitor the output, recognizing that this is an expected occurrence.

45. For the patient with an ileostomy, the critical element is:
    a. skin care.
    b. odor control.
    c. stoma irrigation.
    d. infection prevention.

46. For patients with hypercalcemia, the nurse should implement measures to prevent:
    a. gastric upset.
    b. malabsorption.
    c. constipation.
    d. fluid secretion.

47. The appropriate amount of fluid to prepare for an enema to be given to an average size adult is:
    a. 250 to 350 mL.
    b. 300 to 500 mL.
    c. 500 to 750 mL.
    d. 750 to 1000 mL.

48. A patient who is going to have a colostomy done asks the nurse if a "bag" will have to be worn. The nurse recognizes that which of the following ostomies may not require an externally worn appliance?
    a. Transverse colostomy
    b. Ascending colostomy
    c. Sigmoid colostomy
    d. Loop colostomy

49. The nurse is instructing the patient in stomal care for an incontinent ostomy. The nurse evaluates achievement of learning goals if the patient:
    a. cuts the opening 1/16 inch larger than the stoma.
    b. uses peroxide to toughen the periostomal skin.
    c. applies commercial deodorant around the stoma.
    d. uses alcohol to cleanse the stoma.

50. The nurse is aware that normal bowel sounds are:
    a. high-pitched and irregular.
    b. occur every 5-10 minutes.
    c. absent between meals.
    d. loud and slow.

51. A small-volume enema that is used to provide relief from gastric distention and stimulate peristalsis is a(n):
    a. hypertonic enema.
    b. carminative enema.
    c. oil retention enema.
    d. medication enema.

52. The nurse instructs the patient that, before the fecal occult blood test (FOBT), she may eat:
    a. whole wheat bread.
    b. a lean steak.
    c. grapefruit.
    d. beets.

Practice Situation

The patient with colorectal cancer had a permanent sigmoid colostomy created. She tells you that she doesn't think she can manage this, stating that she "looks awful" and "doesn't think her husband will want to look at her." When you start to talk to her about the ostomy care, she tells you that, "I have no idea how to manage this."
   Use the conceptual care map to document the following:
a. Identify two priority nursing diagnoses.

b. For those nursing diagnoses, indicate patient goals/outcomes.

c. Specify the nursing interventions to assist the patient to achieve the outcomes.

REVIEW QUESTIONS

- How does the physiology of the GI tract function to form, store and eliminate waste products?
- What are some common alterations in bowel function?
- How does the nurse integrate components of a comprehensive patient assessment to identify issues with bowel elimination?

- Which nursing diagnoses related to bowel elimination?
- What are some goals for patients experiencing alterations in bowel elimination?
- Which nursing interventions may be used to maintain normal bowel elimination?

41 Urinary Elimination

CHAPTER REVIEW

Match the description/definition in Column A with the correct term in Column B.

Column A

_b_ 1. Output of 50-100 mL in 24 hours

_g_ 2. Sudden strong desire to void, followed by rapid bladder contraction

_j_ 3. Excessive urination at night

_i_ 4. A constant dribbling of urine or frequency in urination

_h_ 5. Painful urination

_a_ 6. The involuntary passing of urine

_d_ 7. Output of 100-500 mL in 24 hours

_f_ 8. Blood in the urine

_c_ 9. Loss of urine control during activities that increase intraabdominal pressure

_e_ 10. Excessive production and excretion of urine

Column B

a. Enuresis

b. Oliguria

c. Stress incontinence

d. Anuria

e. Polyuria

f. Hematuria

g. Urge incontinence

h. Dysuria

i. Overflow incontinence

j. Nocturia

Complete the following:

11. An average daily urine output is _____ mL.

12. What factors can influence urinary output?

13. For the patient with anuria or oliguria, dialysis may be indicated.
    a. Describe the difference between hemodialysis and peritoneal dialysis.

    b. What is the goal of dialysis?

14. Cautious monitoring by the nurse of the patient with a renal disorder includes:

15. Dysuria is often associated with:

16. Which of the following individuals may be more prone to episodes of urinary incontinence? *Select all that apply.*
    a. Women _____
    b. Men _____
    c. School-aged children _____
    d. Older adults _____
    e. Pregnant women _____

17. Identify at least three factors that may contribute to urinary retention.

18. The patient with an enlarged prostate may exhibit which signs and symptoms?

19. Indicate how the following influence urinary elimination:
   a. Dehydration

   b. Diuretics

   c. Paraplegia

   d. Renal calculi

20. The patient asks why women experience more frequent urinary tract infections (UTIs). How does the nurse respond?

21. What specific aspects of the physical assessment are conducted to determine renal and bladder status?

22. Indicate the expected findings from the physical assessment of the urinary system. *Select all that apply.*
   a. Distention over the suprapubic area _____
   b. Bruit heard over the left renal artery _____
   c. Discomfort on percussion of the kidney _____
   d. Soft abdomen _____
   e. Bilateral ecchymosis to the lower abdominal quadrants _____
   f. Absence of indentation and scarring _____

23. Identify what the following can do to the appearance of a patient's urine:
   a. Beets and blackberries—

   b. Warfarin—

   c. Liver failure—

24. What are the expected characteristics of urine? *Select all that apply.*
   a. Pale yellow color _____
   b. Cloudy _____
   c. Fruity odor _____
   d. pH = 6 _____
   e. Protein present _____
   f. No glucose _____

25. What blood tests are used to evaluate renal function?

26. Diagnostic testing may be done to evaluate the status of the urinary system.
   a. What preparation is necessary for an intravenous pyelogram (IVP)?

   b. Pregnant women should *not* have tests with:

27. Indicate which of the following is/are expected with a cystoscopy: *Select all that apply.*
   a. A biopsy may be performed. _____
   b. The patient is NPO for 8 to 12 hours before. _____
   c. The test will take 1 to 2 hours. _____
   d. An urge to void may be felt. _____
   e. Bladder puncture occurs frequently. _____
   f. Urine may be pink-tinged for several days after the procedure. _____

28. Identify at least three strategies that should be included in patient teaching in order to promote urinary function and prevent infection.

29. A goal is to provide the patient in the acute care setting with optimum conditions for voiding. How can the nurse achieve this goal?

30. What are the indications for the use of a commode?

31. To assist the patient with functional incontinence to void, the nurse may initiate a toileting schedule. Provide an example of this type of schedule.

32. What can the patient do to decrease the occurrence of nocturia?

33. How can the patient prevent UTIs? *Select all that apply.*
   a. Take bubble baths. _____
   b. Wear cotton underwear. _____
   c. Cleanse the perineum from front to back. _____
   d. Drink at least 1500 mL of fluid/day. _____
   e. Urinate as infrequently as possible. _____
   f. Cleanse the genital area before intercourse. _____

34. How does the nurse minimize the risk of a UTI with an indwelling catheter?

35. For the indwelling catheter shown, which lumen is used to inflate the balloon?

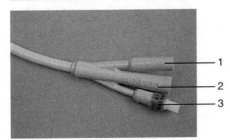

     1

     2

     3

36. Straight catheterization is done to: *Select all that apply.*
    a. Obtain urine samples _____
    b. Drain residual urine _____
    c. Provide continuous bladder drainage _____
    d. Allow for bladder irrigation _____
    e. Pass through a constricted urethra _____
    f. Empty a continent urinary diversion _____

37. What is included in the instruction to the UAP about routine catheter care?

38. Condom catheters are kept in place with:

39. For routine perineal care, cleansing should be done with:

40. For female catheterization, identify the correct sequence of steps in this portion of the skill:
    a. Insert the catheter 2 to 3 inches, advancing after urine appears. _____
    b. Inflate the balloon. _____
    c. Prepare the sterile field and catheter. _____
    d. Connect the drainage system.
    e. Cleanse the perineal area. _____
    f. Release the labia. _____

41. Why is bladder irrigation performed?

42. Identify the nursing actions in response to the following during urinary catheterization:
    a. Resistance is encountered.

b. No urinary drainage occurs.

c. Lidocaine 2% gel is available to use as a lubricant.

d. Contamination of the equipment is suspected.

Select the best answer for each of the following questions:

43. An assessment is completed by the nurse, and a nursing diagnosis for the oriented adult female patient is identified as *Stress incontinence related to decreased pelvic muscle tone.* An appropriate nursing intervention based on this diagnosis is to:
    a. apply adult diapers.
    b. catheterize the patient.
    c. administer urecholine.
    d. teach kegel exercises.

44. A patient in the hospital has an indwelling urinary catheter, and the nurse is instructing the nursing assistant in the appropriate care to provide. The nurse teaches the assistant to:
    a. empty the drainage bag when ⅔ full.
    b. cleanse up the length of the catheter to the perineum.
    c. open the drainage system to obtain a specimen for culture and sensitivity.
    d. place the drainage bag on the patient's lap while transporting the patient to testing.

45. The nurse suspects that the patient has a bladder infection on the basis of the patient exhibiting:
    a. nausea.
    b. hematuria.
    c. flank pain.
    d. incontinence.

46. The patient has an indwelling catheter. The nurse should obtain a sterile urine specimen by:
    a. disconnecting the catheter from the drainage tubing.
    b. inserting a needle into the catheter tubing.
    c. opening the drainage bag and removing urine.
    d. using a syringe to withdraw urine from the catheter port.

47. A patient with an excessive alcohol intake has a reduced amount of antidiuretic hormone (ADH). The nurse anticipates the patient will exhibit:
    a. hematuria.
    b. an increased blood pressure.
    c. dry mucous membranes.
    d. a low serum sodium level.

48. A patient is going to have an IVP. Which of the following reflects the most critical assessment question for this patient before the procedure?
   a. "Are you allergic to iodine?"
   b. "Did you remove all metal?"
   c. "Have you had this procedure before?"
   d. "When did you last have a procedure that required sedatives?"

49. A postpartum patient has been unable to void since her delivery of her baby this morning. Which of the following nursing measures would be beneficial for the patient initially?
   a. Increase fluid intake to 3500 mL
   b. Insert an indwelling catheter
   c. Rinse the perineum with warm water
   d. Apply firm pressure over the bladder

50. The nurse is visiting the patient who has a nursing diagnosis of *Alteration in urinary elimination, retention*. On assessment, the nurse anticipates that this patient will exhibit:
   a. a loss of the urge to void.
   b. severe flank pain and hematuria.
   c. pain and burning on urination.
   d. a feeling of pressure and voiding of small amounts.

51. The unit manager is evaluating the care of a new nursing staff member. Which of the following is an appropriate technique for the nurse to implement in order to obtain a clean-voided urine specimen?
   a. Apply sterile gloves for the procedure.
   b. Restrict fluids before the specimen collection.
   c. Place the specimen in a clean urinalysis container.
   d. Collect the specimen after the initial stream of urine has passed.

52. In an assessment of a patient with overflow incontinence, the nurse expects to find that the patient has:
   a. a constant dribbling of urine.
   b. no urge to void and an unawareness of bladder filling.
   c. an uncontrollable loss of urine when coughing or sneezing.
   d. an immediate urge to void but not enough time to reach the bathroom.

53. In determining the patient's urinary status, the nurse anticipates that the urinary output for an average adult should be approximately:
   a. 400 mL/day.
   b. 800 mL/day.
   c. 1400 mL/day.
   d. 2000 mL/day.

54. A timed urine specimen collection is ordered. The test will need to be restarted if the:
   a. patient voids in the toilet.
   b. urine specimen is kept cold.
   c. first voided urine is discarded.
   d. preservative is placed in the collection container.

55. The nurse is working with a patient who has an incontinent urinary diversion. Included in the plan of care for this patient is instruction that:
   a. special clothing is necessary.
   b. careful skin care is a priority.
   c. a stoma bag will only need to be worn at night.
   d. a strict reduction in physical activity will be planned.

56. The nursing instructor is evaluating the student during the catheterization of a female patient. The instructor determines that the student has implemented appropriate technique when observed:
   a. keeping both hands sterile throughout the procedure.
   b. reinserting the catheter if it was misplaced initially in the vagina.
   c. inflating the balloon to test it before catheter insertion.
   d. advancing the catheter 7 to 8 inches.

57. A patient is receiving closed catheter irrigation. During the shift, 950 mL of normal saline irrigant are instilled, and there is a total of 1725 mL in the drainage bag. The patient's urinary output is calculated by the nurse to be:
   a. 775 mL.
   b. 950 mL.
   c. 1725 mL.
   d. 2675 mL.

58. A toileting program for a patient in an extended care facility should include which of the following?
   a. Providing negative reinforcement when the patient is incontinent
   b. Having the patient wear adult diapers as a preventative measure
   c. Putting the patient on a q2h toilet schedule during the day
   d. Promoting the intake of caffeine to stimulate voiding

59. A sample is obtained from the patient for a routine urinalysis. After reviewing the results of the test, the nurse notes that an expected finding of the urinalysis is:
   a. pH 8.0.
   b. specific gravity 1.018.
   c. protein amounts to 12 mg/100 mL.
   d. WBCs of 5 to 8 per low-power field casts.

60. An order is written for the patient's indwelling urinary catheterization to be discontinued. The unit manager is observing the new staff nurse provide care to this patient and implement the prescriber's order. The unit manager determines that further instruction is required for the new staff nurse in catheter removal if he is observed:
   a. draping the female patient.
   b. obtaining a specimen before removal.
   c. cutting the catheter to deflate the balloon.
   d. checking the patient's output carefully for 6 to 8 hours after removal.

61. A condom catheter is to be used for an adult male patient in the extended care facility. In the application of the condom catheter, the nurse employs appropriate technique when:
    a. using sterile gloves.
    b. wrapping adhesive tape securely around the base of the penis.
    c. leaving a 1- to 2-inch space between the tip of the penis and the end of the catheter.
    d. taping the tubing tightly to the thigh and attaching the drainage bag to the side rail.

62. The patient has a suprapubic catheter in place. Which of the following is correct for this type of catheterization?
    a. Irrigation is required for urine to drain.
    b. The catheter is secured with adhesive tape.
    c. Lotions or creams are used around the site to protect the skin.
    d. It is usually placed 4 to 5 centimeters above the symphysis pubis.

63. Urinary elimination may be altered with different pathophysiological conditions. For the patient with diabetes mellitus, the nurse anticipates that an initial urinary sign or symptom will be which of the following?
    a. Urgency
    b. Polyuria
    c. Dysuria
    d. Hematuria

64. The nurse recognizes that postrenal failure is associated with:
    a. renal damage.
    b. low cardiac output.
    c. vascular collapse.
    d. functional obstruction.

65. Which of the following urinary diversions requires that the patient has a stoma created?
    a. Ileal conduit
    b. Kock pouch
    c. Mainz pouch
    d. Ileal neobladder

Practice Situations

You are the home care nurse who is visiting the 25-year-old patient with paraplegia. The patient has just come home after a long rehabilitation period following an auto accident.
a. What concerns do you have for this patient's urinary elimination?

b. What specific areas will you need to assess?

For the following patient data, identify the intake and output for your 12-hour shift and indicate whether it is a positive or negative fluid balance.

8:00 A.M.	1 cup of black decaf coffee, 1 scrambled egg, 1 glass of juice, 2 pieces of toast, IV—800 mL left in bag, 400 mL of urine
10:00 A.M.	½ glass of water taken with medication, 1 tablespoon of cough medicine administered
12:00 P.M.	1 cup of decaf coffee, ½ glass of ginger ale, 1 turkey burger on a roll with a side salad, ½ cup of Jell-o IV—400 mL left in bag, 350 mL of urine, 50 mL drainage in Hemovac
2:00 P.M.	1 cup of tea, ½ glass of water with medication
4:00 P.M.	IV bag changed with 50 mL left in bag, new 1 L bag hung, 350 mL of urine
6:00 P.M.	1 hamburger, mashed potatoes, green beans, 1 cup of decaf coffee, 1 glass of water, IV 800 mL left in bag, 350 mL urine
8:00 P.M.	½ glass of water with medication, IV 600 mL left in bag, 400 mL urine, 30 mL in Hemovac

Cup = 240 mL, glass = 120 mL

REVIEW QUESTIONS

- What are the anatomic and physiological processes of the urinary system?
- What are abnormal patterns of urinary elimination and causative factors?
- How does the nurse carry out a comprehensive assessment of the patient with urinary elimination problems?
- Which nursing diagnoses are related to urinary elimination?
- How can the nurse create collaborative patient-centered care plans for patients experiencing alterations in urinary elimination?
- What interventions should be implemented to address altered elimination concerns?

42 Death and Loss

CHAPTER REVIEW

Match the description/definition in Column A with the correct term in Column B.

Column A

_____ 1. Occurs when the behaviors of the survivor interfere with normal functioning, but the person who is grieving is not aware that these behaviors are concealing the actual grieving process

_____ 2. Occurs when the survivor is overwhelmed by grief and cannot function in daily life

_____ 3. The cognitive, affective, cultural, and social reactions *to an expected death,* felt by the patient, as well as family members and friends

_____ 4. Characterized by suppression of the grief reaction while the grieving individual consciously or unconsciously avoids the pain that has occurred with the loss

_____ 5. Characterized by grief reactions that do not diminish over time and continue for an indefinite period or very long period of time

_____ 6. Encountered when a loss happens that cannot be openly acknowledged or publicly shared by the grieving individual

Column B

a. Exaggerated grief

b. Disenfranchised grief

c. Chronic grief

d. Masked grief

e. Anticipatory grief

f. Delayed grief

Complete the following:

7. Briefly describe the following:
   a. Loss—

   b. Grief—

   c. Mourning—

   d. Bereavement—

8. Identify ways in which the nurse can help the individual who is grieving.

9. The nurse is caring for a Jewish patient who has died. Although individuals and families can practice differently, the nurse anticipates that which of the following may occur? *Select all that apply.*
   a. The person will be buried quickly. _____
   b. A shrine will be displayed at home. _____
   c. Incense will be burned in the room. _____
   d. Autopsy is discouraged. _____
   e. Cremation is preferred. _____
   f. Visitors will come and prayers will be said for the sick. _____

10. How is Worden's first task in the process of grieving similar to the first stage identified by Kübler-Ross?

11. Identify at least three examples for each of the following reactions to loss:
   a. Physical—

   b. Emotional—

   c. Cognitive—

   d. Behavioral—

12. What are two examples of end-of-life ethical issues that the nurse may encounter in practice?

13. Indicate how the following factors may influence the grieving process:
   a. Relationship of the deceased—

   b. Available support systems—

   c. Other stressors—

   d. Type of loss—

14. The nurse suspects dysfunctional grieving is occurring. What questions will help to confirm this assessment?

15. The nurse should make which assessments for the person who has been the caregiver of a terminally ill family member for many months?

16. What happens in the body with each of the following?
   a. Algor mortis—

   b. Livor mortis—

   c. Rigor mortis—

17. Which of the following is/are specifically indicative of imminent death? *Select all that apply.*
   a. Cold, mottled extremities _____
   b. Decreased blood pressure _____
   c. Increasing periods of apnea _____
   d. Drowsiness _____
   e. Sleeping more _____
   f. Fatigue _____

18. What is the difference between hospice and palliative care?

19. Provide the order of actions that will occur for the pronouncement of a patient's death.
   a.
   b.
   c.
   d.
   e.

20. Postmortem care includes which of the following? *Select all that apply.*
   a. Placing the patient in a prone position. _____
   b. Leaving the eyes open. _____
   c. Replacing dentures and other prosthetics. _____
   d. Allowing the family to spend time with the patient. _____
   e. Removing all clothes and jewelry. _____
   f. Providing a full bath. _____

21. What are key elements in the nursing care of individuals and families who are experiencing loss and grief?

Select the best answer for each of the following questions:

22. The nurse is discussing future treatments with a patient who has a terminal illness. The nurse notes that the patient has not been eating and asks the patient about her appetite. The patient responds by saying, "What does it matter?" Which is the most appropriate nursing diagnosis for this patient?
   a. *Social isolation*
   b. *Spiritual distress*
   c. *Denial*
   d. *Hopelessness*

23. The nurse recognizes that anticipatory grieving can be most beneficial to a patient or family because it can:
   a. be done in private.
   b. be discussed with others.
   c. promote separation of the ill patient from the family.
   d. help a person or family start to develop coping skills.

Chapter **42**   **Death and Loss**

24. A newly graduated nurse is assigned to his first dying patient. The nurse is best prepared to care for this patient if he:
   a. has developed a personal understanding of his own feelings about death.
   b. completed a course dealing with death and dying.
   c. is able to control his own emotions about death.
   d. experiences the death of a loved one.

25. An identified outcome for the family of a patient with a terminal illness is that they will be able to provide psychological support to the dying patient. To assist the family to meet this outcome, the nurse plans to include in the teaching plan:
   a. application of oxygen devices.
   b. demonstration of bathing techniques.
   c. recognition of patient needs and fears.
   d. information on when to contact the hospice nurse.

26. The nurse is assigned to a patient who was recently diagnosed with a terminal illness. During morning care, the patient asks about organ donation. The nurse should:
   a. have the patient first discuss the subject with the family.
   b. suggest the patient delay making a decision at this time.
   c. contact the physician so that consent can be obtained from the family.
   d. assist the patient to obtain the necessary information to make this decision.

27. A patient has been diagnosed with terminal cancer of the liver and is receiving chemotherapy on a medical unit. In an in-depth conversation with the nurse, the patient states, "I don't think that the test results could be right." According to Kübler-Ross, the nurse identifies that this stage is associated with:
   a. anxiety.
   b. denial.
   c. bargaining.
   d. depression.

28. A patient who practices Islam has just died on the unit. The nurse is prepared to provide after death care to the patient and anticipates the probable preferences of a family from this cultural background will include:
   a. pastoral care.
   b. preparation for organ donation.
   c. time for the family to bathe the patient.
   d. preparation for quick removal out of the hospital.

29. Which of the following is the primary concern of the nurse for providing care to a dying patient? The nurse should:
   a. encourage optimism in the patient.
   b. promote dignity and self-esteem.
   c. intervene in the patient's activities of daily living.
   d. allow the patient to be alone most of the time.

30. Hospice nursing care has a different focus for the patient. The nurse is aware that patient care provided through a hospice is:
   a. designed to meet the patient's individual wishes, as much as possible.
   b. usually aimed at offering curative treatment for the patient.
   c. involved in teaching families to provide postmortem care.
   d. offered primarily for hospitalized patients.

31. The nurse is preparing to assist the patient in the end stage of her life. To provide comfort for the patient in response to anticipated symptom development, the nurse plans to:
   a. limit the use of analgesics.
   b. decrease the patient's fluid intake.
   c. provide larger meals with more seasoning.
   d. determine valued activities and schedule rest periods.

32. The nurse is working with a patient on an inpatient hospice unit. To demonstrate caring and maintain the patient's sense of self-worth during the end of life, the nurse should:
   a. leave the patient alone to deal with final affairs.
   b. call upon the patient's spiritual advisor to take over care.
   c. plan regular visits throughout the day.
   d. have a grief counselor visit.

33. A nursing intervention to assist the patient with a nursing diagnosis of *Sleep pattern disturbance related to the loss of spouse and fear of nightmares* should be to:
   a. administer sleeping medication per order.
   b. refer the patient to a psychologist or psychotherapist.
   c. have the patient complete a detailed sleep pattern assessment.
   d. sit with the patient and encourage verbalization of feelings.

34. To promote comfort for the terminally ill patient specific to nausea and vomiting, the nurse should:
   a. provide prompt mouth care.
   b. offer high protein foods.
   c. increase the fluid intake.
   d. place the patient supine.

35. A nurse-initiated or independent activity for promotion of respiratory function in a terminally ill patient is to:
   a. limit fluids.
   b. elevate the head of the bed.
   c. reduce narcotic analgesic use.
   d. administer bronchodilators.

36. The nurse is using Bowlby's phases of mourning as a framework for assessing the patient's response to the traumatic loss of her leg. During the "searching and yearning" phase, the nurse anticipates that the patient may respond by:
    a. acting stunned by the loss.
    b. becoming angry at the nurse.
    c. withdrawing from outside contact.
    d. discussing the change in role that will occur.

37. The nurse prepares for which of the following after the family's home is totally lost in a tornado?
    a. Chronic loss
    b. Unresolved loss
    c. Complicated loss
    d. Perceived loss

38. The patient who is in Kübler-Ross's bargaining stage is likely to state:
    a. "I just want to be able to see my son graduate from school."
    b. "This just can't be the only treatment that is available!"
    c. "I don't believe that the MRI results were actually mine."
    d. "It's going to be okay for me."

Practice Situations

The daughter of a patient who is at home on hospice care tells you that her mother has been having seizures, going in and out of consciousness, and crying most of the afternoon. When the daughter touches her, the mother draws away and moans.
a. What is your assessment of this patient?

b. How can you assist the daughter?

A 62-year-old woman was waiting for her 30-year-old son to come over for dinner. She was informed by the police that there had been an auto accident and her son was killed. The mother keeps saying over and over again that "it can't be true." When you make a follow-up visit, the mother appears fatigued and responds little to questions.
a. What other grieving behaviors do you expect?

b. Identify a possible nursing diagnosis and goal/outcome for this woman.

c. Which interventions are appropriate for this individual?

REVIEW QUESTIONS

- What is the process of grief, loss, and bereavement?
- How can you describe dysfunctional loss and grieving?
- What are the factors affecting the grief and bereavement process?
- What is included in a nursing assessment of individuals and their families who are experiencing loss, death, grief, and bereavement?
- Which nursing diagnoses are appropriate for persons experiencing death and the grieving process?
- What are appropriate goals and outcomes for dying patients and their families?
- How would you implement nursing care plans with interventions that are appropriate for individuals and families experiencing grief?
- What are the effects of death and loss on nurses and which coping strategies may be used?

Answer Key

CHAPTER 1: NURSING, THEORY, AND PROFESSIONAL PRACTICE

1. c
2. d
3. e
4. a
5. b
6. Common concepts include protection, promotion, and optimization of health and abilities; prevention of illness; and the care of ill, disabled, and dying.
7. a. Educator, b. Leader, c. Collaborator, d. Researcher
8. a. Florence Nightingale, b. Dorothea Dix, c. Clara Barton, d. Linda Richards
9. The concepts are optimal functioning of the person, or patient, how people interact with the environment, illness and health promotion, and nursing's role.
10. A model is a collection of interrelated concepts that provides direction for nursing practice, research, and education. A nursing theory represents a group of concepts that can be tested in practice and can be derived from a conceptual model.
11. a. Florence Nightingale—Environmental adaptation with appropriate noise, hygiene, light, comfort, socialization, hope, nutrition, and conservation of patient energy.
    b. Roy—The human being as an adaptive open system.
    c. Rogers—Human beings and their environments are interacting in continuous motion as infinite energy fields.
    d. Orem—The goal of nursing care is to help patients perform self-care by increasing their independence.
    e. Watson—Caring, with nurses dedicated to health and healing.
12.

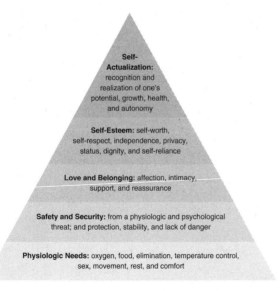

13. Criteria for a profession include altruism, a body of knowledge and research, accountability, higher education, autonomy, a code of ethics, professional organizations, licensure, and diversity.
14. a. Assessment, b. Education, c. Outcomes identification/collaboration, d. Communication, e. Resource utilization
15. The core beliefs are a, c, e.
16. Nurse practice acts provide the scope of practice defined by each state or jurisdiction and are the legal limits of nursing practice.
17. LPNs complete an educational program consisting of 12 to 18 months of training, and upon completion they must pass the National Council Licensure Examination for Practical Nurses (NCLEX-PN) to practice as an LPN/LVN. LPNs are under the supervision of an RN in most institutions, are able to collect data, but usually cannot perform an assessment requiring decision making, cannot formulate a nursing diagnosis, and cannot initiate a care plan. They may update care plans and administer medications, with the exception of certain IV medications.
18. Certification is a voluntary process in a specialty area. Licensure is mandatory in order to practice.
19. The observations include a, b, c.
20. a. Patients should be identified at least two ways—name band and asking them to state their names.
    b. Hand washing is the main way to prevent infection, along with careful medical and surgical asepsis.
    c. Prevention of mistakes in surgery with the "time out" to review the procedure to be done.
21. Characteristics of collaboration among health care professionals include:
    • Clinical competence and accountability.
    • Common purpose.
    • Interpersonal competence and effective communication.
    • Trust and mutual respect.
    • Recognition and valuation of diverse complementary knowledge and skills.
    • Humor.
22. Cultural competency:
    a. For the patient who speaks another language, the nurse obtains an interpreter and health information in the language used by the patient.
    b. After determining the patient's preferences, the nurse investigates how they can be integrated into the patient's diet while in the hospital. Work with the nutritionist.
23. a
24. c
25. a
26. b

Practice Situation

a. Education to become a Registered Nurse may be completed at a diploma school associated with a hospital and/or college (not as common today), associated degree program at a college (usually a 2-year community college), or a 4-year institution for a baccalaureate degree.

b. The nurse in the clinic appears to be an advanced practice nurse/nurse practitioner. This level of practice requires a minimum of a master's or doctoral degree.

CHAPTER 2: VALUES, BELIEFS, AND CARING

1. d
2. f

3. c
4. a
5. b
6. e
7. Many value conflicts can arise between the nurse and patient. One may be that the patient values home remedies while the nurse feels strongly about the use of available prescription medications. The patient may be having a termination of a pregnancy and the nurse could have a religious background that bans the practice.
8. The appropriate interventions are a, d, and e.
9. The appropriate interventions are a, c, and e.

10.

Theorist	Concept	Practice Example
a. Madeline Leininger	Nursing is a transcultural care profession and the concept of care is at its center.	Care related to the recognition of and accommodation for the individual's cultural background and practices, such as praying at particular times during the day.
b. Jean Watson	Belief that health care needs to move from a total disease-cure focus based solely on scientific inquiry to a more holistic approach that incorporates values, beliefs, intentions, and the caring consciousness.	Care that is not just task based but incorporates the overall patient, such as making time for the patient to talk about his or her thoughts about the value of continuing chemotherapy with a late-stage cancerous growth.
c. Joyce Travelbee	The purpose of nursing is achieved through human-to-human relationships.	Care that recognizes the human condition and addresses responses to both positive and negative events, such as the birth of a child with a congenital anomaly.
d. Kristen Swanson	Five processes characterize caring: knowing, being with, doing for, enabling, and maintaining belief.	Care that incorporates actions that demonstrate caring, such as providing a soothing bath to a patient confined to bed.

11. Behaviors associated with codependency include direct control over the dependent person, by making excuses for the dysfunctional behavior or by protecting the person from negative consequences.
12. a. Presence—This is being with the patient/family at some of life's most important events, such as a birth or a death, in a preoperative room before surgery, or as they go through a life-changing illness.
    b. Consistency and predictability—The patient has an expectation for ongoing competent and compassionate care, that is delivered in a timely manner and according to a known schedule.
    c. Touch—The physical contact used by the nurse to demonstrate a connection and establish trust.
13. The factors related to the development of compassion are:
    • the ability to numerous instances when the care provided made a difference in patients' lives.
    • the recognition in childhood that one wanted to become a nurse.
    • the ability to relate some incident in one's life, such as caring for an ill family member.
    • the ability to identify both positive and negative role models that inspired greater compassion.

14. a. Life Span
    Families and cultures have attitudes about what and how to eat that they transmit in the form of values. Some of the strategies include limiting the purchase of unhealthy foods, involving children in shopping and meal preparation, and engaging children in ongoing conversations about healthful eating and the value of weight control.
    b. Cultural, Ethnicity, and Religion
    In some cultures, parents may arrange marriages for their children. Pharmaceutical treatment may be rejected by individuals from some cultures on the basis of traditional beliefs and values. Exploring the implementation of alternative or complementary therapies may help to meet patient needs while demonstrating respect.
    c. Disability
    Persons with disabilities note that a problem is often the feeling of being excluded by society. Nurses demonstrate respect for individuals with disabilities by including them in their care as much as possible and seeking to understand what works best for each individual rather than generalizing treatment modalities.
15. First-order beliefs are derived from life experiences and respected authorities.

16. b
17. a
18. c

Practice Situation

a. The caring behaviors being used are knowing-assessing and listening.
b. The next step is to find out more about how the patient is feeling and if she is having specific difficulty (i.e., pain, emotional issues).

CHAPTER 3: COMMUNICATION

1. g   5. c   9. a
2. j   6. d   10. b
3. e   7. i
4. h   8. f

11. The findings that prompt further investigation are a, c, d, and e.
12. Emotions conveyed through inflection include anger, joy, depression, anxiety, tension, and confusion/questions.
13. The nurse can use positive self-talk to assist a patient to get through painful procedures or treatments or reduce anxiety.
14. Strategies to promote patient safety include clear and concise written and verbal reporting, regular patient rounds or conferences, and prompt referrals and notification of changes in the patient's status.
15. The appropriate actions are c and e.
16. The essential components of professional nursing communication are respect, assertiveness, collaboration, delegation, and advocacy.
17. a. Orientation phase
    • Making introductions, establishing professional role boundaries (formally or informally, as needed) and expectations, and clarifying the role of the nurse
    • Observing, interviewing, and assessing the patient, followed by validation of perceptions
    • Identifying the needs and resources of the patient
    b. Working phase
    • Development of a contract or plan of care to achieve identified patient goals
    • Implementation of the care plan or contract
    • Collaborative work among the nurse, patient, and other health care providers, as needed
    • Enhancement of trust and rapport between the nurse and the patient
    • Reflection by the patient on emotional aspects of illness
    • Use of therapeutic communication by the nurse to keep interactions focused on the patient
    c. Termination phase
    • Alerting the patient to impending closure of the relationship
    • Evaluating the outcomes achieved during the interaction
    • Concluding the relationship and transitioning patient care to another caregiver, as needed
18. a. Location—If the patient is in an area where there is a lot of noise or other distractions, it will be difficult to conduct a discussion. The temperature and lighting may also be uncomfortable. If the location is not conducive, the nurse should seek out another place.
    b. Pain—Patients who are having discomfort will not be able to focus during an interview. It may be helpful to medicate the patient in advance.
19. The following are examples of how the nurse's statements may be altered to be more therapeutic:
    a. "I noticed that you haven't been taking your medications. Are you having any questions about them that I can answer for you?"
    b. "Here is the call bell. If you push this button, the aide or I will come."
    c. "It sounds like you are concerned about the test results."
    d. "Mrs. Jones, I'm here to help you with your bath. Is there a particular way that you like to have me help you?"
20. For the acronym SOLER, the actions are:
    S—sit facing the patient
    O—open stance when listening
    L—lean toward the speaker
    E—eye contact
    R—relax
21. The plate is described as follows: Potato at 12 o'clock, bread at 10 o'clock, butter at 9 o'clock, meat between 6-7 o'clock, and vegetables between 3-4 o'clock.
22. For a patient with expressive aphasia, the nurse can work with the person to have a series of gestures, use a photo/alphabet board, or use a notepad or erasable whiteboard to convey messages.
23. SBAR communication requires the sharing of clear information focused on the four topical areas:
    • **S**ituation: What is happening right now?
    • **B**ackground: What led up to the current situation?
    • **A**ssessment: What is the identified problem, concern, or need?
    • **R**ecommendation: What actions or interventions should be initiated to alleviate the problem?
24. Nonverbal communication involves body language (posture, stance, gait), facial expressions and eye movement, touch, gestures, and symbolic expression (appearance).
25. The therapeutic statements are d, e, and f.
26. One of the top causes of sentinel events was poor communication.
27. d
28. d
29. b
30. a
31. c
32. a

Practice Situation

a. Nonverbal communication is powerful. Patients may perceive this symbolic expression as the nurse being unprofessional and unprepared to provide safe care. This will interfere with the development of a helping, trusting relationship.
b. As the observer, you can approach the nurse to ask how she is doing and if there is anything that she needs. This may stimulate a conversation about concerns that may be occurring in her personal life. It is not your role to be her counselor, but you can provide support and help her to obtain appropriate assistance. If this is not effective, you may need

to discuss your observations with the nurse manager on the unit. You demonstrate caring by going to the new nurse first and offering yourself.

CHAPTER 4: CRITICAL THINKING IN NURSING

1. c
2. d
3. e
4. a
5. b
6. Critical thing traits include thinking independently, fairness, responsibility and accountability, risk taking, discipline, perseverance, creativity, curiosity, integrity, and humility.
7. Information gathering assists the nurse to collect relevant, precise, and accurate data. Because clinical decisions are often based on such data collection, it is important that the nurse utilize critical-thinking skills during these assessments.
8. The critical thinking errors are:
   a. Close mindedness
   b. Lack of information
   c. Bias and/or erroneous assumption
   d. Illogical thinking
9. Critical thinking is instrumental in providing safe patient care (QSEN):
   • Optimal patient management requires critical thinking through collaboration with all disciplines involved in the patient's care. Interdisciplinary clinical rounds are an effective approach to management of complex patient problems related to discharge planning, end-of-life decisions, and other ethical issues.
   • Critical thinking is used by the registered nurse to guide decisions related to delegation of assignments and tasks. Before delegation of a task, the nurse must be knowledgeable about the role, scope of practice, and competency of the person who is to receive the delegated task.
   • When developing preoperative plans of care, nurses use critical thinking, collaboration, and communication to develop individualized plans of care. Critical thinking helps the nurse to identify missing data.
10. a. Concept maps help to provide a way to organize and visualize data in order to identify relationships and solve problems.
    b. Simulation experiences enable the student to apply previously learned content in a safe and realistic environment that allows time for questioning, clarifying, and feedback. This builds confidence that can be applied to actual patient care experiences.
    c. Discussion with colleagues allows for the sharing of best practices and creative ideas for patient care. A cognitive process takes place that identifies and corrects knowledge gaps, erroneous assumptions, and biases.
11. Critical thinking is used as follows:
    a. Assessment—Use of critical thinking skills helps the nurse to identify data gaps and focus on relevant information. Skills can also be used to determine the best way in which to obtain critical patient data.

b. Implementation—Nurses can use critical thinking skills to provide the best type of care for individual patients. They can also adapt care to meet specific needs or when current interventions are not effective.
12. b
13. c
14. a
15. d
16. b
17. c

Practice Situation

a. You can apply critical thinking skills as follows:
   • Obtain as thorough a handoff report as possible.
   • Review the patient assignment in advance and determine the priorities for the shift on the basis of the nursing diagnoses and goals.
   • Determine what care will be delegated.
   • Schedule your activities for the shift, as much as possible, such as medication administration, patient instruction, and admissions/discharges.
b. To maintain patient safety, you will want to know which patients should be seen first and what interventions will be required to prevent injury. Knowledge of the treatments, especially medications, is essential in order to provide safe and effective care. Seek assistance to perform techniques that you have not done before or that may require more than one person to complete. Share assessment findings that are outside of the expected range with your colleagues. Involve the patient in your care.

CHAPTER 5: INTRODUCTION TO THE NURSING PROCESS

1. d
2. e
3. a
4. c
5. b
6. The nursing process is the foundation of professional nursing practice. It is the framework within which nurses provide care to patients in an organized and effective manner.
7. The nursing process requires that nurses think critically. It is dynamic, organized, and collaborative, and it is universally adaptable to various types of health care settings.
8. The primary source of data is the patient.
9. Objective data are b, c, e, and f.
10. The components of the nursing diagnoses are as follows:
    • Actual—This includes (1) the patient's identified need or problem (NANDA-I nursing diagnostic label), *related to* (2) the etiology or underlying cause and *manifested by* (3) signs and symptoms.
    • Risk—A two-part risk nursing diagnostic statement contains only (1) the patient's identified need or problem (NANDA-I nursing diagnostic label) *related to* (2) factors indicating vulnerability.
    • Health promotion—A two-part health-promotion nursing diagnostic statement contains (1) the nursing diagnostic

label and (2) defining characteristics. It always begins with the words *Readiness for Enhanced.*

11. Collaborative care for the patient can involve the patient, family, and nurses; the patient's PCP; medical or surgical specialists; respiratory therapists; a dietician; a physical therapist; occupational, music, or art therapists; a spiritual adviser; and social workers.

12. The essential qualities of patient goals are patient focused, realistic, and measurable.

13. Clinical pathways are multidisciplinary resources designed to guide patient care. Standing orders are written by physicians and list specific actions to be taken by a nurse or other health care provider in instances when access to a physician is not possible or when care is common to a certain type of situation.

14. a. Fluid volume, deficient related to inadequate intake as evidenced/manifested by dry mucous membranes and poor skin turgor.
    b. Urinary retention related to consequence of abdominal surgery (blockage from scar tissue) as evidenced by decreased urinary output, bladder distention, and sensation of fullness.
    c. Risk for injury related to inner ear equilibrium problem and resulting dizziness.

15. a. Patient will verbalize a decrease in pain to less than 3 on a scale of 10 following administration of analgesic medication.
    b. Urine output will be at least 30 mL/hour throughout the day.

16. Pressure ulcer clean, dry with reduction in size by 1 cm and approximation of wound edges within 24 hours.

17. Goal not met. Patient experiencing a pain level above 3 and demonstrating objective signs of discomfort.

18. d	21. b	24. d
19. a	22. c	25. a
20. c	23. a	26. d

Practice Situation

a. Examples of other information to assess include:
   • Does the patient have any additional health problems?
   • Will the patient be the person responsible for the medications and cooking?
   • Is the patient motivated and able to learn?
   • What is the home environment like?
   • Is the patient working?
   • How will the change in diet and addition of daily medication influence his lifestyle?
b. Put the assessment information from the situation into the map to show relationships between the data.

CHAPTER 6: ASSESSMENT

1. e	4. f	7. h
2. a	5. c	8. b
3. g	6. d	

9. The nurse may use the following methods for assessment: observation; the patient interview, including the completion of a health history and review of systems; and a physical examination.

10. a. Sight—physical appearance, movement, gait, coloration, skin integrity, fluid balance—moisture/dryness/edema, facial expressions, posture
    b. Hearing—inflection in the voice, wheezing, coughing, crying, cardiopulmonary and abdominal sounds
    c. Touch—skin temperature and moisture, edema, discomfort, abnormal growths
    d. Smell—body and breath odors associated with hygiene or pathology, bodily elimination

11. Family history:
    • Age and health status of living parents, grandparents, siblings, and children
    • Age at death and cause of death of deceased immediate family members
    • Genetic diseases or traits, familial diseases (e.g., cardiovascular disease, high blood pressure, stroke, blood disorders, cancer, diabetes, kidney disease, seizure disorders, drug or alcohol dependencies, mental illness)

12. The interview should be conducted in an area that is free from as many distractions as possible, ensuring that the patient is comfortable and relaxed. The patient should feel safe because the questions raised may cause stress and anxiety. When feasible, the nurse and the patient should be seated at eye level with each other.

13. The health history includes demographic data, which is collected during the orientation phase of the interview; a patient's chief complaint, or reason for seeking health care; the history of present illness; allergies; medications; adverse reactions to medications; past medical history; family and social history; and health promotion practices.

14. The nurse can use inspection and palpation to see and feel if the patient's abdomen is distended. Percussion may also be used to hear if there is fluid present.

15. The nurse should explain to the patient what will happen during the assessment, then prepare the environment for patient comfort, including privacy, appropriate temperature, and safe and comfortable examination area/table.

16. In an emergency assessment, attention is paid to the ABCs—airway, breathing, and circulation. The nurse quickly assesses the extent of patient injuries and determines care priorities.

17. Information cannot be obtained from the unconscious patient, so the nurse will have to rely on friends and/or family members (secondary sources).

18. The nurse will collect information about the patient's emotional and psychological state, sociocultural background and practices, as well as other personal family, employment, and financial concerns.

19. The actions included in the orientation phase are a and d.

20. Examples of possible questions include: "Have you ever had any difficulty with breathing/chest pain/urination, etc.?" "Are you able to walk on your own?" and "Do you wear glasses?"

21. If diagnostic tests, such as blood tests or x-rays, were ordered before the patient is seen, the results are reviewed by the nurse. Privacy for the patient is ensured; good lighting is

established; and the equipment and instruments needed, such as a stethoscope, sphygmomanometer, and pulse oximeter, are gathered before the physical examination is started. A pen light, otoscope, and ophthalmoscope may be required, depending on the type of physical assessment being conducted. Hand hygiene is performed, and clean gloves are worn if contact with body fluids is anticipated.

22. The three kinds of physical assessments are comprehensive/ complete, clinical/focused, and emergency.
23. Validation is conducted by checking the patient's blood pressure upon the position changes.
24. Body systems—
    a. Chest pain—cardiovascular
    b. Decreased range of motion—musculoskeletal
    c. Periodic epigastric distress—gastrointestinal
25. The nurse should obtain assistance from a co-worker to assist the patient to move to the examination table safely.
26. Examples of questions include: "Have you been told about the low salt diet?", "How long have you had diabetes?", and "What do you do to treat your arthritis?"
27. Demographic data are a, c, and d.
28. a
29. d
30. d
31. b
32. c
33. b

Practice Situation

The data collected should be organized into the functional health patterns as follows:

Health perception and health management	Active social life—spending time with friends
Nutrition and metabolism	Caloric intake is appropriate for his size
Activity and exercise	No difficulty breathing No cardiovascular symptoms
Cognition and perception	Vision and hearing are acute

CHAPTER 7: NURSING DIAGNOSIS

1. d
2. c
3. e
4. b
5. a
6. Actual nursing diagnoses identify existing problems or concerns of a patient. Risk nursing diagnoses apply when there is an increased potential or vulnerability for a patient to develop a problem or complication. Health-promotion nursing diagnoses are used in situations in which patients express interest in improving their health status through a positive change in behavior.
7. Medical diagnoses identify and label medical (physical and psychological) illnesses. Nursing diagnoses consider a patient's response to medical diagnoses and life situations, in addition to making clinical judgments on the basis of a patient's actual medical diagnoses and conditions.
8. NANDA is the North American Nursing Diagnosis Association. The initial goals were to generate, name, and implement nursing diagnostic categories. These goals exist today, in addition to the goals of revising the taxonomy, promoting research to validate diagnostic labels, and encouraging nurses to use the taxonomy in practice.
9. Fluid volume, deficient
10. The errors to avoid include clustering of unrelated data, accepting erroneous data, using medical diagnoses as related factors within the nursing diagnosis statement, missing the true underlying etiology of a problem, and identifying multiple nursing diagnosis labels in one nursing diagnostic statement.
11. The appropriate defining characteristics include b, c, and f.

12. d
13. a
14. b
15. c
16. b
17. d
18. c

Practice Situation

a. The key pieces of data are recent diagnosis, no prior family history, unfamiliar with treatment regimen, and requires oral hypoglycemic and therapeutic diet.
b. A nursing diagnosis for this patient can be:
    Knowledge deficit related to lack of exposure/unfamiliarity as evidenced by "I don't have any idea of what I will have to do."

CHAPTER 8: PLANNING

1. Short-term goals are usually achievable within an immediate time frame of less than approximately 1 week, whereas goals that will take a longer time to achieve—weeks or a month or more—are long-term goals.
2. The first step in the planning phase is to set priorities among nursing diagnoses.
3. By involving the patient and/or family members in the development of the care plan, the patient is more likely to understand and accept the goals and treatment plan, which can contribute to achieving the expected outcomes.
4. The priority order is c, e, b, d, and a.
5. The ABCs of life support are airway, breathing, and circulation.

6. Examples of conflicting priorities may include: The patient may want to have financial concerns addressed before learning injection technique or have the arthritis pain resolved before treatment of an asymptomatic heart disease. The nurse recognizes the importance of the patient's compliance with the therapeutic diet, while the patient may have cultural preferences that make maintaining the diet difficult and undesirable.

7. Characteristics that make goals most effective are mutually acceptable to the nurse, patient, and family.
   • Appropriate in terms of nursing and medical diagnoses and therapy.
   • Realistic in terms of patient capabilities, time, energy, and resources.
   • Specific enough to be understood clearly by the patient and other nurses.
   • Measurable enough to facilitate evaluation

8. a. Body temperature will range between 98.3° and 99° F during the day.
   b. Patient will ambulate up and down the hallway to the room at least tid during hospital stay.
   c. Patient will be able to verbalize the foods allowed on the therapeutic diet by tomorrow.

9. Outcome indicators:
   a. Vital signs—body temperature
   b. Activity/mobility
   c. Appetite

10. The five key elements for nursing interventions are:
    • Patient assessment findings indicating signs and symptoms that have resulted from or in response to an illness or life experience.
    • The underlying etiology or related factor identified in each nursing diagnosis.
    • Realistic patient outcomes in light of the patient's health status and resources for improvement.
    • Evidence-based interventions aligned with patient acceptance and practicality.
    • Expertise of the nurses and other health care professionals and agencies involved in the patient's care.

11. a. Independent—providing patient education or emotional support, assessing status, instituting preventive measures
    b. Dependent—administering medications, performing wound care
    c. Collaborative—physical therapy, hospice care, spiritual or financial counseling

12. Discharge planning should begin when the patient is admitted to the acute care facility and continue until he or she goes home.

13. The patient's disability can influence the way or the time frame in which the goals can be achieved.

14. The measurable verbs are b, d, and f.

15. Nurses are faced with a significant population of adults who are health illiterate. They have difficulty completing routine health tasks such as understanding a drug label or vaccination table.

16. Goal statements
    a. Body weight (indicator): Patient will lose at least 1 lb per week.
    b. Vital sign assessment—pain (indicator): Patient will express less than a pain level of 3 on a scale of 10 following medication administration.

17. d   19. a   21. a
18. b   20. d   22. a

Practice Situation

a. Nursing diagnosis—*Knowledge deficit*
b. Short-term goal examples—Patient will be able to discuss the dietary requirements for the therapeutic diet by the next clinic visit. Patient will describe the dosage, action, and side effects of the prescribed medication by 9/3.

CHAPTER 9: IMPLEMENTATION AND EVALUATION

1. Implementation consists of both the performance of a nursing task and the documentation of the intervention.

2. Direct care involves having personal contact with patients. For example, direct-care interventions include cleaning an incision, administering an injection, ambulating with a patient, and completing patient teaching at the bedside. Indirect care includes nursing interventions that are performed to benefit patients but do not involve face-to-face nurse-patient contact. Examples of indirect care include making the change-of-shift report, communicating and collaborating with members of the interdisciplinary health care team, and ensuring availability of needed equipment.

3. Asking a patient to state his or her name and birth date while cross-checking what the patient says with the patient's armband information are the two most common ways to verify patient identity.

4. Continual reassessment of the patient detects noticeable changes in the patient's condition, requiring adjustments to interventions outlined in the plan of care.

5. Activities of daily living (ADLs) include tasks that are undertaken on a regular basis: eating, dressing, bathing, toileting, and ambulation.

6. Nurses may teach patients and/or families about medications, wound care, use of assistive devices, diets, postoperative cautions, pain relief measures, and many other areas related to their physical, mental and emotional health.

7. Referral can occur when more specific patient concerns arise, such as extreme anxiety, dietary requests, and discharge/home care needs.

8. Evidence-based practice information can be found in recent literature. Accurate communication of care plans among health care team members and the use of resources to locate relevant research information and treatment options support the implementation of best practices.

9. Nurses advocate for patients by coordinating care and supporting changes necessary to improve patient conditions and outcomes.

10. The five rights of delegation are:
    • *Right task:* Is this a task that can and should be delegated?
    • *Right circumstance:* Is this appropriate, at this time, with what is going on?
    • *Right person:* Does this person have the skills, scope of practice, understanding, and expertise to perform this task?

- *Right direction/communication:* Has proper information about what tasks need to be completed been shared so that what needs to be done is clear?
- *Right supervision/evaluation:* Has the nurse followed up to ensure that care was adequate to meet the needs of the patient?

11. Examples of prevention-oriented nursing interventions include patient education, immunization programs, cleansing an incision, and placing infants on their backs to sleep.
12. The independent nursing actions are c, e, and f.
13. False
14. c, d, f
15. False
16. Patient care is influenced as follows:
    a. Life span:
       - Interventions must always be age or developmental-level appropriate.
       - Individuals with cognitive deficits may require care that would typically be provided only for people who are much younger.
       - Encouraging patients of all ages to actively participate in their care provides them with a sense of control, even in the most serious circumstances.
    b. Gender:
       - Identify gender roles that may impact care delivery.
       - Some patients may prefer care from nurses of the same gender. This preference may stem from generational norms, personal comfort, or cultural considerations.
    c. Culture:
       - Culture plays an important role in communicating with patients. Professional interpretation services should be implemented when detailed care information is to be shared.
       - It is important to know whether eye contact or physical contact should be avoided.
       - Proper explanation of all procedures is essential for individuals of all cultures.
       - Asking patients to share their understanding of a procedure that has just been explained is a valuable way to verify that communication has been successful.
17. Electronic health records often include care plan formats that enhance nurses' ability to formulate individualized plans of care and facilitate coordination of care. Documentation of evaluative criteria and data in a patient's EHR allows nurses and other health care providers to collaborate electronically while responding to changes in a patient's health status.
18. c
19. d
20. b
21. c
22. a

Practice Situations

a. Nursing diagnosis—*Knowledge deficit*
b. Short-term goal examples—Patient will be able to discuss the dietary requirements for the therapeutic diet by the next clinic visit. Patient will describe the dosage, action, and side effects of the prescribed medication by 9/3.

c. Interventions—Instruct the patient about diabetes, the dietary requirements and the prescribed medication. Provide informational materials for the patient to review. Refer the patient to a nutritionist for follow-up with the diet.
a. If the nurse does not document the patient's allergy, the information will not be available to the rest of the health care team, the patient could receive the drug and suffer a severe adverse reaction.
b. The assessment of the patient's drug allergy should have been recorded/reported immediately.

CHAPTER 10: DOCUMENTATION, ELECTRONIC HEALTH RECORDS, AND REPORTING

1. a. APIE—assessment, problem, intervention, evaluation
   b. MAR—medication administration record
   c. EHR—electronic health record
   d. SBAR—situation, background, assessment, recommendation
   e. HIPAA—Health Insurance Portability and Accountability Act
   f. BCMA—bar-coded medication administration
   g. POMR—problem-oriented medical record
2. The purpose of documentation is the facilitation of information flow that supports the continuity, quality, and safety of care.
3. The guidelines for documenting require accessible, accurate, timely nursing documentation that is clear, concise, complete, and objective (ANA, 2010). Documentation should be factual and nonjudgmental, with proper spelling and grammar. Sequencing of events should be in the order they happened, and documentation should occur as soon as possible after assessment, interventions, condition changes, or evaluation. Each entry should include the date, time, and signature with credentials of the person documenting. Double documentation of data should be avoided because legal issues can arise due to conflicting data.
4. The advantage of a paper record is that no special technical training is required. Disadvantages include that it can be difficult to locate a particular chart because it is in use by someone else, is in a different department, or is misfiled. The paper chart is available to only one person at a time, and paper is fragile, is susceptible to damage, and can degrade over time. Handwriting may be illegible. Storage and control over paper records can be a major problem. Electronic records can demonstrate major cost savings, through gains in productivity, reduction of errors, and an improvement in health status. The most common benefits from electronic records are an increase in delivery of guideline-based care, better monitoring, a reduction of medication errors, and a decrease in utilization of care (Chaudhry et al., 2006). Movement toward electronic health records (EHRs) can reduce storage space, allow simultaneous access by multiple users, facilitate easy duplication for sharing or for backup, and increase portability in environments using wireless systems and handheld devices. A disadvantage of the EHR is the need for special technical training of

the users, concern over privacy, initial cost of installation, and possible failure with power losses.

5. The major components of the electronic health record (EHR) are health information, diagnostic test results, an order-entry system, and decision support.

6. Patient data can be put into the electronic health record (EHR) via keyboard, dictated voice recordings, light pens, or handwriting and pattern recognition systems. Computer programs can convert these types of data entry into text.

7. Example of a QSEN competency and the relationship of documentation:
   Safety—Accurate and prompt recording of patient information can be shared with other members of the health care team so that appropriate care is provided and errors are avoided.

8. Point-of-care documentation is done at the patient's bedside with a mobile computer station or handheld device.

9. Confidentiality of electronic records is maintained by not sharing one's password with others or leaving the patients' computer records open to scrutiny by others.

10. The do-not-use abbreviations are a, c, and e.

11. Charting by exception records only abnormal or significant data. It reduces charting time by assuming certain norms. In this type of charting each facility must define what is normal. Any assessment finding outside normal is charted as an exception.

12. a. Ate all of her sandwich, 120 mL of orange juice, 1/2 of the fruit cup.
    b. Stated that he "wasn't feeling like doing anything today."
    c. T—98° F, P = 78, R = 18, BP = 118/72

13. An admission summary includes the patient history, a medication reconciliation, and an initial assessment that addresses the patient's problems, including the identification of needs pertinent to discharge planning and formulation of a plan of care based on those needs. The discharge summary addresses the patient's hospital course and plans for follow-up, and documents the patient's status at discharge. It includes information on medication and treatment, discharge placement, patient education, follow-up appointments, and referrals.

14. The correct guidelines are b and e.

15. Protected health information may be used only for treatment, payment, or health care operations.

16. Handoffs can be oral, as in a face-to-face meeting or telephone communication, or can be written or taped. The information exchange can take place between providers, between shifts, and at the time of unit transfer or discharge referral.

17. ANTICipate:
    Administrative data
    New clinical information to be updated
    Tasks to be performed
    Illness severity
    Contingency

18. If a verbal or phone order is necessary in an emergency, the order must be taken by a registered nurse who repeats the order verbatim to confirm accuracy and then enters the order into the paper or electronic system, documenting it as a verbal or phone order and including the date, time, physician's name, and RN's signature. Most facility policies require that the physician cosign a verbal or telephone order within a defined time period.

19. When an unusual and unexpected event involving a patient, visitor, or staff member occurs, an incident report is completed. An incident might be the occurrence of a fall, a medication error, or an equipment malfunction. The purpose of this report is to document the details of the incident immediately to ensure accuracy.

20. d
21. a
22. b
23. d
24. b

Practice Situations

Using PIE/DAR

Problem/Data: Recently diagnosed with hypertension. Anxious about learning how to manage his blood pressure medications and new diet restrictions. Stated that he has never had to take medications regularly and does not really understand the diet.

Intervention/Action: Instructed about the treatment plan, including medications and diet. Referred to the nutritionist.

Evaluation/Response: Able to verbalize accurately about his diet and medications.

The handoff report should include information about the patient's current status (VS), including fluid intake and output, medications and their effectiveness, dietary intake and preferences, and body weight.

CHAPTER 11: ETHICAL AND LEGAL CONSIDERATIONS

1. f	5. h	9. b
2. d	6. e	10. a
3. j	7. c	
4. i	8. g	

11. Ethics are the standards of moral conduct within a society. Family, friends, beliefs, education, culture, and socioeconomic status all influence the development of ethical behavior. Behaviors that are judged as ethical or unethical, right or wrong, reflect a person's character.

12. a. Deontology stresses the rightness or wrongness of individual behaviors, duties, and obligations without concern for the consequences of specific actions.
    b. Utilitarianism maintains that behaviors are determined to be either right or wrong solely on the basis of their consequences.

13. a. Advocacy—Supporting or promoting the interests of others or of a cause greater than ourselves.
    b. Autonomy—The importance of allowing patients to make their own health care decisions.
    c. Beneficence— Defined as "doing good." Nurses demonstrate beneficence by acting on behalf of others and placing priority on the needs of others rather than on personal thoughts and feelings.

d. Confidentiality—Limits the sharing of private patient information. Maintaining the confidentiality of patient information means that its disclosure will be limited to only authorized individuals and agencies.

e. Veracity—Truthfulness defines the ethical concept of veracity. Honesty promotes unrestricted communication among individuals, demonstrates respect for others, and builds trust.

14. Accountability is demonstrated by the nurse admitting his or her error and taking steps to report and correct the mistake.

15. Nonmaleficence may be in conflict with health care delivery when treatments are given that are painful or interfering with the patient's quality of life. "The cure being worse than the disease."

16. The student should talk to the classmate about the plagiarism and how it can be seen as a lack of integrity by the faculty. Talking about the consequences of being caught might be helpful in preventing the peer from continuing on this path. If the classmate is unreceptive, then it is a responsibility of the other student to inform the faculty.

17. Ethics committees:
    - Provide educational resources on ethical issues to committee members and institutional staff.
    - Establish policies that govern health care decision making.
    - Review cases in which clarity is necessary.
    - Identify sets of values relevant to cases requiring consultation.
    - Determine any values conflicts that may exist.
    - Interview key individuals impacting the case being reviewed.
    - Provide unbiased input that is not possible from a patient, family members, or close caregivers.
    - Clarify potential legal implications of the medical or nursing interventions.

18. Civility (acting politely) is essential in all interactions among faculty and nursing students. Respectful interaction between students and faculty members establishes professional communication patterns and affects the way in which students interact with patients.

19. The four major sources of law are:
    - Constitutional law is derived from a formal written constitution that defines the powers of government and the responsibilities of its elected or appointed officials. Constitutional law in the United States is based on the U.S. Constitution. Each state has a constitution that must be consistent with the U.S. Constitution.
    - Statutory law is created by legislative bodies such as the U.S. Congress and state legislatures. Statutory laws are often referred to as *statutes*. State statutes must be consistent with all federal laws.
    - Regulatory law—State legislatures give authority to administrative bodies, such as state boards of nursing, to establish regulatory law, which outlines how the requirements of statutory law will be met. Nursing rules and regulations are categorized as regulatory law.
    - Case law—Judicial decisions from individual court cases determine case law. In contemporary society, case

law is established by judicial decisions based on the outcome of specific court cases.

20. The Code of Ethics is a powerful mandate for all nurses to communicate and act professionally to prevent inflicting physical or emotional pain on others while pursuing nursing education and engaging in nursing practice.

21. Student nurses are held to the same ethical standards as professional nurses. This requires that students pursuing nursing education behave responsibly and respectfully toward all people, be accountable for their actions, develop professionally, and strive to learn all that is necessary to safely care for patients and their families.

22. Bioethical challenges include genetic testing, cloning and embryonic stem cell research, end-of-life care, and resource allocation and access, including organ transplants.

23. Examples of felonies include practicing nursing without a license, child abuse, and illegal drug dealing.

24. Negligence:
    - *Duty:* It must be proved that the nurse or other health care provider owed a duty of care to the accusing patient.
    - *Dereliction:* There must be evidence that the nurse's actions did not meet the standard of care required or that care was totally omitted.
    - *Damages:* Actual injury to the accusing patient must be evident.
    - *Direct cause:* A causal relationship must be established between harm to the accusing patient and the actions or omitted acts of the nurse.

25. Actions especially helpful in avoiding charges of malpractice include maintaining (1) current professional practice knowledge, (2) competent practice skills, and (3) professional relationships with patients and their families. In addition, the nurse should:
    - Maintain confidentiality.
    - Follow legal and ethical guidelines when sharing information.
    - Document punctually and accurately.
    - Adhere to established institutional policies governing safety and procedures.
    - Comply with legal requirements for handling and disposing of controlled substances.
    - Meet licensure and continuing education requirements.
    - Practice responsibly within the scope of personal capabilities, professional experience, and education.

26. False

27. The violations of professional boundary are b, d, and e.

28. In addition to professional boundary violations, nursing practice misconduct may include illegally obtaining patient medication (including narcotics), engaging in drug abuse, or practicing incompetently. All of these are serious offenses punishable by law.

29. The individuals who are unable to give consent are a and e.

30. Documentation errors include: (1) omitting documentation from patient records, (2) recording assessment findings obtained by another nurse or unlicensed assistive personnel (UAP), and (3) recording care not yet provided. Sometimes nurses will document that a patient has received medication before its administration. This is a serious violation of the law and becomes a medication error of omission if the nurse is

distracted before actually administering the patient's medication. A second major legal concern related to documentation is the issue of timeliness and not charting information promptly and at the time interventions occurred.

31. In 1968 the Uniform Anatomical Gift Act was approved to allow people older than the age of 18 to donate their bodies or body parts, after death, for transplantation, deposit in tissue banks, or research. Consent for organ donation must be in writing. In many states, licensed drivers are permitted to sign organ donation forms on the back of their licenses. Adults who do not have driver's licenses can obtain a separate organ donation card to carry in their wallets. However, having a signed form indicating desire to be an organ donor is not enough in most states. It is imperative that individuals make their desire to donate organs known to family members before their death to ensure that their wishes are fulfilled. In some states, regardless of the existence of signed organ donation forms, final permission for organ and tissue donation must be received from family members of the deceased.

32. Per the Patient's Bill of Rights, patients should expect: (1) excellent care, (2) a safe environment, (3) participation in planning their care, (4) privacy, (5) help with discharge arrangements, and (6) assistance with fulfilling financial responsibilities.

33. Advance directives consist of three documents: (1) living will, (2) durable power of attorney, and (3) health care proxy, commonly referred to as *durable power of attorney for health care.*

34. Protected health information (PHI) includes physical or mental health data, health care treatment locations and occurrences, and payment information related to all health care treatment.

35. a. Standards of care are the minimum requirements for providing safe nursing care.
    b. Standards are established by federal and state laws, rules and regulations, accreditation standards, and institutional policies and procedures. Institutional policies and procedures must be consistent with state laws, rules, and regulations, which in turn must comply with federal law.
    c. The American Nurses Association (ANA) identifies standards for safe practice and regularly releases policy statements and current practice information to guide and update the standards of care for nurses.

36. Licensure—The laws of each state require that graduates of accredited nursing schools and colleges pass the National Council Licensure Exam (NCLEX) before beginning professional practice. Not required by law, specialty certification seeks to ensure safe, competent nursing practice.
    Certification (voluntary) is available to nurses in a wide variety of specialties including critical care, gastroenterology, oncology, pediatrics, and education. Becoming certified in a nursing specialty requires years of practice, a recognized level of expertise, and a commitment to excellence, in addition to the time and financial resources needed to prepare for and successfully complete the certification examination.

37. The Privacy Rule allows for individuals to control how their health information is shared. The Privacy Rule limits disclosure of patient health care information to the patient and only those people and health care agencies to which the patient has granted specific permission. Confidential treatment of patient records involves limiting access to documentation of interactions between patients and health care providers.

38. Accurate statements are a, c, d, and e.

39. Determination of death—There are two criteria on which death can be established, either when all spontaneous respiratory and circulatory function stops or when all brain function ends, including in the brainstem.

40. Natural Death Acts exist in some jurisdictions that permit competent patients to make health care decisions that may result in their deaths. This includes nursing actions such as discharging patients who are likely to die without acute care and withholding or withdrawing life-sustaining treatments under the direction of a physician when requested by a competent patient. The acts prevent civil liability, criminal liability, and professional sanctions against health care providers who explain the medical risks associated with the decisions before their initiation. Assisted suicide and euthanasia are illegal in many places, even if the patient involved is competent.

41. The ADA provides protection against discrimination for individuals who have a physical or mental impairment that interferes with one or multiple life activities, have a history of impairment, or are perceived as having a disability. Life activities are identified by the ADA (2008) as difficulty performing activities of daily living (ADLs), "seeing, hearing, eating, sleeping, walking, standing, lifting, bending, speaking, breathing, learning, reading, concentrating, thinking, communicating, and working" [Section 12102, (2) (A)].

42. Restraints—Federal and state laws and guidelines from The Joint Commission have mandated that physical restraints be used only in the event that alternative, less restrictive interventions to prevent patient injury have been unsuccessful and a written order for restraints is in place. The written order must include dates, indicating the start and stop times for physical-restraint usage, and it must be updated frequently according to institutional policies.

43. The accurate statements about HIPAA are a, c, and e.

44. a	48. c	52. a
45. c	49. b	53. b
46. d	50. c	54. a
47. a	51. d	55. c

Practice Situations

a. The ethical principles involved are veracity (telling the truth to the patient) and advocacy (supporting the patient's decision regarding the care).

b. This could be an ethical dilemma if you believe that the patient should try everything possible to treat the disease. It is also a concern that the oncologist may not be willing to share the information with the patient, even if you think it should be offered.

c. You should first determine what your feelings are so that they will not interfere with what is best for the patient. You should also find out what the patient knows and how she feels about what is happening. A discussion from the oncologist about futile care and the patient's quality of life might be beneficial.

a. First, verify that the provider wants to give that dose and identify what the normal range is for the medication.

Depending on your experience and the provider's degree of insistence, you may want to contact the nurse manager or supervisor for support. Refusing to give the medication is the best option to reduce the potential for a patient injury.

b. You are liable if you administer the medication and the patient suffers a reaction to the high dosage.

CHAPTER 12: LEADERSHIP AND MANAGEMENT

1. e
2. b
3. d
4. a
5. c
6. Leadership is the ability to influence, guide, or direct others. Leadership focuses on relationships, using interpersonal skills to persuade others to work toward a common goal. Leaders may or may not have the authority that comes with a formal position in an organization; their power lies in their ability to form relationships and alliances with those around them.

   Management is the process of coordinating others and directing them toward a common goal. Management is focused on the task at hand. A manager holds a formal position of authority within an organization; with that position comes both the accountability and the responsibility for accomplishing the tasks within the work environment.
7. a. Trait theory—Assumed that leaders were born with the personality traits necessary for leadership
   b. Behavioral theory—Assumed that leaders learn certain behaviors. These theories focus on what leaders do, rather than on what characteristics they innately possess.
   c. Situational theory—Suggests that leaders change their approach depending on the situation.
8. a. The autocratic leader would give out the staff assignments and expectations and not want much input from anyone.
   b. The democratic leader would invite the staff members to work with him or her to consider the assignment and patient goals for the day.
   c. The laissez-faire leader would provide the assignments and let the staff figure out how to schedule and achieve goals.
9. Examples of how the qualities of effective leaders are exhibited are:
   a. Integrity—being a good role model and maintaining policies/procedures and ethics
   b. Dedication—staying and finishing patient care activities
   c. Magnanimity—giving credit to the staff for instituting an effective infection control policy
   d. Humility—treating the staff with respect
   e. Openness—taking staff member suggestions into consideration
   f. Creativity—implementing a new staff scheduling plan
10. Formal leadership is part of an official position, which may or may not be in a management role. Informal leadership comes from outside of a formal position and is demonstrated when stepping up and leading others.
11. The functions of management are planning, organizing, directing, and controlling.
12. At the People Level, the manager focuses on b and f.
13. Competencies of effective managers are:
    • Communication and relationship building
    • Knowledge of the health care environment
    • Leadership
    • Professionalism
    • Business skills
14. Theory Y style managers believe that satisfied workers are capable of self-direction, self-control, and initiative. They believe that, given the proper conditions, employees will accept and seek out responsibility on the job. Theory X–style managers are more autocratic and do not see employees as being motivated to be productive.
15. a. Patient advocate—speaking on the patient's behalf and protecting his or her interests.
    b. Case manager—helping the patient through the process, beginning discharge planning upon admission.
16. The nurse manager uses business skills to ensure that patient care is cost-effective. The individual must understand budgeting, staffing, marketing, and information management, along with human resources.
17. a. Resources about delegation can be found in the state's nurse practice act, the health care organization's policies and procedures, the National Council of State Board's (NCSBN) website, and nursing journals.
    b. First principle of delegation: Nurses must have knowledge of the nurse practice act in the state where they are licensed.
       Second principle of delegation: The RN cannot delegate assessment, planning, evaluation, or accountability for the assigned task.
       Third principle of delegation: The person to whom the assignment was delegated cannot, in turn, delegate that assignment to someone else.
18. The quality indicators and standards put forth in the Magnet Recognition Program are designed to create a professionally satisfying environment for nurses. By enacting nurse-friendly policies and programs, Magnet hospitals are able to recruit and retain nurses at higher rates than non-Magnet organizations. Patients benefit, as well, since Magnet organizations, with more stable staffing patterns, are better able to consistently provide safe, competent patient care.
19. The appropriate diversity considerations are:
    a. Communication—Be aware of racial, ethnic, and gender differences. Males and females transmit and interpret messages differently. In addition, the influence of culture in the form of race and ethnicity affects both verbal and nonverbal communication. Eye contact, posture, and use of assertive or passive terms are all influenced by these factors and must be considered in communicating to staff.
    b. Time—Cultural groups are past, present, or future oriented. Past- and present-oriented cultural groups tend not to focus on long-range goals.

c. Environmental factors—Cultural groups and individuals with an internal locus of control have a need to feel in control of their environment and will focus on planning. Those with an external locus of control believe that fate or chance plays a role in life events and will focus more on the obstacles they face.

20. d
21. a
22. b

Practice Situation

For the Five Rights of safe delegation

Right task: For the unstable patients, specific aspects of care may not be delegated, such as vital signs.

Right circumstances: With the patient admission, you will benefit from the UAP's assistance in performing appropriate care to the patients. The unstable patients, however, will require more supervision.

Right person: Having never worked with this UAP before, you will need to determine that she is able to perform the care safely.

Right direction/communication: It is extremely important to communicate clearly with this UAP about your expectations, especially since you have not worked with her before. You will want her to know what she should and should not do for the patients and what the goal is for the shift.

Right supervision: With the unstable patients and unfamiliar UAP, you will need to periodically monitor your patients' status and how the UAP is proceeding with the care that has been delegated.

CHAPTER 13: EVIDENCE-BASED PRACTICE AND NURSING RESEARCH

1. e	5. h	9. b
2. d	6. f	10. i
3. g	7. a	
4. j	8. c	

11. Evidence-based practice is the integration of best research evidence with (1) clinical expertise, (2) patient values and needs, and (3) the delivery of quality, cost-effective health care. The ultimate goal is to promote positive outcomes for the patient.

12. Research is the structured process of investigation that is used to generate and test theories. Evidence-based practice is the use of this information in patient care.

13. Quantitative research usually results in data in the form of numbers. Qualitative research usually results in data in the form of words, often in the form of a narrative.

14. The order of the research steps is e, c, a, d, b, and f.

15. A hypothesis is a statement about two or more variables and their relationship to each other.

16. Nurses are expected to use research findings in practice and participate in research activities that are appropriate for their position and level of education. Activities may include identifying problems in the clinical setting to be researched; participating in data collection; participating as a member of a research committee or a research program; sharing research findings; conducting research; critiquing research; using research findings to develop policies, procedures, and standards for patient care at health care facilities; and incorporating research as part of ongoing learning.

17. For this example, the independent variable is the anti-itch medication, the dependent variable is the itching, and the control is Group B (no treatment received).

18. The ethical principles are beneficence (minimize harm), justice (fair and equal treatment), and autonomy/respect (decision-making capability).

19. Protection of human subjects in research involves informed consent, confidentiality, and anonymity. Participants are made aware of the study and what is involved, information is only shared with those who require access, and personal identity and information are not used. Written and electronic documents need to be secured, including computer passwords and any paper copies.

20. Outcomes can be disseminated by publication in a journal or through a poster, an oral presentation, or a workshop at a conference. Study findings can also be shared with colleagues in more informal settings.

Nursing research with practical implications may need to be reported to agencies and health care providers to initiate necessary change. If the research is to have a large-scale impact, study results should be disseminated to the community, those who funded the research, and policy makers. Research reports can be published by a university on a website or in printed newsletters to provide more public dissemination. A dissemination plan should be devised at the beginning of the research.

21. The IRB is established to help protect the rights and welfare of human research subjects.

22. Quantitative analysis is usually completed with appropriate statistics. Qualitative analysis involves review of narrative content, such as verbal information from participants.

23. a. Filtered sources include Cochrane Reviews, Joanna Briggs Institute Library of Systematic Review.
    b. Unfiltered sources include MEDLINE/PubMed, PsychINFO, and CINAHL.

24. Internal validity is evident with a, c, and f.

25. Criteria for Magnet status include excellent patient outcomes due to nursing, a high level of nursing job satisfaction with a low nurse turnover rate, and appropriate resolution of any grievance.

26. The vulnerable individuals are a, b, c, and e.

27. Evidence-based practice (EBP) is incorporated delegation by educating unlicensed assistive personnel, before delegating care, on the importance of EBP for positive patient outcomes, and encouraging colleagues to use research when caring for the same patient on various shifts and days.

28. c
29. b
30. a
31. d
32. a

Practice Situation

Assess the problem: You have begun to do this by identifying that there is a discrepancy in the patients' ability to maintain the diet. Develop the question:

P—Adult patients at the clinic who have diabetes and are not following their diabetic diets

There is inconsistency in the type of information and method of transmission.

I—Provision of written dietary resource materials alone

C—Provision of the written materials and follow-up with the nurse and dietitian

O—Patients' ability to maintain the diet successfully

Search the databases: Investigate other studies regarding patient instructional strategies that have been successful in promoting compliance. Review for specific studies on patients with diabetic diets.

Critically appraise the information: Determine if the studies have validity and the results can be applied to your practice area.

Design a practice change: Based on the search, it was determined that both written resources and in-person consultation were most successful. Prepare written materials on the diet and arrange for the nurse and/or dietitian to meet with the patients during their clinic appointments.

Maintain the change and reevaluate: Implement the intervention and collect data on the effectiveness of the strategy to see if there is a significant change in the dietary compliance of the patients.

CHAPTER 14: HEALTH LITERACY AND PATIENT EDUCATION

1. Health literacy is the unique ability of the patient to understand and integrate health-related knowledge.

2. Components of patient education are preventing disease, promoting health, providing treatment instructions, clarifying information, and teaching patients to cope with limitations.

3. Examples of literacy/education gaps include providing the patient with important instructions to follow for medication administration and finding that the patient is unable to read English, or identifying when the patient should come back if complications arise and the caregiver cannot follow the verbal directions.

4. It is expected that the patient will be able to:
   • Read and identify credible health information.
   • Understand numbers in the context of the patient's health care.
   • Make appointments.
   • Fill out forms.
   • Gather health records and ask appropriate questions of physicians.
   • Advocate for appropriate care.
   • Navigate complex insurance programs, Medicare/ Medicaid, and other financial assistance programs.
   • Use technology to access information and services (U.S. Department of Health and Human Services [USDHHS], 2010a).

5. Teaching is imparting knowledge or giving instruction, while learning is acquiring knowledge or skills through instruction or experience.

6. Cognitive domain learning comprises knowledge and material that is remembered. Memorization and recall of information is necessary for the learner to progress and comprehend, apply, analyze, synthesize, and evaluate the new material. Examples—patients verbalizing about prescribed medications, diets, complications of treatments, when to notify the prescriber about status changes, etc.

The psychomotor domain incorporates physical movement and the use of motor skills into learning. Examples—patients demonstrating colostomy care, wound care, injection technique, crutch walking, etc.

Affective domain learning recognizes the emotional component of integrating new knowledge. Taking into account the patient's feelings, values, motivations, and attitudes. Examples—patients inquiring about ways to add new things to the diet, demonstrating positive reactions to their treatment success, joining support groups, etc.

7. a. Age-appropriate teaching strategies need to be implemented for children. Older adults may suffer from cognitive and physical changes that affect their learning.
   b. Environment—private, quiet and with minimal interruptions, good lighting, and a comfortable temperature.
   c. Timing—consider rescheduling teaching sessions for patients who are in pain, experiencing distress, or fatigued. Teach the most important/key concepts at the beginning of the sessions.

8. Indications that the patient has less than adequate health literacy:
   • Patient asks health care provider to read information aloud, stating, "I left my glasses at home."
   • Registration or other forms are incomplete or inaccurate.
   • Patient frequently misses appointments.
   • Patient does not comply with medication regimens.
   • Patient does not follow through with laboratory tests, imaging tests, or referrals to consultants.
   • Patient says he or she is taking medication, but laboratory tests or physiologic parameters do not change in the expected fashion.
   • Patient asks to bring a written document home to discuss it with a spouse or child.

9. Nursing diagnosis—Deficient Knowledge (wound care) related to new surgical incision as evidenced by patient's verbalized and demonstrated lack of knowledge.
   Goal statement—Patient will discuss and demonstrate the correct technique for wound care within 48 hours.
   Nursing intervention—Instruct the patient in the wound care procedure. Ask the patient to demonstrate and explain the procedure.

10. Examples of teaching strategies include verbal instruction, media such as computer-assisted programs, videotapes or audiotapes, demonstration, return demonstration, and written instructions.

11. Patient education is coordinated by the nurse but involves other members of the health care team. Teamwork is demonstrated when the nurse collaborates with the primary care provider, therapists, dietitians, and social workers to promote patient learning and outcomes.

12. Documentation includes a detailed description of the goals, what was taught, how it was taught, and the patient's reaction to the teaching.

13. The accurate statements are b, d, e, and f.

14. Some individuals are visual (seeing) learners, whereas others are auditory (hearing) or kinesthetic (doing actively). Visual

learners do better with information presented in words or pictures. Auditory learners do better by listening to a presentation. Kinesthetic learners benefit from manipulating materials. The nurse may find that the patient is a multimodal learner or can work with different types of strategies.

15. d	18. d	21. a
16. b	19. a	22. d
17. b	20. c	23. c

Practice Situation

a. Questions that you could ask to determine the patient's comfort with English include:
"What is your preferred language?", "Do you read the local newspaper, books, or magazines?"
"What language is spoken at home?"

b. In planning teaching sessions, you will want to have written information in the patient's language and photos or drawings. There may also be a need for an interpreter. Family members who will be involved with the patient's care should be included in the teaching, if the patient approves.

c. In addition to asking the patient to explain the procedure, you will want the patient to demonstrate their ability to do the colostomy care (psychomotor learning). Again, an interpreter may be necessary to assist in evaluating the patient's cognitive learning.

CHAPTER 15: NURSING INFORMATICS

1. Informatics is a broad academic field encompassing artificial intelligence, cognitive science, computer science, information science, and social science. Nursing informatics is a specialty area of informatics that addresses the use of health information systems to support nursing practice.

2. Nursing informatics can enhance patient care by decreasing the time spent on documentation, reducing the potential for errors, and supporting improved assessment and data communication. There is evidence of improved organization, improved communication, improved information access, safer medication administration, reduction of duplicate orders and paperwork, better decision making, reduced charting time, and improved administrative functions.

3. Technological tools used include computer access at every bedside (mobile devices and workstations on wheels [WOW]) and cell phones with cameras, global positioning systems, and Internet connections. Mobile devices (phones, tablets) are all being used in health care for communication, reference, and documentation. Many mobile devices include handwriting recognition software, some support voice recognition, and some have an internal cell phone and modem to link with other computers or networks.

4. Telehealth nursing is the transmission by a nurse of electronic data, images, or audio from a patient's bedside or home to other health providers for the purpose of providing care and improving outcomes. Patients may have telehealth hardware in their homes to provide in-home monitoring and direct reporting to their health care providers.

5. Computerization can promote patient safety through a bar-code medication administration system, safe practice alerts, direct order entry to improve sharing of information, and elimination of legibility issues of handwriting.

6. The electronic medical record (EMR), which is the documentation of a single episode of care (outpatient visit or inpatient stay), becomes a part of the electronic health record (EHR), which is a longitudinal record of care. The term *electronic health record* is becoming widely accepted for both individual health care encounters and for maintaining patients' health records over a long period of time.

7. Some of the advantages of the electronic record include provider order entry, progress notes for all disciplines, computerized medication profiles, access to diagnostic test results on a timely basis, decision support systems, and online clinical reminders and alerts. Nurses have access to health care resources, so the latest literature on a specific medical problem is readily available. Patient data can be searched for cases, trends, and outcomes that can be analyzed to determine the best evidence for practice. The ability to quickly review a patient's longitudinal data at the point of care supports the improved management of each patient. Work lists can be created so that nursing measures can be carried out at the appropriate times. Captured health data can be used for nursing research.

8. Beginner skills include a and e.

9. Computer literacy is knowledge of computers and the ability to use them efficiently. Information literacy is the ability to recognize when information is necessary and to locate, evaluate, and effectively use the needed information.

10. A standardized nursing terminology is a structured vocabulary that provides a common means of communication among nurses. A standardized language ensures that when a nurse talks about a specific patient problem, another nurse fully understands what the first nurse is describing.

11. Nurses can use electronic communication and social media, such as E-mail, listserv, internet, blogs, and social media sites, to provide health information and connect groups of patients with common problems. It can also be used to network nurses in order to share evidence-based practice information.

12. Specific aspects of informatics in the eHealth Code of Ethics are privacy (electronic), professionalism in online health care, and responsible partnering.

13. c

14. d

Practice Situation

When reviewing a website, the following questions should be asked in order to determine if it is a legitimate site to recommend. Websites sponsored by established institutions or agencies tend to be more reliable. Sites offered by profit-based entities, such as pharmaceutical companies, may have information that supports their business, so care should be taken in only using that type of resource.
Who is the sponsor/publisher? Is this a personal page? Where does it come from? Is the author or organization listed? What are the author's credentials?
Does the site inform? Explain? Share? Disclose? Sell? What is the intended audience?
Are citations correct? Is there a balance of text and images?
When was the site created? How often is it updated?

What are the goals and objectives of the site? Is there evidence of bias? Is bias explicit or hidden?

Are there footnotes or links to information sources?

Can the information be found in other sources?

Website example:

http://www.mayoclinic.org/diseases-conditions/thrombocytopenia/basics/definition/CON-20027170

CHAPTER 16: HEALTH AND WELLNESS

1. c
2. e
3. b
4. f
5. d
6. a

10.

Theory/Model	Primary Concept
Basic Human Needs	The interrelationship between the elements of basic requirements for survival and the desires that drive personal growth and development. The model is most often presented as a pyramid consisting of five levels—the lowest level is related to physiological needs, whereas the uppermost level is associated with self-actualization.
Health Belief Model	It explores the relationship between patient attitudes and beliefs and how those factors predict health behavior. There are three primary components: (1) perception of susceptibility to illness, (2) perception about the seriousness of the illness, and (3) probability that the individual will act to prevent avoidable health risks.
Holistic Health	Based on the philosophy that a synergistic relationship exists between the body and the environment. Holistic care is not solely a method of healing but also an approach for how healing therapies can be applied. Holistic concepts focus on the interrelatedness of the physical body and the psyche. Incorporating features of spirituality, emotional security, and environment into natural, holistic care supports the premise that the body knows how to heal itself given the proper support systems needed to do so.

7. The ethical concern for nurses is balancing the need to assist patients to receive optimum care while considering the cost of that care.

8. Holistic strategies include the use of natural remedies, art and guided imagery, therapeutic touch, music therapy, relaxation techniques, reminiscence, and referral for acupuncture, yoga, and tai chi.

9. The levels of prevention are:
   a. Tertiary
   b. Primary
   c. Secondary
   d. Primary

11. Health promotion activities include routine exercise, meeting nutritional and vitamin requirements, maintaining a body mass index within acceptable range, good sleep habits, and stress reduction.

12. Examples of risk-reduction activities are smoking cessation, beginning an exercise regimen, eating less salt and saturated fat, using stress-reducing techniques, and avoiding excessive alcohol consumption.

13. Healthy People 2020 is designed to track the risk factors and personal behaviors related to physical activity, access to health services, tobacco use, substance use, responsible sexual behavior, mental health, immunizations, and injury and violence prevention (U.S. Department of Health and Human Services, 2010).

14. a. Response to illness is influenced by an individual's cognitive and emotional development, as well as the body's physiological reaction to the stress.
    b. Examples of responses to illness include denial, anger, frustration, withdrawal, depression, and acceptance.

15. The behaviors associated with Stage IV are d and f.

16. a. acute
    b. chronic
    c. chronic
    d. chronic
    e. acute

17. a. Individuals with chronic illnesses need to adapt their lives to incorporate medication therapy, health care provider visits, laboratory testing/radiologic studies, dietary intake, activity restrictions or requirements, and other ongoing treatments (e.g., colostomy care, diabetic foot care).
    b. The nurse can use strategies to help patients cope with feelings of anger, frustration and depression, and provide measures to promote comfort and symptom management.

18. a. Age—young children and older adults more susceptible to illness
    b. Gender—susceptibility to reproductive-specific diseases, pregnancy and childbirth issues
    c. Lifestyle– smoking, poor diet, physical inactivity, substance abuse, high-risk hobbies (e.g., rock climbing), extended sun exposure, and excessive drinking
    d. Environment—indoor exposure to household cleaning agents, chemicals, tobacco smoke, microwave use, mold, household pests, and unsanitary living conditions; outdoor exposure to areas of sanitation and waste disposal, water quality, air quality, and safety issues (gang activity, sexual predators, or heavy traffic)

19. Individuals see themselves in relation to social character or abilities, physical appearance, body image, and ways of thinking. This entails the person's mental image of himself or herself in relation to others.

20. Cultural practices can influence how patients approach their treatment regimen and adapt their lifestyles to meet their health needs. Examples include a resistance to dietary changes, the need for family support in decision making, the refusal of traditional medical treatments, and an inability to integrate the regimen into daily life.

21. Patients in rural areas with limited health care access have the following challenges: time needed to travel to the nearest health care provider or facility, delayed treatment for so long that a non-life-threatening, minor, treatable disease becomes a severe, life-threatening, systemic infection requiring hospitalization and intravenous drug therapy. It is not uncommon to address patients' multiple problems of differing levels of severity that have been saved up for the trip to a distant provider.

22. c　　　　25. b　　　　28. b
23. b　　　　26. c　　　　29. d
24. d　　　　27. a

Practice Situation

a. This individual is most likely in stage IV as a result of recognizing that he is in the patient role and requires treatment. His affect is demonstrating that he knows that he has to incorporate the treatment regimen into his life, but he is not happy about having to do it.

b. You will want to provide emotional support for him and education about the disease and treatments. You can provide strategies to assist with coping, including relaxation techniques, imagery, exercise (as permitted), massage, and music therapy. The cardiac rehabilitation program may offer a schedule of support group meetings so that he can be with others who are experiencing the same issues. If this individual continues to struggle emotionally or psychologically, a referral to a mental health provider may be indicated.

CHAPTER 17: HUMAN DEVELOPMENT: CONCEPTION THROUGH ADOLESCENCE

1. f　　　　5. i　　　　9. c
2. h　　　　6. e　　　　10. a
3. g　　　　7. b
4. j　　　　8. d

11. Growth is the increase in height and weight of a child. Growth proceeds in an orderly, predictable pattern, from head to tail (cephalocaudal) and in proximal to distal direction. Development is the increasing maturation of physical ability, thought processes, and behaviors of a child.

12. This concept is whether development is predetermined at birth (nature) or whether the child's environment (nurture) controls how development progresses. Current belief is a mixture of the two.

13.

Theorist	Type of Theory	Major Concept(s)
Freud	Psychosocial/Psychosexual	3 basic concepts of the personality: id, ego and superego, stages of psychosexual development: oral, anal, phallic, latency, and genital
Erikson	Psychosocial	A series of psychosocial crises that shape personality, 8 stages (Trust vs. Mistrust through Integrity vs. Despair)
Piaget	Psychosocial/Cognitive	4 stages of development: sensorimotor, preoperational, concrete operational, and formal operational
Kohlberg	Moral Development	3 levels of moral reasoning, divided into sublevels: preconventional, conventional, and postconventional
Westerhoff	Faith Development	4 styles of faith: experienced, affiliative, searching, and owned

14. The developing fetus is susceptible to a variety of substances from the outside environment called teratogens. Teratogens include certain medications, illegal drugs, alcohol, infectious agents, and certain diseases.

15. Information that can be provided to the parents includes expectations for infant development, safety measures ("back to sleep," hand washing, eliminating suffocation risks, using car seats), need for sleep, hygienic care, and nutritional needs for breastfeeding or bottle feeding (iron and vitamin supplements).

16. The nurse instructs the parents to place the infant on the back for sleep to reduce the chance of SIDS.

17. Foods that can create a choking hazard include hot dogs, hard candy, fruit with pits, and large pieces of meat.

18. Examples of some of the characteristics of growth and development for the following ages:
   a. Newborn—adapts to the environment, depends on the caregiver, grows rapidly, lifts the head, looks at people, sleeps a lot
   b. Infant—smiles, responds to and imitates sound, reaches and holds objects, progresses during the stage from rolling to sitting to standing, triples birth weight by 12 months
   c. Toddler—becomes picky about food, demonstrates negativism and ritualism, has improved visual acuity and fine motor skills, walks, talks, throws balls
   d. Preschool—gains about 5 lbs and grows about 3 inches per year, becomes less rounded (toddler shape), draws, prints, dresses self, rides a tricycle, runs, jumps, climbs, plays with others, toilet trained

e. School age—grows at a slower pace, becomes slimmer and more graceful, has more mature body systems and less caloric needs, likes new skills and collecting, plays organized games

f. Adolescent—goes through puberty with all of the associated body changes, has the final growth spurt, body systems grow to adult size, nutritional needs increase, experiences emotional upheaval and peer pressure, wants to fit in, engages in risk behaviors (substance abuse, smoking, unsafe sex), socialization is critical

19. The correct order is d, e, c, b, and a.

20. The nurse reminds the parents to order car seats when renting the car on vacation.

21. Lifestyle risks in the prenatal period can be assessed with questions like: "Do you drink alcohol? If so, how many drinks do you have per week?", "Do you use illegal or street drugs?", "Do you smoke?", and "What kind of activities or hobbies do you do?"

22. Screening tests done are fetal chromosome screening, ultrasound, chorionic villi sampling, amniocentesis, quad screening, blood test for Tay-Sachs, and hemoglobinopathies.

23. Expectations for an infant at 4 to 6 months are c and e.

24. To reduce or eliminate the aggressive behavior, the nurse suggests that the mother reduce the amount of time spent watching TV or playing video games, have the child do other things (music, art, singing), and discuss how there are other options for problem solving (in a way that the child can understand).

25. For an adolescent patient:
    a. The Freudian stage is Genital, which is associated with sexual reawakening and gratification.
    b. The Erikson stage is Identify vs. Role Confusion where the adolescent explores and integrates multiple roles, has emotional fluctuations, and struggles to sort out the identity.
    c. Puberty, with its hormonal changes, brings about the following:
    For females—
    • Breast enlargement
    • Increased height and weight
    • Growth of pubic and axillary hair
    • Menstruation
    In males, changes include:
    • Enlargement of testicles
    • Growth of pubic, axillary, facial, and body hair
    • Rapid increase in height
    • Changes in larynx, causing lowering of the voice
    • Nocturnal emissions
    d. Adolescents face many challenges, which include fitting into peer groups, dealing with physical and emotional changes, dealing with the need to move away from the parents but still needing support, avoiding the temptations of alcohol, smoking and illegal substances, and having safe and satisfying sexual encounters.

26. The expectations for development at age 2 are d, e, and f.

27. The nurse can support ritualistic behavior by finding out what the child usually does at home for meals, hygiene, and bedtime. For example, if the parents read to the child at bedtime at home, this could be something that will help the child to feel more comfortable.

28. An example of magical thinking is hoping that it will rain or become sunny and having that happen. The child then associates the wish with the occurrence. They may blame their illness on something they perceive they did wrong.

29. Besides the physical signs of bruises, burns, scratches, and fractures, the nurse is alert to signs of withdrawal, fear of going home, prior injuries, a vague explanation of how an injury occurred, or no explanation offered at all, an explanation that is inconsistent with the pattern, age, or severity of the injuries or markedly different stories from different witnesses about how an injury occurred.

30. d	36. b	42. b
31. a	37. b	43. d
32. b	38. c	44. c
33. a	39. d	45. c
34. b	40. d	46. d
35. c	41. d	

Practice Situation

a. For this situation, the priority is safety for the two children. Toddlers are curious and can get into dangerous situations by falling and ingesting dangerous substances. The availability of prescription drugs can be a safety hazard for the adolescent. There is also a concern regarding the nutritional intake of the family and how often fast food and bad snacks are consumed.

In the teaching plan, you should include the following information:

Safety—locking cabinets with hazardous materials, objects and medications, placing gates on the stairwells, covering wall sockets, keeping small items and food sources of choking out of reach

Nutrition—using MyPlate guidelines for the children and adults, choosing alternative high-quality, good-tasting snacks

b. You will want to find out the following from the adolescent:
• Self-image—feelings of depression
• Peer group interactions
• Presence of risk behaviors—substance abuse, smoking, unsafe sex practices
• Activities—safe driving/driver's education, bicycle riding with a helmet
• Nutritional intake

CHAPTER 18: HUMAN DEVELOPMENT: YOUNG ADULT THROUGH OLDER ADULT

1. g	5. b	9. c
2. i	6. j	10. e
3. h	7. f	
4. a	8. d	

11. Changes associated with aging are a, b, d, e, and f.

12. Young adults face many challenges, including leaving home, getting an education, finding employment, establishing healthy personal relationships, taking on marital and parental responsibilities, planning for the future, and dealing with physiological concerns from childhood (e.g., obesity, diabetes, eating disorders).

13. Delirium is a transient, usually reversible, cause of cerebral dysfunction (acute confusion), whereas dementia has a gradual onset and is not reversible (chronic confusion).

14. The most common causes of death for older adults are heart disease, cancer, cerebrovascular accident (stroke), lower respiratory disease, pneumonia, influenza, and complications from diabetes mellitus.

15. The accurate statements about older adults are b, c, and f.

16. a. Young adults: 18 to 34 years
    b. Middle adults: 35 to 65 years
    c. Older adults: 66 years +

17.

Theory	Concept(s)
Wear and Tear	The body wears out from hard use. Organs and organ systems are worn down by toxins in the diet and in the environment; by the excessive consumption of fat, sugar, caffeine, alcohol, and nicotine; by the ultraviolet rays of the sun; and by the many other physical and emotional stresses to which the body is subjected.
Cross-Linking Theory	Protein fibers that make up the body's connective tissue form bonds, or links, with one another. When these normally separate fibers cross-link, tissue becomes less elastic, leading to negative outcomes such as loss of flexibility.

18. Emerging adulthood is associated with a much slower transition to adulthood, marked by indecision and lack of commitment to one fixed goal in life. There is a delay in marriage and parenting, extension of education, and job switching.

19. Lifestyle assessment of the young adult should include sexual orientation, safe-sex practices, sexually transmitted diseases (STDs), pregnancy prevention, domestic and intimate partner violence, and substance use and abuse. In addition, identification of other risk behaviors, such as hazardous hobbies and practices (e.g., sunbathing, rock climbing).

20. In addition to those noted, lack of exercise, adequate sleep, and poor dietary habits can have an influence on overall health.

	Developmental tasks	Health risks
Young adult	Establishing healthy interpersonal relationships, succeeding in school, and making their way in the workforce.	Domestic violence, increased alcohol use, illicit drug use, and frequent sexually transmitted diseases.
Middle adult	Reevaluating their lives, looking for meaning in their existence, refining and strengthening their identities, reaching out to younger generations, and making adjustments in their daily lives, their outlook on life, and their goals.	Cancer and cardiovascular disease, along with type 2 diabetes and the beginning of other chronic illnesses.
Older adult	Adjusting to decreasing physical strength and health, retirement and reduced income, death of a spouse, and the processes of establishing an explicit affiliation with their age group, adopting and adapting to social roles in a flexible way, and establishing satisfactory physical living arrangements.	Cardiovascular disease, cancer, stroke. Increased susceptibility to infectious diseases, chronic illnesses—osteoporosis, osteoarthritis, rheumatoid arthritis, chronic obstructive pulmonary disease, hearing and visual alterations, and cognitive dysfunctions such as dementia. Pneumonia, fractures, and trauma from falls and motor vehicle accidents.

21. Screenings should include:
    a. Young adults—Pap smears for sexually active women, breast self-examination, testicular examination, and skin assessment
    b. Middle adults—blood pressure checks, colonoscopies, prostate examinations for men, mammograms and Pap smears for women, and blood work for diabetes
    c. Older adults—blood pressure checks, colonoscopies, prostate exams for men, and mammograms for women, and blood work for diabetes
    Note—screening for mental illness and domestic violence should be done for all ages

22. Exercise helps decrease the risk of heart disease, obesity, diabetes, and cancer. It strengthens the heart, reduces anxiety, improves mood, and enhances overall well-being in individuals.

23. Depression is being seen across the adult life span.

24. The accurate statements about middle adults are a, b, c, e, and f.

25. True

26. Primary prevention for the older adult includes exercise, adequate rest and sleep, good nutrition, positive relationships, leisure activities/hobbies, screenings, vaccinations (flu, pneumonia), and social activity.

27. Signs and symptoms for the following are:
   a. Cardiovascular—chest pain, shortness of breath, palpitations, fatigue, decreased sensation to the extremities, edema, leg pain
   b. Respiratory— dyspnea, shortness of breath, coughing, excess sputum, pallor, fatigue, orthopnea
   c. Endocrine—polyuria, polydipsia, polyphagia, glycosuria, hypo/hyperglycemia, changes in vision or peripheral sensation

28. To assess/respond for domestic violence, the nurse should:
   • Ask about abuse.
   • Identify barriers for detection of abuse.
   • Facilitate screening.
   • Provide training on signs and symptoms and detection of abuse.
   • Provide services.
   • Empower patients.

29. Behaviors associated with anxiety disorders are nervousness, fidgeting, pacing, wringing the hands, talking a lot, or being unable to sit still.

30. To reduce the incidence of the following, the nurse teaches the patient the following:
   a. Sexually transmitted disease (STD)
      • Teach patients the signs and symptoms of common sexually transmitted diseases.
      • Ask patients to verbalize an understanding of the importance of practicing safe sex.
      • Teach patients that latex condoms, when used consistently and correctly, are highly effective in preventing the sexual transmission of HIV, the virus that causes AIDS, and reducing the risk of other STDs, including diseases transmitted by genital secretions and, to a lesser degree, genital ulcer diseases.
      • Demonstrate proper condom application to both males and females, with a return demonstration to assess knowledge.
   b. Cancer—inform patients to:
      • Know the symptoms of cancer.
      • Perform self-examinations.
      • Get regular checkups, screenings, and immunizations.
      • Avoid tobacco, sun exposure, pollutants, and x-ray exposure.
      • Eat a healthy diet and maintain a healthy weight.
      • Drink alcohol only in moderation.
      • Exercise daily.

31. The QSEN competency of teamwork and collaboration is exhibited in the home environment by connecting patients to available services, including skilled nursing care, physical therapy, occupational therapy, and speech-language services, medical social services, and home health aide services. Coordination of health care personnel and services helps to determine that the patient is able to perform ADLs independently. Patient and family education is provided so that proper care continues even when the agency is not present.

32. Recommendations for exercise:
   • Teach patients that most adults need at least 30 minutes of moderate physical activity such as brisk walking or bicycling at least 5 days per week.
   • Encourage patients to find an exercise that they enjoy and to start slowly if they have not been exercising regularly. Walking with a friend or joining a class may help to keep them motivated.
   • Advise patients that adding stretching and weight training to their routine will improve strength and fitness.

33. Respiratory depression occurs with b and d.

34. b	41. d	48. c
35. c	42. b	49. a
36. c	43. b	50. a
37. a	44. a	51. d
38. c	45. b	52. c
39. b	46. d	
40. c	47. d	

Practice Situation

a. Your concerns for this patient center on the need for her to adapt to the new diagnosis of diabetes. She will probably have to incorporate medication (oral or injectable) and/or dietary restrictions. There will be a need for her to establish an exercise plan, foot care, and regular checkups. On top of this, the patient's mother is in a period of rehabilitation and living with the daughter. With the mother, three children, and diabetes, the patient is going to have to deal with a lot.

b. For this situation, you will want to provide support for the middle adult parent who is "sandwiched" between the care of the aging parents and the support and supervision of their children.
   There are going to be considerations for the diabetic care, as well as stress reduction activities. Personal health issues, ongoing responsibility of the mother, respite care needs, and financial concerns will have to be addressed. The children can be brought into the discussion at a level that is understandable and appropriate for their ages. You can help the patient find local support groups or a counselor, if she needs to talk about her issues. Providing information about her care and opportunities for assistance with her family responsibilities is crucial.

CHAPTER 19: VITAL SIGNS

1. d	5. b	9. f
2. a	6. j	10. e
3. g	7. c	
4. i	8. h	

11. The expected vital signs are a, b and f.
12. The apical pulse is found at the fifth intercostal space at the midclavicular line.
13. Tachycardia can be caused by c, d, and e.

14.

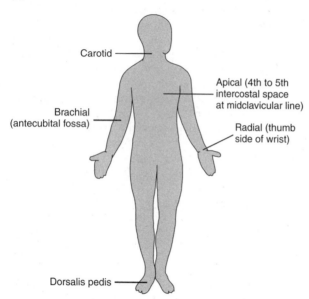

Carotid

Apical (4th to 5th
intercostal space
at midclavicular line)

Brachial
(antecubital fossa)

Radial (thumb
side of wrist)

Dorsalis pedis

15.

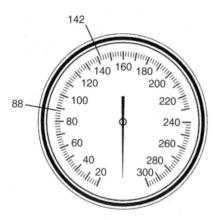

16. The blood pressure should not be monitored on the upper extremities, but the legs can be used (popliteal artery).
17. The accuracy of pulse oximetry can be affected by cold or injured extremities, peripheral edema, jaundice, movement where the sensor is attached, shivering, and some types of nail polish.
18. The signs of a fever include b, d, and f.
19. The tympanic thermometer is used on an adult by pulling the pinna of the ear up and back, placing the covered probe snugly into the ear canal, and angling it toward the jaw line before activating. If the patient has been lying down, use the ear that has not been against the pillow.
20. Examples of nursing diagnoses, goals, and interventions include:
    a. Hyperthermia
       Goal—Patient will exhibit temperature within normal range 1 hour after receiving antipyretic medication.
       Intervention—Administration of acetaminophen per order
    b. Ineffective breathing pattern.
       Goal—Patient will exhibit regular respiratory rate and depth after nebulizer treatment.

Intervention—Assess respiratory function after respiratory therapist provides treatment.
21. The correct statements about the pulse are a, d, e, and f.
22. Rectal temperatures are contraindicated for newborns and patients with neutropenia, spinal cord injuries, diarrhea, rectal disease/surgery, and quadriplegia.
23. Vital sign measurement is usually done every 4 to 8 hours for stable patients.
24. Hypoventilation is associated with drug overdose, obesity, COPD, and cervical spine injury.
25. An electronic device should not be used for patients with low blood pressure, irregular heart rates, shivering, or seizure activity.
26. Some general guidelines include making sure that the equipment is functioning correctly, accurate skills are used, changes in patient findings are compared and reported, measurements are conducted as often as needed and appropriate to the patient's condition, factors are considered that may alter the readings; only delegating when the patient is stable; and ensuring the environment is conducive to privacy and hearing.
27. The assessment of a patient's pain includes SOCRATES—site, onset, character, radiation, associated signs and symptoms, time pattern, exacerbating/relieving factors, and severity.
28. Examples of nonverbal indications of pain are grimacing, pulling away from touch, changes in vital signs, agitation, and restlessness.
29. The temporal artery measurement is taken in the center of the forehead and then moved across to the hairline by the temple. If there is perspiration present, the probe should be touched to the skin behind the earlobe over the mastoid process.
30. Irregular and apical pulses are counted for a minute (60 seconds).
31. The correct order for the pulse oximetry steps are e, d, a, f, b, and c.
32. The popliteal pulse is used for the measurement.
33. The correct order for the two-step blood pressure is e, c, a, d, f, b, and g.
34. The nurse needs to apply a small amount of special gel to the skin or the tip of the ultrasound probe in order to transmit and amplify the sound waves.
35. The nurse advises the patient to:
    • Dress in layers, even while at home. Long underwear may be worn under clothing, along with socks and slippers.
    • Use a blanket or afghan to keep legs and shoulders warm.
    • When outside in cold weather, wear a scarf and gloves. A hat is especially important to maintain body heat.
    • Keep extremities covered to prevent heat loss.
    • Keep the thermostat at a minimum of 68° F.
36. For a dual-head stethoscope:
    a. Antimicrobial wipes can be used before and after use. It cannot be sterilized with steam heat and should not be submerged in water.
    b. Higher-pitched sounds are best heard with the diaphragm of the stethoscope.
37. True

38. Orthostatic hypotension is assessed by measuring the patient's blood pressure in the supine, sitting, and standing positions, immediately after the patient changes position.

39. c	47. a	55. c
40. c	48. c	56. b
41. d	49. d	57. d
42. a	50. a	58. c
43. d	51. c.	59. b
44. c	52. b	60. c
45. b	53. b	61. a
46. b	54. c	

Practice Situation

For the Conceptual Care Map, information is documented as follows:
Admission Diagnoses/Chief Complaint
Shortness of breath, dizziness, green-tinged sputum, and pain with deep inspiration. He started sleeping with two pillows 2 nights ago to ease his breathing.
Assessment Data
T 38.89° C (102° F), P 104 regular, R 32 and shallow and labored, BP 160/94, SaO2 89% on RA, and chest pain of 5 out of 10 with deep breathing.
Barrel-shaped chest, crackles bilaterally, diminished lung sounds in the left lower lobe, pedal pulses not palpable—heard on Doppler, and 3+ pedal edema.
Exhibits dyspnea on exertion and when lying flat and use of accessory muscles to breathe.
15-pound weight gain noted as compared with finding at outpatient clinic obtained 1 week ago.
Braden score =17, Morse Fall Scale score = 48.
Treatments
• VS q4h with pulse oximetry
• Fluid restriction of 1200 mL per 24 hours
• No-added-salt diet
• Up with assistance; fall precautions
• Intake and output
• Titrate O_2 up to 4 L to keep SaO$_2$ ≥ 92%
• Incentive spirometer (IS) and coughing and deep breathing (CDB) q2h
Lab Values/Test Results
Chest radiograph shows pneumonia and exacerbation of heart failure.
Arterial blood gas report pending.
Serum K = 3.0 mEq/L and WBCs = 19,000. UA ordered—has not voided.
Past Medical History
Hypertension, high cholesterol, heart failure. Smoked one pack/day x 30 years (quit 20 years ago)
Medications
• Digoxin 0.125 mg PO q day
• Furosemide to 40 mg IV q day
• KCl 40 mEq PO q day
• Levofloxin 750 mg IV q24h x 5 days

CHAPTER 20: HEALTH HISTORY AND PHYSICAL ASSESSMENT

1. a. Alopecia: Permanent or temporary hair loss
   b. Atelectasis: Collapse of all or part of the lung
   c. Bruit: Abnormal swooshing sound
   d. Cerumen: Ear wax
   e. Diplopia: Double vision
   f. Ecchymosis: Bruising
   g. Erythema: Redness of the skin
   h. Jaundice: Yellowish discoloration of the skin, mucous membranes or eyes
   i. Paresthesia: Numbness or tingling
   j. Pruritus: Itching
   k. Tortuosity: Bending and twisting
   l. Vertigo: Disequilibrium, spinning sensation
2. The nurse should provide privacy, ensure a comfortable room temperature, warm the equipment, position the patient comfortably when sitting and laying down, maintain a relaxed atmosphere, and reduce or eliminate distractions.
3. A third person can be present in the room if the patient requests someone else to be there, there is a need for maintaining patient or nurse safety, or the nurse is a different gender than the patient.
4. a. The statement by the nurse may communicate disinterest and the need to get through the examination quickly.
   b. The nurse can take the topic(s) that the patient is talking about and create a question that will direct Mrs. J. back to the interview/examination.
5. a. Vital signs
   Sphygmomanometer with cuff
   Stethoscope with bell and diaphragm
   Thermometer
   Wristwatch
   Pulse oximeter
   b. Oral exam
   Flashlight or penlight
   Tongue depressor
   Gloves
   2 × 2 gauze
   c. Weber test—tuning fork
6. The positions are:
   a. Sitting
   b. Prone
   c. Lithotomy
   d. Supine
7. a. Inspection involves the use of vision and smell to closely scrutinize physical characteristics of a whole person and individual body systems.
   b. Palpation uses touch to assess body organs and skin texture, temperature, moisture, turgor, tenderness, and thickness.
   c. Percussion is an advanced practice examination technique used to assess body tissues and structures. Percussion involves tapping the patient's skin with short, sharp strokes that cause a vibration to travel through the skin and to the upper layers of the underlying structures.
   d. Auscultation is the technique of listening to sounds made by body organs or systems such as the heart, blood

179

vessels, lungs, and abdominal cavity, with and without the assistance of a stethoscope.

For the abdominal assessment, the order of techniques is inspection, auscultation, palpation, then percussion.

8. The nurse should make sure that the diaphragm or bell of the stethoscope is in contact with the skin, ask patients or visitors to refrain from talking, turn down/off TVs and radios, or obtain an amplified stethoscope.

9. The general survey includes age, race, sex and gender orientation, appearance, affect and mood, safety concerns, substance abuse/use, speech, gait, VS, height, and weight.

10. The nurse should obtain and wear gloves for assessment where there is an open lesion.

11. The expected findings on the skin are c, d, and f.

12. The skin lesions are:
   a. Macule/Patch: Flat, not detectable with palpation, changes in color, and < 1 cm. A macule that is > 1 cm is called a patch.
   b. Nodule: This is a raised solid mass with defined borders that extends into the dermis or beyond. It is deeper and more solid than a papule, generally 0.5 to 2 cm.
   c. Papule/Plaque: A solid, raised lesion with distinct borders that present in a variety of shapes including domed, flat-topped, and umbilicated. These are often associated with secondary features such as crusts or scales and are < 0.5 cm. A papule that is > 0.5 cm is referred to as *plaque*.
   d. Wheal: Irregularly shaped area of edema caused by serous fluid in the dermis that varies in color and size.

13. The accurate statements about palpation are b, d, e, and f.

14. The expected findings for the hair and nails are a and b.

15. Changes in hair growth are usually associated with poor nutrition, circulatory insufficiency, hormonal imbalance, chemotherapy, and overuse of dyes/rinses.

16. Examples of areas assessed in the head include positioning of the head, presence of any tremors or tics, contour of the skull, presence of lesions or growths, positioning of the nose, ears, eyes and mouth, and shape and function of the jaw.

17. The expected finding for the eyes is f.

18. The nurse suspects that the patient has ingested an opioid or a medication for glaucoma.

19. PERRLA—pupils equal, round, reactive to light, and accommodation

20. For assessment of visual acuity:
   a. For near vision, have the patient read printed material. If the patient wears glasses, have them worn during the examination. Have the patient stand 20 feet away from the chart.
   b. 20/100 means that this patient can read at 20 feet what the average person can read at 100 feet.
   c. For a patient who does not read English, an E chart can be used.

21. For the nose and ears, the unexpected findings are a, e, and f.

22. For the Romberg test, the nurse should tell the patient to open the eyes if they feel a loss of balance and the nurse should also "spot" the patient in case the patient actually starts to fall.

23. For the mouth, throat, and neck, the unexpected findings are c, e, and f.

24. The carotid arteries are inspected to see if a pulse is visible, palpated one at a time to prevent occlusion, and then auscultated to listen for bruits.

25.

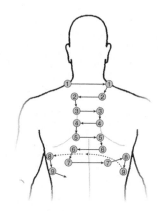

26. For the thoracic assessment, the expected findings are a, b, d, and f.

27.

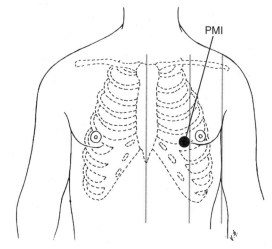

28. Unexpected cardiac-related findings for an over 30-year-old adult are murmurs, thrills, S3 and S4 sounds, friction rubs, clicks, bruit over abdominal aorta, and pulse deficit.

29. A peripheral pulse that is faint but detectable is documented as 1+.

30. For determination of phlebitis: Inspection for heat, swelling, redness and tenderness, along with measuring the circumference of each calf.

31. The pulses being assessed are:
   a. Ulnar
   b. Posterior tibial
   c. Femoral
   d. Brachial
   e. Dorsalis pedis

32. The Allen test is used to evaluate for collateral circulation to determine the patency of the arteries of the hand before arterial blood tests. The Allen test is performed by having the patient elevate the extremity and make a fist. The examiner occludes the radial and ulnar arteries, using pressure. The hand should lose color. The patient then opens the fist, and the pressure is released from the ulnar artery. The normal pink color should return to the hand within 10 seconds, showing good circulation.

33. The first clinical signs of osteoporosis are sudden and severe loss of height and back pain.

34. For the musculoskeletal assessment, unexpected findings are a and d.

35. The Glasgow Coma Scale score is = 13. This is not within normal limits.

36. The questions are:
    - Person: "What is your name?"
    - Place: "Where are you?"
    - Time: "Do you know what day, month, season, and year it is?"
    - Situation: "Can you tell me what happened or what brought you to the hospital?"

37. Long-term memory can be tested by asking the patient to repeat three words or numbers used earlier in the assessment.

38. The notation should be in the lower area on the left hand side of the graphic (this is the right-hand side for anatomic position).

39. For the abdominal assessment, the expected findings are b and d.

40. The nurse should wear gloves for palpation of the mucous membranes and work from front to back.

41. For male and female genital examinations, the expected findings are a, e, and f.

42. Available public and home health services generally include immunizations, environmental surveillance, medical equipment, and medication delivery.

43. Prevention strategies to be taught to the patient include:
    a. Cataracts:
       - Wear sunglasses and hats when outside.
       - Quit smoking and limit alcohol consumption.
       - Increase intake of vitamins E and B.
    b. Glaucoma:
       - Having regular eye examinations by an ophthalmologist.
       - Wearing protective eyewear at work, during construction projects, or while participating in sports to prevent injury.
       - Limiting caffeine intake, increasing water consumption.
       - Engaging in regular physical exercise.

44. Breast cancer risk reduction includes exercise, limit to one glass of alcohol/day, and a low-fat diet with more fruits and vegetables.

45. If the patient begins to experience respiratory distress, the nurse should stop the examination, sit the patient up, apply oxygen if available, and call for help.

46. a	54. d	62. a
47. c	55. d	63. c
48. d	56. c	64. b
49. d	57. a	65. a
50. b	58. b	66. a
51. a	59. c	67. d
52. c	60. b	68. d
53. c	61. a	

Practice Situations

For the Conceptual Care Map:
- Possible nursing diagnoses—Activity Intolerance, Decreased Cardiac Output, Excess Fluid Volume
- Expected treatments—Vital signs, leg elevation, medications—diuretic and cardiac (e.g., Lasix and digoxin), oxygen prn, periods of rest and activity

For the patient who comes to the clinic and answers "yes" to these questions, the follow-up should be to ask for more details about the problem and:
- Inspecting and palpating the eye, doing a visual acuity test, and checking relevant cranial nerve function.
- Inspecting and palpating the oral mucosa and gums and inquiring about medications, dental care, and nutritional intake.
- Performing a respiratory assessment, vital signs, instructing the patient about the hazards of smoking, and referring him or her to supportive resources.
- Inspecting and palpating the abdomen (distended bladder) and the urethral meatus, informing the provider so that laboratory tests can be ordered, and instructing the patient on perineal hygiene.

CHAPTER 21: ETHNICITY AND CULTURAL ASSESSMENT

1. g	5. j	9. i
2. e	6. a	10. h
3. f	7. d	
4. b	8. c	

11. Culture refers to the learned, shared, and transmitted knowledge of values, beliefs, and ways of life of a particular group that are generally transmitted from one generation to another and influence the individual's thinking, decisions, and actions in patterned or certain ways (Leininger). Ethnicity is the individual's identification with or membership in a particular racial, national, or cultural group and observation of the group's customs, beliefs, and language. Ethnicity is based on cultural similarities and differences within a society or nation.

12. Culturally competent care is a complex integration of an individual's knowledge, attitudes, beliefs, skills, and encounters with those of persons from different cultures. To reach cultural competence, one has to engage in a cultural self-assessment.

13. True

14. a. Learned—Culture is passed on through attributes that one acquires by growing up in a particular society and being exposed to traditions. Enculturation begins at birth as parents and other family members begin to teach the child what is expected in terms of familial responsibilities and contributions. This learning process occurs consciously and unconsciously through interactions with other family and community members.
    b. Symbolic—There are signs, sounds, clothing, tools, customs, beliefs, rituals, and other items that represent meaningful concepts. Language is the most important symbolic aspect of culture.

c. Shared—Culture is an attribute of members of a group, not just individuals. People who grow up in a particular culture often have shared values, beliefs, ideals, and expectations. These shared attributes are absorbed and transmitted through generations of teaching and sharing ideas, traditions, and rituals.

d. Integrated—Cultures are integrated, patterned systems. The foundation of culture includes three structural elements that work together to keep the culture strong: An infrastructure provides the basic necessities of life; a social structure determines how people interact with one another; and a superstructure, or worldview, provides a belief system that helps people identify themselves, their society, and the world around them.

15. Stereotypes can lead to false opinions, perceptions, or beliefs and they are developed when there is an unwillingness to obtain all of the information necessary to make fair judgments about particular individuals or situations. In the absence of confirmed knowledge, stereotypes allow individuals to make unfounded assumptions, lead to discrimination, and result in the provision of unequal care.

16. Discrimination can be seen in the harsher treatment that minorities may face from law enforcement agencies or the judicial system. Historically, it was seen by segregation in the United States and apartheid in South Africa. There are also instances in society of discrimination against those with nonheterosexual preferences, women, and disabled individuals.

17. Symbolic characteristics of community include sharing a specific dialect or language, lifestyle, history, art, dress, or music.

18. Schools are places where a society's cultural values, traditions, and official heritage are taught. The school curriculum can reinforce what is learned in the family, but it can also challenge family socialization.

19. Rituals can sustain and provide support for patients during a time of illness or suffering. In caring for patients, nurses need to be aware of their own beliefs and feelings regarding certain rituals, as well as understand how these rituals may affect their patients and families.

20. The goal of transcultural nursing is to provide culturally congruent care, identifying cultures that are neglected or misunderstood, and using knowledge to be creative, sensitive, and safe.

21. CLAS refers to national Culturally and Linguistically Appropriate Standards (CLAS) from the U.S. Department of Health and Human Services, which identify methods for providing culturally competent care and guidelines for their implementation. The standards address language access, organizational support, diverse and culturally competent staff, existing laws, data collection, and information dissemination.

22. The nurse brings the following into the patient relationship: the first culture of the personal self, the second culture of the health care delivery system, and the third culture of the patient.

23. Available assessment tools include Leininger's Transcultural Theory and Assessment Model (the first tool developed), Giger and Davidhizar Transcultural Assessment Model, and the 4 C's of Culture mnemonic.

24. When assessing a dark-skinned patient for oxygenation, it is important to examine the least pigmented areas, such as the buccal mucosa, lips, tongue, nail beds, and palms of the hand. Do not rely on the skin tone alone. Establish a baseline skin color by assessing a patient in direct sunlight or by asking family members.

25. The correct responses for present time orientation are c, d, and f.

26. The following are influenced by cultural background as follows:

a. Hygienic care—Patients may have preferences for the frequency of hygienic care, preference for a same gender care giver, particular soaps/lotions, and showers or baths.

b. Nutrition—Individuals from different cultures have different preferences for food types. They may also have financial constraints that restrict the type of food that may be purchased. Celebrations can be associated with particular food choices as well.

27. Purnell (2012) identified that culture has three levels: (1) At the tertiary level, culture is visible to outsiders and is reflected in things that can be seen, worn, or otherwise observed; (2) at the secondary level, members of a particular group know the rules of behavior and can articulate them; and (3) at the primary level, the group rules are known by all, observed by all, implicit, and taken for granted.

28. True

29. False

30. For a person who comes from a different country and speaks a different language, strategies include:
- Arranging for a professional interpreter to be available by phone in challenging situations.
- Identifying community agencies that work specifically with people of the patient's culture.
- Seeking social service care from a specialist who speaks the patient's language.

31. The nurse should assess the patient's language preference; race; ethnicity; and cultural, spiritual, and religious beliefs. Dietary needs and restrictions are to be assessed and documented in the electronic health record.

32. Cultural beliefs can become challenges to health care delivery when patients are hesitant to seek medical care because of fear, distrust of professionals, learned practices, and fatalistic attitudes. There are also challenges to meet patients' needs for cultural rituals, nutritional preferences, time orientation, and communication.

33. Important aspects of nursing care for culturally diverse individuals are to recognize the nurse's own cultural beliefs, demonstrate respect for patients and their cultures, use knowledge of different cultures, make the patient a part of the care, be creative in communication, and verify preferences, beliefs, and practices.

34. The correct questions for assessment of a patient's space needs and time orientation are d, e, and f

35. The 4 C's of Culture are:
- What do you call your problem?
- What do you think caused your problem?
- How do you cope with your condition?
- What are your concerns regarding the condition and/or recommended treatment?

36. The accurate statements are b, c, d, and f.

37. d	40. c	43. d
38. c	41. b	
39. a	42. c	

Practice Situation

a. While Mr. R. is receiving emergency treatment, communication with him needs to be with gestures, showing him the equipment and reinforcing the care with touch (e.g., holding his hand) and eye/facial contact. Continuing to explain what is happening calmly, even though he may not fully understand, will reinforce that things are being done to help him.

b. As soon as Mr. R. is physically stable, it is important to obtain a translator so that he can be better informed about his condition and treatment.

CHAPTER 22: SPIRITUAL HEALTH

1. Spirituality and religion are complementary yet distinctly different concepts. Spirituality focuses broadly on the meaning of life, death, and existence, while religion is an organized, structured method of practicing or expressing one's spirituality.

2. Spiritual practices promote connecting with oneself through reflection, others through relationships, and a higher power through faith.

3. Examples of rituals associated with religions are baptism, marriage, funerals, communion, and confirmation.

4. The accurate statements about Hinduism are b, e, and f.

5. Actions that the nurse may implement to assist the patient are referring the patient to a chaplain or spiritual advisor, baptizing an at-risk infant in an emergency, praying with patients at their request, and respecting the rituals that the patient needs to integrate into their day.

6. Parish nurses come from many faith traditions, including Jewish Congregational Nurses, Muslim Crescent Nurses, and registered nurses working within a wide variety of Christian traditions. Some roles of a parish nurse are health adviser, health educator, advocate, liaison to faith and community resources, coordinator of volunteers, and developer of support groups. Parish nurses seek to provide holistic care by focusing on the mind, body, and spirit in addition to community wellness. Parish nursing was designated as a specialty by the ANA in 1997.

7. Patients express spiritual needs using both verbal and nonverbal cues. In many cases, patients express spiritual distress through anger, depression, neediness, or crying. Nurses need to be attentive to the patient's health care situation and behavior to determine whether spiritual care is necessary.

   Nurses should be observant of potential religious needs. To promote spiritual health, nurses must be attentive to these verbal, nonverbal, environmental, and situational patient cues indicating a need for spiritual care and must recognize the patient's spiritual or religious orientation.

8. Nursing interventions for spiritual issues include:
   • Allow time and opportunity for self-disclosure by the patient.
   • Be physically present and actively listen when the patient speaks.
   • Support avenues to spiritual growth that are meaningful to the patient, such as praying, meditating, listening to music, viewing or creating art, or reading or writing poetry.
   • Arrange for regular visits from religious advisers.
   • Refer the patient to the agency chaplain, if available.
   • Monitor and promote supportive social contacts.
   • Integrate the family into spiritual practices, as appropriate.
   • Avoid sharing personal beliefs that are in direct conflict with those of the patient.
   • Refer the patient to or arrange for the patient to engage in a support group or counseling, as appropriate.

9. Nurses can attend to their own spiritual health by reflecting, which can be facilitated by journaling, quiet time, gardening, music, artwork, exercise, or prayer and meditation. Reflecting on a patient-nurse encounter can transform a sad, spiritually distressing encounter into a positive spiritual memory, thereby facilitating spiritual growth.

10. The acronym SPIRIT represents:
    S: spiritual belief system
    P: personal spirituality
    I: integration and involvement in a spiritual community
    R: ritualized practices and restrictions
    I: implications for medical care
    T: terminal-events planning (advance directives)

11. The environmental and situational spiritual cues include:
    a. Environmental—The patient has religious objects, books, or jewelry and displays family pictures.
    b. Situational—The patient is informed of a life-threatening diagnosis or life-changing condition or is facing death or treatment decisions.

12. b	15. a	18. c
13. d	16. c	19. b
14. b	17. d	20. a

Practice Situation

Examples include:

Nursing Diagnosis—Moral Distress related to conflict between accepting medical treatment and religious beliefs as evidenced by expressions of concern about rejection by parents and religious community.

Goal/Outcome—Patient will indicate acceptance of medical interventions by second clinic visit.

Patient will discuss treatment choices.

Interventions—Allow time for the patient to express her feelings, investigate support groups or individuals who have experienced similar conflicts, assist the patient in role-playing any discussions she may want to have with her family, be an advocate for her decision.

Note—You may want to obtain permission and refer the patient to the chaplain or another advisor. The patient may not be comfortable discussing her choices with an advisor from her own faith. You will need to determine how the patient wants to proceed.

CHAPTER 23: PUBLIC HEALTH, COMMUNITY-BASED, AND HOME HEALTH CARE

1. b
2. d
3. e
4. a
5. c
6. Public health nurses are required to coordinate services, provide health education, promote healthy lifestyles, consult with government officials, and participate in regulatory activities. Public health nursing focuses on disease prevention, health protection, and health promotion within identified populations.
7. Public health focuses on populations, whereas community-based nursing provides personal care to individuals or families.
8. The social determinants of health are income, education, health literacy, residence, place of employment, early childhood development, social exclusion, family structure, status and role of women, and vaccination compliance.
9. The role of the community-based nurse includes advocating for clients, conducting routine check-ups, caring for the sick, providing client education, and managing chronic client conditions at outpatient, community, or government health care facilities, as well as providing home care, which includes coordinating multidisciplinary health care teams for client care.
10. Used syringes and needles could be discarded into empty soda bottles, plastic closable containers, or metal boxes (e.g., round cookie container).
11. The skilled nursing interventions are b, c, and f.
12. Home health services are funded through Medicare, Medicaid, and private health insurance.
13. End-of-life care for terminally ill patients is called hospice or palliative care.
14. An example for each of the following levels of health care prevention is:
    a. Primary prevention—employee wellness programs, fitness classes, nutrition education, safety workshops
    b. Secondary prevention—health screenings, special diets to treat problems
    c. Tertiary prevention—blood glucose monitoring, follow-up laboratory studies, medication education
15. Examples of intrinsic factors are b, c, and e.
16. Vulnerable populations include:
    - Refugees and immigrants
    - Individuals who have experienced a natural or man-made disaster, such as an earthquake or a terrorist attack
    - Military personnel and veterans
    - Workers exposed to chemicals or radiation
    - Homeless persons or families
    - Minority groups within a larger population, including members of various cultural, racial, religious, age, and gender groups that may be denied equal services on the basis of their differences from the general population
    - Mentally ill and disabled individuals
    - Substance abusers or those with severe chronic illnesses
    - Emotionally, physically, or sexually abused or neglected individuals
    - Age-related populations such as the very young, adolescents, or elderly persons
    - International foreign travelers
17. Available online resources include the following sites:
    a. Centers for Disease Control (www.cdc.gov)
    b. U.S. census data (www.census.gov)
18. A windshield survey includes observations by the community or public health nurse on the following:
    - Whether people are walking or engaged in physical activity.
    - Whether there are single- or multiple-family private and public housing units in good or poor repair.
    - Whether health, safety, and social services agencies are available and are located along a bus or public transportation line.
    - Spiritual or religious places of worship, educational institutions, and news and media services, types of open and closed businesses and industries.
    - Availability of grocery stores.
    - The general climate.
19. Assessment areas on the OASIS form include:
    - Current and past medical and surgical histories
    - Influenza and pneumococcal vaccination status
    - Living arrangements and activities-of-daily-living capability
    - Sensory status and neurologic, emotional, and behavioral status
    - Integumentary status
    - Respiratory and cardiac status
    - Elimination status
    - Medication regimen and client and caregiver understanding of required medications and schedule
    - Therapy needs and schedule
    - Hospitalizations, including admission and discharge plans from inpatient facilities or agencies
    - Plan of care management
20. The stakeholders are the community residents, service providers (e.g., police, fire department, schools) and politicians.
21. A nursing diagnosis could be Deficient Community Health related to increased risk of transmission of disease as evidenced by a nonpurified water source.
22. Readability levels can be assessed with tools, such as the Fry readability formula, which is based on the number of syllables and sentences in 100-word passages or other online tools that assess grammar and word usage.
23. For the QSEN competency of teamwork and collaboration, the nurse may interact with one or more of the following individuals:
    - Nurse educators
    - Exercise physiologists
    - Administrators of child and adult day care centers
    - Primary health care providers
    - Visiting nurse association representatives and leaders
    - Public officials, including governors, mayors, and council members
    - City parks and recreation department officials

- Community hospital administrators and staff
- Public health department officials
- Media outlets (television, radio, newspaper, and online resources, including social media sites)

24. This patient is at the tertiary level of prevention.
25. c
26. d
27. b
28. a

Practice Situation

a. For this patient, your primary concerns are related to her safety within her home and prevention of medical complications. Issues include:
   Possible falls—wooden floors with throw rugs that may not be secure, clutter around the floor, dim lighting in the bathroom
   Burns—a water temperature that is too hot
   Medication dosage errors— inconsistent amount of medication in the bottles
   Medical complications— inconsistent medication administration, frozen meals (usually high in salt and fat content), nutritional insufficiency
b. This patient may benefit from a homemaker to assist with daily activities, like meal preparation and cleanup. If that is not feasible, you will want to see if there are family members to help the patient with shopping, meals, and cleaning. A referral to Meals-on-Wheels can be made. For the medications, there are containers that are labeled for the days of the week and the medications can be placed in one of these to make sure that the correct daily dosages are administered. Lighting can be addressed by checking the wattage of the bulb(s) in the bathroom and having the patient/agency get a more effective light source. There are resources available to assist community residents in obtaining supplies, like smoke detectors.

CHAPTER 24: HUMAN SEXUALITY

1. c	5. j	9. g
2. d	6. h	10. f
3. b	7. a	
4. i	8. e	

11. Methods of contraception are:
    a. Barrier—condoms, spermicidal products
    b. Prescriptive—hormonal (birth control pill, transdermal patch, subdermal implant, vaginal ring), IUD, cervical cap, diaphragm, surgery
    c. Sterilization—tubal ligation, vasectomy
12. Infertility occurs when a couple has not conceived after 12 months of contraceptive-free intercourse for a female younger than age 34 or after 6 months if the female is older than age 35.
13. Areas of concern to sexual education include contraception, unwanted pregnancy, STDs, HIV, sexual abuse, and sexual orientation.

14. Factors that can affect gender identification are family experiences and values, association with or lack of a relationship with the same-sex parent, parental identification of gender from birth, self-concept, and confidence about one's sexuality.
15. a. Possible signs and symptoms of STDs include genital discharge or sores, burning and pain on urination, and CNS manifestations (late-stage syphilis).
    b. Abstinence and the use of condoms reduces the risk of disease transmission.
    c. HIV can also be transmitted through IV needles and transfusion of infected blood products.
16. a. Chronic disease—decreased intimacy, personal stress and/or stress with partner, reduction in the frequency of sexual relations
    b. Work issues—fatigue, decreased intimacy, personal stress and/or stress with partner, reduction in the frequency or satisfaction of sexual relations
    c. Poor body image—lack of intimacy, personal stress, changes in frequency or satisfaction of sexual relations
17. The accurate statements for older adults are a, e, and f.
18. PLISSIT stands for:
    P: obtaining permission from the patient to initiate sexual discussion.
    LI: providing the limited information needed to function sexually.
    SS: giving specific suggestions for the individual to proceed with sexual relations.
    IT: providing intensive therapy surrounding the issues of sexuality for the patient.
19. In the sexual history, the following should also be included: The patient's past and current health and sexual practices, as well as medications that may impact sexual function, the reproductive history, STD history, sexual dysfunction history, sexual health self-care practices, frequency and technique of breast self-examination (BSE) and/or testicular self-examination (TSE), and sexual identity, self-concept, and self-esteem.
20. a. Culture and religious beliefs influence family structure, roles within the family, who the dominant figure is within that structure, and how and whether sexuality is displayed. Guilt and resentment may result from cultural or religious constraints.
    Nursing—Be knowledgeable about cultural and religious variances and expressions of sexuality. Remain nonjudgmental. Teach this information to patients and families.
    b. Environment—Privacy may be an essential element for both sexual discussion and sexual activity.
    Nursing—Comply with all privacy guidelines. Respect the patient. Provide a nonjudgmental environment.
21. Medications that can influence sexual function include anticonvulsants, antidepressants, antihistamines, antihypertensives, antipsychotics, antispasmodics, and narcotics.
22. For SANE and SART:
    a. They collect DNA evidence, seminal fluid evidence, physical injury evidence, blood and urine evidence, and genital-trauma evidence.

b. They provide education and information about STIs, prophylactic treatment against pregnancy, crisis intervention, and comfort measures (bathing, clean clothes, call to family/friends, shelters)

23. The accurate statements about domestic violence are b, c, d, and f.

24. a	27. c	30. a
25. c	28. d	31. d
26. d	29. b	

Practice Situations

a. You will need to bring the patient to a private area to conduct a screening, which will need to include questions about the abuse, the abuser, frequency (cycle of violence), and injuries received. A plan should be developed with the patient for her safety. Emotional support and a nonjudgmental attitude are important.

b. Resources to share with the patient include the addresses and phone numbers of womens' shelters, crisis centers, and local police and emergency services.

For Mr. Wells, the patient in the chapter's case study, the data in the conceptual care map will be:

Admission: Hypertension, mild congestive heart failure

Assessment: BP = 148/86, P = 78, regular & strong, R = 16, eupneic

No health restrictions

States concern over erectile dysfunction (ED)

Medications: ASA 325 mg PO daily, furosemide 20 mg daily, lisinopril 10 mg bid

Laboratory tests: CBC, PSA, urinalysis—results pending

Primary nursing diagnosis: Sexual Dysfunction related to antihypertensive and possible anxiety over ability to perform as manifested by inability to achieve an erection.

Short-term goal: Patient will request further information about ED at next clinic visit.

CHAPTER 25: SAFETY

1. Unintentional injuries result from incidents such as falls, motor vehicle crashes, poisonings, drownings, fire-associated injuries, suffocation by ingested objects, and firearms.

2. The 2014 National Patient Safety Goals are to:
   - Identify patients correctly.
   - Improve staff communication.
   - Use medicines safely.
   - Use alarms safely.
   - Prevent infection.
   - Identify patient safety risks.
   - Prevent mistakes in surgery.

3. a. Musculoskeletal function—Restrictions in range of motion and diminished strength can lead to subsequent loss of balance and unsteady gait. These changes can affect overall mobility, including the ability to transfer, stand, and walk. With limitations in mobility, the propensity for falling is increased.

   b. Neurologic function—Changes in mental status can occur, judgment may become altered, and safety awareness may become compromised. With an alteration in any of the five senses (vision, hearing, touch, smell, taste), a variety of safety risks may result, such as an inability to smell smoke or hear an alarm.

4. Information for infant safety should include placing infants on their backs for sleep, never leaving the baby unattended, correctly using rear-facing car seats and carriers, obtaining approved cribs and toys, childproofing the home, keeping small objects and dangerous substances out of reach, fencing swimming pools, and never leaving children in a car alone.

5. a. Lighting—To safely and successfully navigate pathways and perform various activities while avoiding potential obstacles and hazards, the environment must be well illuminated. Well-lit, glare-free halls, stairways, rooms, and work spaces help to reduce the risk of tripping, slipping, and falling. Night-lights reduce the risk of injuries to children, guests, and older adults.

   b. Workplace hazards—Depending on the occupation, individuals may be exposed to chemicals, fumes, dust, body fluids, repetitive motion, heavy lifting, falls, crushing injuries, needle-sticks, cuts, abrasions, and loss of body parts.

6. Safety hazards in the home include unsafe cooking or storage of foods; transportation injuries (cars, motorcycles, bicycles); electrical equipment; tools; fire; gas; and water (slippery floors, pools). Falls on slippery floors or from the use of ladders/stepstools can occur.

7. Unintentional poisoning can result from the ingestion of chemicals, cleaners, medications, plants, lead, and carbon monoxide.

8. Electrical shock can occur from a, c, e, and f.

9. Common agents for bioterrorism are anthrax and smallpox.

10. Suffocation can result from drowning, choking, and smothering.

11. Safety concerns for older adults include b, d, e, and f.

12. Adolescents are susceptible to the hazards of substance abuse, psychologic issues (e.g., depression), sexually related activities, motor vehicle accidents, and overexposure to TV and Internet.

13. True

14. Negative outcomes from restraint use include compromised circulation, impaired skin and tissue integrity, incontinence, mental status changes, difficulty breathing, pneumonia, impaired hydration and nutrition, aspiration, strangulation, entrapment, muscle atrophy, reduced bone mass, contracture, fractures, and death.

15. Medication errors can be avoided by carefully checking in accordance with the Six Rights, communicating with colleagues, and verifying orders with the providers. Special care must be taken with sound-alike or similarly spelled medications. In addition, identifying the patient (procedural safety) is crucial!

16. Nurses are exposed to radiation when patients are receiving treatments or having diagnostic tests, such as PET or CT scans.

17. The nurse can ask the patient:
    For fire hazards:
    - Do you have adequate outlets for all of your appliances and electronic devices?
    - Do you check for frays or loose wires on electrical cords?
    - Are your appliances working properly and grounded?
    - Do you have smoke detectors? A fire extinguisher? An evacuation plan in case of a fire?
    - How do you heat your home?
    - Do you use an oven and stove?
    - Do you smoke, or does anyone in your home smoke?

    For falls:
    - Have tripping and falling hazards been removed, such as electric cords in walking areas? Clutter on the floor? Toys? Do area rugs have rug pads beneath them?
    - Is there adequate lighting in hallways and on the stairs?
    - Do you have night-lights?
    - If there are children in the house, are gates installed in doorways and at the top and bottom of stairs?
    - Are there handrails on the stairs?
    - Are there grab bars in the bathroom? Is there a rubber mat in the tub and on the shower floor?

18. Examples of nursing diagnoses and goals/outcomes are:
    Risk for Injury, Risk for Falls, Risk for Poisoning, Risk for Infection, and Risk for Aspiration.
    Patient will experience no injuries while hospitalized.
    Patient's risk for falls will be minimized upon discharge home.
    Patient will not be exposed to household chemicals upon discharge home.

19. PASS = pull, aim, squeeze, and sweep

20. Interventions to reduce falls in the health care environment are having the call bell and frequently used items within reach, making hourly rounds, keeping the patient close to the nurses' station, having a 24-hour sitter, making sure that the brakes/locks are in place on beds and wheelchairs, and encouraging the patient to use grab bars near toilets and in showers/tubs.

21. The correct information on the use of restraints is f.

22. Hand washing and hand sanitizing are the most important actions to prevent transmission of infectious organisms.

23. a. Dislodging of a nasogastric tube—make sure that the tube is in the stomach by checking the pH of aspirated contents, along with measuring the length of the tube that is exiting the nose.
    b. Inaccurate readings on glucose meters—check the batteries and calibrate the device in accordance with the manufacturer's instructions.
    c. Radiation exposure—use lead shielding and a radiation-monitoring device or badge.

24. The use of mitt restraints will keep the patient from pulling out IVs, tubes, or drains.

25. Assessment should include the condition of the area with the restraint for skin integrity, sensation, and circulation. Patients with vest restraints need to have their respiratory status evaluated. The mental and emotional condition of the patient should also be checked.

26. a. Occupational therapist—evaluates the patient for safe performance of ADLs and makes recommendations to enhance these activities, such as the use of specialty equipment for dressing or eating.
    b. Social worker—contact insurance companies and other agencies to assist with the financing of recommended therapeutic devices, such as walkers.

27. False

28. a. For prevention of fires, it is recommended that individuals:
    - Do not use stoves for heating the house.
    - Do not use ovens for storing food, such as crackers, cookies, or cereal.
    - Do not leave irons face-down on the ironing board.
    - Properly dispose of or recycle trash, and do not allow it to accumulate.
    - Install smoke alarms on every floor of the house.
    - Change batteries in smoke alarms at least twice per year.
    - Establish fire escape plans, and practice them several times each year.
    - Ensure that all family members know how and when to call emergency telephone numbers.
    - Obtain fire extinguishers, and be sure family members learn how to use them.
    - Consider installing fire sprinklers in the home. (U.S. Fire Administration, 2014)

    b. The CDC (2009a) recommends the use of the following measures in the home or community setting to avoid carbon monoxide poisoning:
    - Scheduling annual checks and service of the heating system, water heater, and any other gas-, oil-, or coal-burning devices by a qualified technician.
    - Installing a battery-operated carbon monoxide detector, and checking or replacing the batteries each spring and fall, along with smoke-detector battery checks.
    - Immediately evacuating and calling 911 if the carbon monoxide detector alarm goes off.
    - Seeking medical attention promptly if carbon monoxide poisoning is suspected (symptoms of nausea, dizziness, light-headedness).
    - Using items such as charcoal grills, camp stoves, and generators outside and not inside the garage or basement.
    - Avoiding running cars or trucks inside a garage attached to the house.
    - Burning objects or materials only in vented fireplaces or stoves.
    - Never heating the house with a gas oven.

29. Breaches in safety standards include:
    - Wrong-side surgeries and amputations.
    - Wrong-patient errors (i.e., medications given to the wrong patients or diagnostic procedures or treatments performed on the wrong patients, having deleterious effects).
    - Medication dosage errors resulting in organ damage or failure or in death (e.g., lack of adjustment or lowering of the dose for children or geriatric patients).

187

- Fall-related injuries and death (particularly in older-adult populations).
- Restraint-related injuries and death.

30. a	34. c	38. c
31. d	35. b	39. d
32. b	36. d	40. c
33. a	37. d	

Practice Situation

a. You should do the following as alternatives to restraints:
- Orient the patient to the surroundings, and explain all care-related interventions.
- Relocate the patient to a room near the nurses' station.
- Use pressure-sensitive and motion-sensitive bed and chair alarms consistently. Tabs and Bed-Check alarm systems can be used in the bed or chair.
- Ensure that alarms and sensors are functioning, and perform battery checks according to facility protocol.
- Encourage the family and significant others to spend time with the patient.
- Minimize environmental stimuli (e.g., noise and bright lights).
- Provide types of distraction on the basis of patient preferences (e.g., music, television, a doll to hold).
- Promote relaxation through gentle massage.
- Use aromatherapy to relax the patient.
- Assess for sources of agitation, and ensure that the patient's basic needs are met (food, fluids, toileting, pain or discomfort relief, sleep, ambulation).
- Obtain an order for a 24-hour sitter (UAP).
- Cover or disguise tubes or drains with clothing, or wrap IV sites with gauze so that they are kept out of the patient's sight.
- Use untied, cloth-padded protective mitts on the patient's hands to prevent the patient from removing tubes or drains.

b. Falls can be prevented or reduced in the home environment by:
- Removing obstacles from walking paths (clutter, throw rugs, and cords).
- Ensuring adequate lighting in areas such as bathrooms, halls, and stairways.
- Keeping assistive devices (canes and walkers) within reach.
- Using assistive devices consistently and properly when moving.
- Repairing loose or uneven floor and stairway surfaces.
- Installing and maintaining handrails and grab bars.
- Utilizing devices such as long-handled grabbers rather than reaching or stooping.
- Keeping frequently used items close by or within reach.
- Maintaining floor surfaces that are dry and free of debris.

CHAPTER 26: ASEPSIS AND INFECTION CONTROL

1. e	5. i	9. g
2. d	6. a	10. f
3. h	7. j	
4. b	8. c	

11. a. Local inflammatory response—redness, heat, pain, and swelling.
    b. Systemic response—fever, chills, increased heart and respiratory rates, anorexia, enlarged lymph nodes, malaise, lethargy, and altered mental status.

12. Passive immunity is acquired in utero or through breast milk and with immunizations when antibodies are introduced through an injection.

13. a. Infectious agent—bacteria, viruses, fungi, and parasites
    b. Source of infection—inanimate objects, human beings, and animals
    c. Portal of exit—emesis, sputum, urine, stool, blood, genital secretions, and wound drainage
    d. Mode of transmission—contact, airborne, vehicle (such as food, water, and objects), droplet, and vector-borne
    e. Portal of entry— the gastrointestinal tract via ingestion, the genitourinary tract via contact with mucous membranes, the respiratory tract via inhalation, the integumentary system via breaks in skin integrity, and the urinary tract via introduction through the urethra
    f. Susceptible host—someone exposed to an infectious disease. Increased susceptibility is associated with people at the extremes of age, those who are nutritionally compromised, and those who have experienced recent trauma or surgery. A lower resistance to infection occurs in those who are immunocompromised through chemotherapy, radiation treatments, long-term use of steroids, or transplantation. Patients with chronic illnesses, such as heart or lung disease, diabetes, liver or kidney disease, and HIV or AIDS have a lower resistance to infection.

14. a. HAIs can be caused by the use of medical devices such as catheters and ventilators, complications following a surgical procedure, contagious transmission between patients and health care workers, and the overuse of antibiotics.
    b. HAIs can best be prevented by hand washing, along with use of PPE and aseptic technique.

15. The correct statements about infection control are a, e, and f.

16. Specific questions for the presence of infection include:
- Do you feel tired or fatigued?
- Do you feel short of breath?
- Do you often feel chilled and require a blanket when others in the room are comfortable?
- How is your appetite?
- Do you have any areas of pain, redness, swelling, and warmth?
- Do you have any rashes, breaks in the skin, or reddened areas?

- Do you have swollen lymph nodes?
- Do you feel that you empty your bladder when you go to the bathroom?
- Do you have a cough or difficulty swallowing?
- Have you had a fever?
- What medications are you on? Have you taken an antibiotic recently?
- Are your immunizations up to date?

17. With an infection, the temperature usually elevates, blood pressure rises, and heart and respiratory rates increase. A late sign of infection, associated with septicemia and shock, is a decreased blood pressure.

18. Surgical asepsis actions are d and e.

19. Nutrients to replace include protein, vitamins, minerals, and water.

20. a. The factors that contribute to resistant organisms include the overprescribing of antibiotics for non-bacterial-based infections, the use of inappropriate antibiotics for the infecting microorganism, and incomplete courses of antibiotics.
    b. Examples of resistant organisms include MRSA, VRSA, VRE, and C-Diff.

21. Impaired Skin Integrity means that there is a break in the skin, which can interfere with one of the body's defenses against infection and create a portal of entry for microorganisms.

22. Web-based sites include:
- Centers for Disease Control and Prevention (CDC): www.cdc.gov
- National Guideline Clearinghouse (NGC): www.ngc.gov
- National Institute for Health and Clinical Excellence (NICE): www.nice.org.uk
- National Resource for Infection Control: www.nric.org.uk/
- The Cochrane Collaboration: www.cochrane.org/

23. Contact precautions are used for a, c, and f.

24. Protective isolation may be used for a patient who is immunocompromised, such as post-transplant, on chemotherapy, or with a disease such as lupus, leukemia, or HIV.

25. PPE is donned as follows c, b, d, and a.

26. The nurse should make sure to wear a waterproof gown, goggles/protective eye shield, cap, and gloves.

27. a. Cuts on the hands—Cover the injuries with appropriate dressing after washing; wear gloves; or delegate the assignment and/or request a different one.
    b. Visible dirt—Use soap and water, not a hand sanitizer.
    c. Artificial nails are in place—Remove artificial nails.

28. The order to open the package is c, d or b, then a.

29. Photo A—The nurse is holding the instrument below the field/waist level and the gloved hand may be touching the uniform.
    Photo B—The sterile field is wet, and the dressing and instrument are on the wet spot.

30. Standard precautions include b, d, e, and f.

31. To pour liquid into a sterile container within the sterile field, hold the lid of the bottle in the nondominant hand with the inside facing up. Hold the bottle in the dominant hand and pour the liquid slowly into the sterile container. Place the bottle on a nonsterile surface, and replace the lid.

32. b	39. b	46. d
33. a	40. b	47. a
34. c	41. c	48. b
35. a	42. a	49. c
36. d	43. b	50. d
37. a	44. c	
38. a	45. b	

Practice Situation

a. The patient with a surgical infection may have a nursing diagnosis of Risk for Infection, with a goal of "incision will remain free of infection throughout hospital stay."

b. You can help to prevent infection for this patient by:
- Washing hands before and after giving care to each patient.
- Educating patients regarding hand washing techniques, factors that increase the risk of infection, and the signs and symptoms of infection.
- Wearing gloves to maintain asepsis during any direct patient care when there is a risk of exposure to blood or other body fluids.
- Monitoring the patient's temperature every 4 hours.
- Monitoring the WBC count as ordered.
- Assisting the patient with oral hygiene every 4 hours.
- Using strict aseptic technique when inserting an IV or Foley catheter and when performing suctioning of the lower airway.
- Changing IV tubing and giving site care every 24 to 48 hours or in accordance with hospital or facility policy.
- Rotating the IV every 48 to 72 hours or in accordance with hospital or facility policy.
- Having the patient perform cough and deep-breathing exercises every 4 hours.
- Turning the patient every 2 hours, and performing skin care, especially over bony prominences.
- Ensuring optimal nutrition by offering high-protein supplements unless contraindicated.

c. When the patient is going to be discharged home, you should:
- For wound care:
  - Teach the patient and family the signs of wound healing and wound infections.
  - Explain the proper technique for changing dressings and disposing of the soiled ones. Reinforce the need to place contaminated dressings and other disposable items containing body fluids in moisture-proof plastic bags.
  - Have the patient and family repeat instructions and demonstrate skills.
- Teach proper hand hygiene (before handling foods, before eating, after toileting, before and after required home care treatment, and after touching body substances such as wound drainage) and related hygienic measures for all family members.

189

- Instruct the patient and family not to share personal care items, such as toothbrushes, washcloths, and towels. Infections can be transmitted from shared personal items.
- Discuss antimicrobial soaps and effective disinfectants.
- Instruct about cleaning reusable equipment and supplies: Use soap and water, and disinfect with a chlorine bleach solution.
- Teach the patient and family members the signs and symptoms of infection, how to avoid infections, and when to contact a health care provider.
- Emphasize the need for proper immunizations of all family members.
- If self-injections are required, advise the patient to put used needles in a puncture-resistant container with a screw-top lid and label the container so that it will not be discarded in the garbage.

CHAPTER 27: HYGIENE AND PERSONAL CARE

1. h	5. i	9. f
2. j	6. b	10. e
3. g	7. c	
4. a	8. d	

11. a. Ulcers—Open areas on the skin provide opportunities for microorganisms to invade the body. Care must be taken to protect the areas and prevent further breakdown and infection.
    b. Decreased sensation—Patients will not be able to feel the temperature of the water and may be burned.
    c. Pediculosis—The nurse uses personal protective equipment when bathing and providing care for patients with pediculosis to avoid spreading the infection. It will require special shampoo to remove the infestation.
12. Bathing or helping the patient bathe provides the nurse with an opportunity to inspect the integument and identify abnormal findings. The nurse may also discuss care with the patient and educate him or her about hygienic care. In addition to cleansing, bathing can promote circulation and range of motion and be soothing and relaxing.
13. Considerations for age and culture/ethnicity are:
    a. Infants and young children are dependent on others to care for their hygienic needs.
    Skin becomes thinner, drier, and less elastic with age, making older adults more susceptible to skin breakdown.
    b. In Hispanic and Arab cultures, male nurses may be prohibited from performing perineal care or examining private areas of a female patient's body. Cultural traditions and religious beliefs affect hygienic practices. North American and many other cultures consider it common to shower or bathe daily. In other cultures, bathing weekly is the norm. A beard in certain religions or cultures indicates that a man is married. Women of some cultures shave their axillae (armpits) and legs. In other regions of the world, women do not shave these areas. The nurse should always consult with the patient or family before shaving or cutting a patient's hair. Persons of African descent tend to have hair that is drier and does not require washing as often.

14. To assess the patient's ability to perform hygienic care, the nurse can observe how the patient manages basic ADLs—bathing, oral care, dressing, grooming. In addition, the nurse can ask questions to get the patient's perspective, such as:
    - Are you able to bathe yourself?
    - Do you become short of breath during your bath?
    - Has there been a change in your ability to take care of yourself?
15. The anticipated findings are b and f.
16. The ethical considerations include maintaining the patient's privacy, dignity, and value, along with recognizing and implementing the patient's preferences for care, as able.
17. a. Massage can provide relaxation, relief of pain and depression, and stimulation of circulation and sensation. Agitation can be reduced for patients with dementia.
    b. The nurse may massage the arms, hands, feet, neck, shoulders, and back, down to the buttocks, unless a condition exists that would contraindicate the procedure. Reddened areas and the calves/legs are never massaged.
    c. Effleurage, petrissage, and tapotement may be used, depending on the patient's condition and preference.
18. a. Complete bath—for patients who are completely bedridden or totally dependent
    b. Partial bath—when the patient can complete some of the care and only a portion of the body is washed
    c. Shower—for ambulatory patients who are capable of being independent
19. The temperature for the water should be from 105° to 110° F.
20. For a patient with a cognitive impairment, routine is beneficial. Techniques that are effective and preferred by the patient should be part of the routine. Playing soothing music, speaking softly, using gentle touch, and keeping the room comfortably warm can help to promote a calm and secure environment.
21. Perineal care for a female patient requires that the area be cleaned from front to back, privacy is maintained, and determination be made to see if the patient needs a same-sex caregiver. Gloves should be worn by the nurse.
22. A Sitz bath may be used to cleanse the perineal area.
23. Documentation of hygienic care includes the date, time, procedure performed, any problems noted during the procedure including reddened or tender areas, sores, skin breakdown, any odors present, and the patient's response to the procedure.
24. Foot care includes inspecting and cleaning the feet and nails. The feet may be soaked, unless the patient is diabetic. If the agency allows for nurses to trim toenails, then care should be taken to not injure the surrounding skin. A podiatrist may do the toenails of the patient with diabetes or other peripheral neuropathies or circulatory insufficiencies.

25. a. Options for a shampoo include no-rinse shampoos, shampoo cap, and shampoo basin.
    b. For tangled hair, the nurse can apply warm water and a conditioner or detangler. A comb and/or fingers can be used to work through the tangles. For matted hair, a solution of 25% hydrogen peroxide and 75% saline can be applied to the matted area with cotton balls to dissolve the mats. A comb or gloved fingers can be used to work through the matted tangles individually before shampooing.
26. The nurse should suggest rinsing the oral cavity often, taking frequent sips of water or sucking on ice cubes, and applying a lip balm.
27. Patients on anticoagulants should not use hard-bristle toothbrushes or shave with anything other than an electric razor.
28. The correct techniques for care of the eyes, nose, and ears are a, e, and f.
29. The correct order for the bath is e, g, b, f, a, c, and d.
30. Upon completion of the bath, safety measures to implement include leaving the bed in the lowest position, raising the top side rails, making sure that the call light is within reach, discarding used equipment and supplies properly, and performing hand hygiene.
31. For male and female perineal care, nonsterile gloves should be worn, cleansing should be done from front to back for a female and from the tip of the penis to the scrotum and anus for a male, and different areas of the washcloth should be used for each wipe (or individual disposable cloths, if available).
32. For oral care of a comatose patient, a bulb syringe and/or suction equipment should be available and the patient's head should be lowered (as appropriate) and the patient turned to the side facing the nurse. Disposable oral swabs should be used, with the minimal amount of fluid necessary to clean the oral cavity.
33. To prevent damage, the nurse should use a 4 x 4 gauze pad to grasp the dentures and clean them over a towel in the sink.
34. The correct techniques are a, d, and e.
35. The important actions when making a bed are to keep the bed at working height to avoid back strain, hold linens away from the body and dispose of them properly, avoid shaking out the linens, keep the patient warm and covered, obtain assistance to move the patient, provide comfort with toe pleats and smooth linens, and clean the mattress if the linens are wet/soiled. Nonsterile gloves and waterproof pads are applied in the presence of bodily fluids.

36. a	40. b	44. b
37. b	41. d	45. c
38. a	42. c	46. d
39. d	43. d	47. a

Practice Situations

a. The UAP should be taught:
- The type and time of bath for the patient.
- Any special hygienic care that should be performed with the bath, such as foot and hand care or shampoo.
- Appropriate encouragement of the patient's abilities to assist with the procedure.
- Positioning concerns specific to the patient.
- Appropriate care and positioning of specialized medical interventions for the patient during the procedure (e.g., a Foley catheter, IV catheter, casts, traction).
- Positioning concerns specific to the patient.
- Cultural, privacy, and ethical concerns.
- Avoidance of pressure over bony prominences.
- Appropriate care, including trimming and filing of nails, if allowed by facility policy.
- The type of shampoo for the patient and the appropriate time for hair care.
- The patient's abilities to assist with the procedure, such as combing and styling.
- Positioning concerns specific to the patient.
- Appropriate care and positioning of specialized medical devices needed by the patient during the procedure (e.g., hearing aid).
- Ethnic hair variations and specific interventions (such as use of a wide-tooth comb).
- Appropriate adaptations and emergency care for patients at risk for choking.
- Appropriate encouragement of the patient's abilities to assist with the procedure.
- Positioning concerns specific to the patient.
- Appropriate care and positioning of specialized dental devices for the patient during the procedure, such as braces, full or partial dentures, or retainers.
- Conditions specific to the patient (such as bleeding tendencies), as well as training for interventions and reporting concerns.
- Appropriate positioning specific to the patient and diagnosis.
- Ethnic and cultural variations and concerns, such as differences in hair texture.
- Consent for and desires regarding care of mustache and beard.
- Appropriate documentation according to facility policy.

b. The UAP should report:
- Sores, wounds, irritations, lesions, redness, or rashes noted on the patient.
- Concerns regarding the procedure or patient.
- Episodes of incontinence (urinary or fecal, quantity, unusual characteristics).
- Patient discomfort reported during the procedure.
- Nails that are thick, yellowed, or otherwise unusual.
- Patient complaints regarding neck or back discomfort.
- Coughing or choking symptoms (report immediately).
- Sores, wounds, irritations, lesions, or bleeding in and around the mouth.
- Complaints of discomfort related to teeth, such as sensitivities that might indicate cavities or other dental concerns.
- Discomfort or refusal related to denture wear or any damage noted to dentures.
- Lost or missing dentures.

- Obvious tooth decay or dental problems.
- Difficulties during the procedure.
- Any nicks or cuts that occur during the procedure.
- A general narrative regarding the experience.

For the patient in the case study, a sample plan for the day is:

7:10 A.M.—Visit Mr. Randall, assess his status, take vital signs, check the oxygen, evaluate the IV access site for infiltration or phlebitis, make sure that the patient was weighed by the UAP, set up the Intake & Output sheet, provide urinal.

8:00 A.M.—Check on the hygienic care provided by the UAP and completed by the patient, including shaving, oral care, and shampooing. Verify that the patient received the no-added salt diet, and determine the amount of breakfast consumed.

9:00 A.M.—Administer Lisinopril and Ipratropium inhaler (document).

9:35 A.M.—Return to the room to check on the patient and assess his respiratory status and I&O.

11:00 A.M.—Take vital signs and compare them to prior readings, determine effectiveness of medication and oxygen use, teach use of pursed-lip breathing, effective coughing, and energy conservation.

11:30 A.M.—Speak with the UAP about having a chair in the shower to reduce Mr. Randall's activity intolerance.

12:00 P.M.—Check on the lunch provided and the amount consumed by the patient. Assist patient to bathroom with UAP assistance. Measure output.

1:00 P.M.—Administer medications (document).

2:00 p.m.—Assess patient's status, determine if he has questions or concerns he wishes to discuss.

3:00 P.M.—Take vital signs, check the oxygen, evaluate the IV status, and calculate I&O. Provide SBAR report to oncoming staff.

Note—Documentation of care is done consistently throughout the day after assessments and interventions.

CHAPTER 28: ACTIVITY, IMMOBILITY, AND SAFE MOVEMENT

1. j	5. c	9. g
2. e	6. i	10. b
3. f	7. a	
4. h	8. d	

11. a. Musculoskeletal
   - Impairment or injury—affects the body's ability to move.
   - Inadequate dietary intake of calcium and vitamin D or impaired calcium metabolism—osteoporosis, which increases bone fragility and may lead to fractures.
   - Decreased physical exercise contributes to bone deterioration, loss of strength, or hypotonicity.
   - Rheumatoid arthritis and osteoarthritis—inflammation of joints, pain, and limited joint mobility.

   - Genetic disorders (e.g., muscular dystrophy)—muscle weakness and gradual muscle wasting, difficulty with maintaining posture and impairing mobility.
   b. Neurologic
   - Damage to the cerebrum or cerebellum of the brain and spinal cord injury—directly affects ability to ambulate and control movement.
   - Cerebrovascular accidents (CVAs or strokes) and traumatic brain injuries—hemiparesis, hemiplegia
   - Spinal cord injury—lower and/or upper-body paralysis, difficulty with breathing.
   c. Cardiopulmonary
   - Compromised cardiac function, decreased tissue perfusion, and diminished respiratory capacity—affect ability to perform activities of daily living (ADLs) and exercise.
   - Congestive heart failure (CHF), peripheral vascular disease, and chronic obstructive pulmonary disease (COPD)—decrease ability to deliver oxygen and nutrients to body organs and tissues, diminished capacity for exercise.

12. Assessment questions may include:
   - Are you experiencing any stiffness, joint discomfort, or pain with movement?
   - Have you noticed any difficulty with dizziness or balance?
   - Do you become short of breath or easily fatigued when completing your activities of daily living?
   - How is your appetite? What is your typical dietary intake in a day?
   - What is the frequency of your bowel movements?
   - Describe your normal sleep pattern.
   - Do you exercise?

13. Effects of immobility on the following body systems include:

Complications of Immobility	Nursing Interventions/ Recommendations
a. Musculoskeletal—weakness, decreased muscle tone, decreased bone (disuse osteoporosis) and muscle mass, potential muscle atrophy, contractures (foot drop)	Range of motion, exercise, ambulation Foot board, trochanter roll, hand rolls Turning, positioning Calcium supplements, as indicted
b. Cardiopulmonary—atelectasis, orthostatic hypotension, increased cardiac workload, decreased lung capacity, circulatory stasis (DVT)	Deep breathing and coughing, incentive spirometer Gradual position changes Exercise, fluids (within any restriction) Antiembolism hose (stockings), sequential compression device (SCD)

Complications of Immobility	Nursing Interventions/ Recommendations
c. Gastrointestinal—decreased peristalsis: indigestion, anorexia, constipation, distention, impaction	Fluids (2 L/day), fiber, nutrients Positioning on bedpan, use of commode Exercise, turning, ambulation
d. Integumentary—tissue ischemia, pressure ulcers	Frequent turning, positioning, support mattresses, heel and elbow protectors/cushions

14. Muscle strength is assessed by asking the patient to squeeze the nurse's hands and having the patient plantar-flex the feet against resistance by the nurse's hands. Nurses must evaluate muscle symmetry by comparing one side of the patient's body with the other.
15. In the presence of resistance or pain during range of motion, the activity should be stopped.
16. Dangling can prevent postural hypotension and syncope (fainting) by allowing patients to sit with their legs in a dependent position for a few minutes before standing.
17. Examples of special mattresses include surface redesign, foam, gatch, gel, low air-loss, and air-fluidized.
18. The correct body mechanics are c, e, and f.
19. Reducing friction includes slightly lifting rather than pulling patients, using a trapeze bar, transfer/slide board, or friction-reducing sheets. The patient may also benefit from the use of heel and elbow protectors.
20. a. Range of motion is usually performed twice daily.
    b. Each joint is moved 3 to 5 times.
21. The correct use of a mechanical lift involves b, c, d, e, and f.
22. The nurse can include patients in the decision making for their care, encourage visits from family and friends, spend time with the patient, explain procedures, institute reality orientation (clocks, calendars), and have books, TV, pictures available in the environment.
23. For logrolling, three people are recommended and the use of a mechanical or assistive device should be determined. The goals are to prevent injury to the patient and nurse(s), maintain the patient's body alignment, and keep all tubes, etc. intact.
24. The nurse can obtain an order for an analgesic and premedicate the patient before the activity.
25. The patient needs to be able to raise the legs 1 inch off of the bed in order to have strength for ambulation.
26. General safety measures for the use of assistive devices for ambulation include checking if they are sturdy and intact, correctly fitted for the patient, able to fit through doors, appropriate for the need of the patient. Patients should have nonskid and well-fitting shoes, and the route for ambulation should be free of clutter. There should be sufficient personnel for assistance to prevent patient injury.
27. The correct order is c, b, d, and a.
28. The appropriate use of antiembolism hose includes a, d, and f.

29. a
30. d
31. b
32. c
33. c
34. d
35. a
36. c
37. d
38. b
39. d
40. a
41. b
42. c
43. a
44. b
45. a
46. c
47. c
48. d
49. b
50. d
51. b
52. d
53. a

Practice Situations

a. You should conduct a fall risk assessment with the agency's tool. In addition, a thorough health history and physical assessment should be completed to determine the patient's current status and a possible etiology for the vertigo (e.g., orthostatic hypotension, medications, fluid loss).
b. A nursing diagnosis based on the data presented is "Risk for Falls. Goals/outcomes—Patient will not experience any falls or injuries during the hospital stay, Patient will ambulate with assistance within 24 hours."
c. Interventions include vital signs, observation of mental status and level of consciousness, caution in transfers, and education about safety.

Specialized and general fall prevention actions to implement include:
- Repeating the fall assessment daily.
- Frequently observing the patient.
- Placing the patient in a room near the nurses' station.
- Using a low bed.
- Using a mattress or wheelchair seat with pressure alarms.
- Using upper side rails.
- Always returning the bed to its lowest position.
- Keeping the call bell within reach of the patient.
  - Remind the patient about how to use the call bell.
  - Immediately answer the call bell if it is sounded.
- Keeping the wheels of any wheeled device (bed, wheelchair) in the locked position.
- Leaving lights on or off at night depending on the patient's cognitive status and personal preference.
- Keeping patient belongings (tissues, water, urinals, personal items) within the patient's reach.
- Frequently orienting and reorienting the patient.
- If the patient is ambulatory, requiring the use of nonskid footwear.
- Clearing any potential obstructions from the walking areas.
- Ensuring that patient clothing fits properly; improper fit can cause tripping.

CHAPTER 29: SKIN INTEGRITY AND WOUND CARE

1. e
2. h
3. c
4. j
5. i
6. a
7. b
8. f
9. d
10. g

11. a. Vascular disease—impacts the skin's ability to obtain required oxygen and nutrients
    b. Malnutrition—inadequate intake of proteins, cholesterol and fatty acids, vitamins and minerals leads to weight loss and the decreased ability of the tissue to withstand pressure, shear and infection.
    c. Aging—Older adults may have comorbidities such as diabetes or cardiovascular disease, be on medications that impact their skin, and have increased exposure to the damaging effects of ultraviolet light. Aging leads to a thinning of the epidermis, dermis, and subcutaneous layers, with a resultant reduction in elastin, collagen fibers, sweat glands, and sebaceous glands. This leads to sagging or wrinkling of the skin and to the dry, paper-thin appearance seen in the skin of elderly individuals. It contributes to a reduction in the skin's ability to serve as both insulation and cushioning, thereby increasing the elderly person's vulnerability to trauma and temperature extremes. A loss of melanocytes after age 40 leads to the graying of hair and an increased susceptibility to the development of skin cancers. With the decrease in Langerhans cells, there is a corresponding decrease in the elderly person's resistance to infections. The skin becomes more susceptible to mechanical trauma, shearing forces, and skin tears.
12. Examples of open wounds are abrasions, puncture wounds, and surgical incisions.
13. Surgical incisions or traumatic wounds heal by primary intention.
14. Effect on wound healing:

Decreased oxygenation	Chronic tissue hypoxia is associated with a reduction in collagen formation, a decrease in the action and proliferation of fibroblasts, a reduction in leukocytes, and an impairment of the cell's ability to migrate.
Diabetes	Changes in the microvascular and macrovascular systems lead to a thickening of the vessel wall and occlusion of blood flow with its needed nutrients and oxygen. For a diabetic patient, the presence of a wound is accompanied by a reduction in collagen synthesis, a decrease in the strength of that collagen, impaired functioning of leukocytes, and a reduction in the number and action of macrophages.
Infection	A prolongation of the inflammatory phase occurs, with delayed collagen synthesis, prevention of epithelialization, and additional tissue destruction. Infection contributes to a wound's failure to progress through the phases of wound healing and leads to the development of chronic wounds.

Spinal injury	The patient is unable to feel pain (the warning sign of tissue ischemia), respond appropriately, and/or move or maintain position independently.

15. The nurse can prevent dehiscence and evisceration by teaching the patient to "splint" the incision with a pillow or folded blanket or to use an abdominal binder for comfort while coughing and deep breathing and during movement.
16. A fistula can result in fluid and electrolyte loss, nutritional deficits, and alterations in skin integrity.
17. a. Full-thickness pressure ulcers are stages III, IV, and unstageable.
    b. True
18. A focused wound assessment includes an evaluation of the wound's location, size, and color; presence of drainage; condition of the wound edges; characteristics of the wound bed; and patient's response to the wound or wound treatment. In addition, the nurse will ask the patient:
    • How long has this wound been present? What do you think caused this wound? Have you ever had a wound like this before?
    • What are you doing for this wound at home? What are you using to clean the wound? What have you put on it?
    • Have you noticed any changes in the appearance of the wound or the skin around it?
    • How much wound drainage is there? Has the amount, color, or odor of the drainage changed? How often do you need to change the bandage at home?
    • Do you live alone? Do you have anyone who helps you at home?
    • Is the cost of caring for this wound difficult for you to manage?
19. The Braden score is 17, which indicates a mild risk for pressure ulcer development but should prompt preventive measures.
20. The photos indicate (a) an incision closed with staples and (b) a Jackson-Pratt drainage system.
21. a. Pressure ulcers develop primarily as a result of tissue ischemia from pressure, but moisture, immobility, poor nutrition, and comorbidities contribute to their development.
    b. Sites marked should include: occipital bone (1), scapula (2), spine (3), elbow (4), iliac crest (5), sacrum (6), ischium (7), Achilles tendon (8), heel (9), and sole of the foot (10).

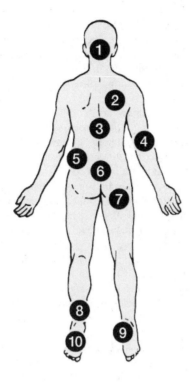

22. a. 4.3 cm × 2 cm
    b. The wound has serosanguineous drainage with undermining.
23. a. For maceration, the wound will appear pale, soft, or wrinkled skin
    b. Redness, warmth and induration are seen with an infection, along with purulent drainage that may appear yellow, greenish or beige.
24. The appropriate interventions to prevent pressure ulcers are a, b, d, and f.
25. Wound debridement can be done by mechanical, enzymatic, biologic, autolytic, and sharp methods.
26. a. A simple, dry wound—gauze dressing
    b. A wound with a moderate to heavy amount of exudate—foam or alginate dressing
27. Placement of a drain in a wound prevents excess blood, serum, or pus from collecting in the surgical area.
28. For a T-tube or Penrose drain, nurses should protect the surrounding skin with barrier ointments and frequent dressing changes and be careful not to dislodge or compress the drain tubing.
29. The correct actions for removal of sutures and staples are a, c, and e.
30. The five P's of circulation are pain, pallor, pulselessness, paresthesia, and paralysis.
31. The correct actions for application of heat are b, d, and e.
32. a. Irrigation is used to:
    • Clean a wound.
    • Apply heat, which promotes healing.
    • Apply medication such as antibiotics.
    • Remove debris and exudates.

• Remove bacterial colonizations.
• Prevent skin from healing over a deeper wound that must remain open.
b. The solutions that can be used are:
    • Sterile normal saline solution
    • Lactated Ringer solution
    • Ordered antibiotic solution
c. The necessary pressure is provided by a 30- to 50-mL syringe and an 18-gauge catheter.
33. The order of the steps for wound irrigation with a dressing is d, c, a, e, and b.
34. The unlicensed assistive personnel (UAP) should be instructed to report:
    • Pain before, during, or after the procedure
    • Appearance of bleeding or signs of infection
    • Difficulties in performing the procedure
35. General principles of asepsis that are used for wound care include:
    • Use of clean or sterile gloves, as appropriate
    • Cleansing from least to most contaminated
    • Appropriate preparation of sterile fields
    • Disposal of soiled dressings and materials in waterproof bags
    • Avoiding personal exposure with the use of gowns, gloves, masks, and eyewear
36. a. What equipment is needed for a wound culture?
    • Sterile culturette swabs
    • Waterproof trash bags
    • Patient labels
    • Laboratory requisitions
    • Clean or sterile gloves, depending on the wound
    • Sterile normal saline solution
    • Irrigation syringe
    • Personal protective equipment, as needed
b. This skill should not be delegated to the UAP.
c. The sample should be taken from actively draining tissue.
37. The nurse should discontinue wound care if the patient develops new pain, other physical distress, or unexpected bleeding.
38. a. Before wrapping a limb with a bandage, the nurse should elevate the extremity for 15 to 30 minutes.
    b. Limbs are bandaged from distal to proximal.
    c. After application, the nurse should assess the circulation to the area.
    d. Bandages should be removed at least once every 8 hours, or as ordered.

39. c	50. d	61. c
40. c	51. c	62. d
41. b	52. a	63. c
42. c	53. c	64. a
43. a	54. c	65. c
44. a	55. d	66. a
45. b	56. a	67. d
46. d	57. a	68. b
47. d	58. b	
48. a	59. a	
49. c	60. d	

a. For this patient, possible nursing diagnoses are:
- Acute pain related to open wound on heel manifested by rating pain as a 5 out of 10.
- Impaired skin integrity related to prolonged pressure and tissue ischemia as manifested by a 5 cm x 3 cm stage III ulcer on the right heel.

b. Short-term goals include:
- Patient will report a pain of 3 out of 10 or less by the next shift.
- Patient's wound will remain free of infection during hospitalization.
- Granulation tissue will form in the wound within 14 days.
- No additional ulcers will form during hospital stay.
- Patient will participate in turning and positioning q2h.
- Patient will consume a diet high in fiber, vitamin C, and protein by the end of the week.

Interventions include:
- Pain assessment and administration of prescribed analgesics
- Premedication before dressing changes, if indicated
- Assessment of the patient's skin and wound (measurement, observation of drainage and signs of healing)
- Care and dressing of the wound, as ordered
- Instructing and reminding the patient about turning and positioning q2h or more often
- Pad the heels or elevate them above the mattress
- Speak with the dietician about the diet and observe the patient's intake

c. Evaluation of the goals includes:
- Monitoring the patient's level of pain—asking the level
- Measuring the wound and observing for signs of healing or infection
- Determining the patient's frequency of turning and positioning off of susceptible sites

For the patient requiring wound care at home, the following are some ideas for saving money on supplies:
- Determination of the patient's insurance coverage to see what supplies are covered.
- Use of sanitary napkins or diapers as absorptive dressings.
- Creation of homemade saline: 1 quart of boiled water (5 minutes) with 2 teaspoons of salt dissolved in the water. Let the water cool.
- Use of clean technique, rather than sterile, which eliminates the need for sterile gloves, drapes, etc. that can be costly.
- If a syringe is used for irrigating, a plastic soda bottle can be used for disposal.

CHAPTER 30: NUTRITION

1. b	4. f	7. h
2. e	5. c	8. g
3. a	6. d	

9. Nutrients are necessary substances obtained from ingested food that supply the body with energy; build and maintain bones, muscles, and skin; and aid in the normal growth and function of each body system. Macronutrients are water, carbohydrates, fats, and proteins. Micronutrients are vitamins and minerals.

10. a. Simple carbohydrates are broken down and absorbed quickly, providing a quick source of energy. Complex carbohydrates are composed of starches, glycogen, and fiber. They take longer to break down before absorption and utilization by the body's cells.
   b. Simple carbohydrates are sugars such as those derived from fruit (fructose), table sugar (sucrose), milk products (lactose), and blood sugar (glucose). Complex carbohydrates include bread; rice; pasta; legumes such as dried beans, peas, and lentils; and starchy vegetables such as corn, pumpkin, green peas, and potatoes.
   c. Carbohydrates provide the body with 4 kcal/g.

11. a. Fats include fatty acids, cholesterol, and phospholipids.
   b. Total fat intake should be between 25% and 35% of total caloric intake daily.
   c. Fat-soluble vitamins are A, D, E, K.
   d. Examples of essential fatty acids include linolenic (omega-3) and linoleic (omega-6).

12. Examples of saturated fats are b, c, and f.

13. Proteins are necessary in the body for the development, maintenance, and repair of the body's tissues, organs, and cells. Hemoglobin (protein) is responsible for transporting oxygen throughout the body. Prothrombin is the protein necessary for clotting blood. Other tasks include the production of hair and nails, muscle movement, nerve conduction, digestion, and defense against bacteria and viruses.

14. An individual with a water (fluid) deficiency is anticipated to have signs of dehydration—headache, loss of concentration, dry mucous membranes, decreased blood pressure, and decreased urinary output.

15. Foods high in vitamin A include a, c, and e.

16. The nurse can help the patient to eat healthier foods by:
- Determining the patient's knowledge about nutrients and food sources
- Having the patient examine his or her dietary habits
- Teaching about reading food labels
- Using fresh rather than processed foods
- Eating smaller portions
- Eating fruits, vegetables, whole grains, and lean meats
- Drinking water

17. Vitamin C is important in the body for synthesizing protein collagen (wound healing, repair of bones), antioxidant effects, and antibody production.

18. The general role of the B complex vitamins is to form red blood cells, act as coenzymes, and facilitate energy production in the body.

19. Coffee contains a large amount of vitamin B3 (niacin).

20. Intake should include: b, c, and d. Dietary sources of potassium include milk, bananas, legumes, green leafy vegetables, orange juice, tomatoes, vegetable juice, avocados, and cantaloupe.

21. a. Antioxidants may prevent development of heart disease, cancer, and diabetes.
    b. Food sources of vitamin E are olives, soybeans, corn oil, nuts, whole grains, legumes, and dark leafy vegetables.
22. For the child with a milk allergy or digestive problem, a soy-based or hydrolyzed protein formula is recommended.
23. Culture influences nutritional intake by affecting a person's food preferences. Foods traditionally consumed by various cultural/ethnic groups may contribute to the development of chronic illnesses. Individuals may consume large amounts of salted products or higher levels of carbohydrates, which can lead to an increased incidence of obesity, heart disease, and/or diabetes.
24. a. Musculoskeletal—softening of the bone due to vitamin D deficiency (osteomalacia), osteopenia, or osteoporosis, with increased bone fragility and greater risk of fractures.
    b. Cardiopulmonary—atherosclerotic heart disease (ASHD), with the potential for cardiac damage or heart attack.
25. The patient who is lactose intolerant should avoid dairy products.
26. The correct information is found in b, d, and f.
27. The primary treatment is counseling to assist individuals with eating disorders to develop a sense of control and a positive body image, build relationships, and improve nutritional intake.
28. Information can be obtained on the patient's food intake through a 24-hour recall or a 3- to 5-day journal of foods eaten, amounts, and how the foods were prepared.
29. Physical assessment focused on nutritional status includes measurement of height and weight, calculation of body mass index (BMI), review of laboratory values, and identification of unanticipated findings (poor skin condition, etc.). In addition, waist circumference, vital signs, medical history, medications, and activity level can determine risk factors.
30. When repeated measurements of the patient's weight are necessary, make sure the patient is weighed at the same time of day, on the same scale, and in the same clothing (if possible) for each measurement. Instruct the patient to remove his or her shoes; assist if needed. Follow the manufacturer's directions for the scale used (electronic, platform, stretcher, chair, bed).
31. a. BMI 22.4 kg/m²—normal weight
    b. BMI 22.2 kg/ m²—normal weight
    c. BMI 32.9 kg/m²—obese, class 1
32. Metabolic syndrome includes:
    • Insulin resistance
    • Obesity
    • Abdominal fat
    • Increased blood glucose, triglycerides, serum cholesterol
    • Hypertension
33. Malnutrition is associated with a, c d, and e.
34. The nurse can prevent aspiration by:
    • Following orders for dietary consistencies and textures.
    • Following the manufacturer's instructions and facility policies and procedures for thickening of liquids as ordered.
    • Elevating the head of the bed to 45 degrees or higher during eating and for a minimum of 45 minutes after eating.

• Keeping the head of the bed elevated to 30 degrees at all other times, including during enteral feeding.
• Encouraging slow eating patterns.
• Instructing the patient to avoid eating or drinking for 2 to 3 hours before sleep.
• Administering gastrointestinal (GI) medications as ordered.
• Inspecting the patient's mouth for pocketing of food.
• Observing the patient for swallowing between bites of food and fluids.
• Instructing the patient to alternate between bites of food and sips of fluids to facilitate swallowing.
• Maintaining the patient's status of no food or fluids by mouth (NPO) following procedures in which the throat was anesthetized, until a gag reflex has been verified.
35. Iron is found in liver, dark-green leafy vegetables, seafood, and bran.
36. For the Quality and Safety Education for Nurses (QSEN) competency of teamwork and collaboration, the planning should include the nutritionist or registered dietitian, case manager, speech therapist (patient with impaired swallowing), psychologist (eating disorders), and UAPs.
37. A vegetarian should make sure to include cereals, dried beans and peas, and a variety of vegetables. Soy products are often added to the diet.
38. a. Signs and symptoms of dysphagia are coughing, incomplete lip closure, poor tongue control, excessive chewing, gagging before swallowing, failure to swallow, foods held in the cheek, or refusal to eat.
    b. The following are measures to take to assist an adult patient with feeding.
       • Provide oral care before and after feeding.
       • Ensure that dentures, if worn, are in place and well fitted.
       • Elevate the patient's head at least 30 to 45 degrees unless contraindicated.
       • Special caution should be taken if the patient has impaired swallowing.
       • If the patient has one-sided muscle weakness, have the patient turn the head to the affected side to assist in airway protection.
       • Chin-tucking may help to prevent aspiration.
       • Follow the occupational or nutrition therapy guidelines or the manufacturer's instructions for use of any assistive devices.
       • Position yourself so that the patient can see you.
       • Allow at least 30 minutes for each meal. Offer small bites (½ to 1 tsp).
       • Wait at least 10 seconds between bites.
       • Alternate food with fluids.
       • Avoid unnecessary use of straws to prevent air ingestion.
       • Observe for the rise and fall of the patient's larynx to verify swallowing.
       • Check the patient's mouth frequently to prevent retention of food in the cheeks (pocketing).
39. The nurse can flush the percutaneous endoscopic gastrostomy (PEG) tube with a small amount of air. If this does not work, then use a 50- to 60-mL syringe to flush the tube with 20 to 30 mL of warm water, carbonated beverages, or pineapple juice (if not contraindicated).

197

40. a. Patients who can benefit from total parenteral nutrition (TPN) are those who do not have a functioning GI tract or are unable to ingest, digest, or absorb essential nutrients due to conditions such as some stages of Crohn disease or ulcerative gastritis, GI obstruction, diarrhea unresponsive to treatment, abdominal trauma, or postoperative status.

   b. Monitoring should include weight, complete blood cell count (CBC), electrolytes, and blood urea nitrogen (BUN), plasma glucose and electrolytes, intake and output, and presence of complications.

   c. Complications include: site infections, air embolism, catheter-related infections, and dislodgment or occlusion of tubing. Metabolic complications can range from common glucose abnormalities to adverse reactions to the lipid formula, liver dysfunction, metabolic bone disease, gallbladder dysfunction (cholelithiasis, choleocystitis), and other metabolic abnormalities.

41. a. The patient should be placed in high-Fowler position (or as far as the patient can tolerate up to that position).

   b. If resistance is felt, the procedure should be stopped and the following done:
   - Rotate the tube because this may enable easier insertion.
   - Ensure that the patient is swallowing when the tube is being inserted.
   - Ensure proper positioning of the patient and the tube.
   - Withdraw the tube, and reapply water-soluble lubricant.
   - Attempt insertion in the other naris.
   - If indicated, the tube may be placed orally.
   - Notify the primary care provider (PCP) if the tube cannot be placed properly.

   c. To anchor the tube:
   - If using tape, apply a skin prep or adhesive if needed. Attach one end of the prepared piece of tape at a time to secure the ends of the tape on the bridge of the nose, forming a sling for the tube. Secure the tube away from nasal mucosa.
   - If using a tube fixation device (a winged bandage is described here), apply a skin prep or adhesive if needed; remove the backing from the bandage, and place it over the bridge of the nose. Insert the tube into the clamp of the fixation device, and close the clamp.

42. a. The residual needs to be less than 100 mL.

   b. Continuous feedings are usually administered with the use of a feeding pump.

   c. Gravity feedings, in addition to the formula, require the use of a 50- to 60-mL syringe and graduated container.

43. b	49. c	55. d
44. b	50. a	56. a
45. d	51. d	57. b
46. c	52. a	58. a
47. a	53. c	59. b
48. b	54. c	

Practice Situation

a. You should start by asking questions about the patient's intake, such as:
   - What was your dietary intake for the past 24 hours?
   - While eating, do you experience any difficulty chewing or swallowing?
   - Have you gained or lost weight in the past month? Collection of a diet history will allow you to analyze data regarding the type and quantity of foods consumed, establish baseline values for identifying any health problems that may adversely affect the patient's nutritional status, and identify the need for nursing interventions.

   A thorough physical assessment with a focus on nutritional status includes height and weight measurements; determination of body mass index; evaluation of laboratory values; notation of any adverse signs and symptoms typical of malnourished individuals (poor dentition, poor skin turgor, or dull, thinning hair); and recognition of any existing physical and psychological illness. Assessment of a person's waist circumference, vital signs, past medical history, current medications, and activity level are essential in identifying the potential risk factors for cardiovascular diseases. Assessment of the older adult (age 65 and older) must include close attention to the mouth, teeth, and gums. Consideration must be given to the decrease in organ function related to aging, such as changes in the ability to smell, taste, chew, and digest food. Other physiological changes may include increased fat stores, limited activity, decreased bone mass, decreased kidney function, and a decline in the immune system. Tools such as the Mini Nutritional Assessment (MNA) or the DETERMINE self-assessment are helpful in screening for malnutrition in older adults. The acronym DETERMINE stands for "disease, eating poorly, tooth loss, economic hardship, reduced social contact, multiple meds, involuntary weight loss, needs assistance in self-care, and elderly above age 80."

b. A possible nursing diagnosis is *Risk for or Actual Imbalanced Nutrition related to intake of foods high in sodium and saturated fat and inadequate nutrient dense foods.*

   Possible goal: Patient will verbalize knowledge of nutrient-dense foods by next visit.

   Long-term goal: Patient will purchase and consume foods that are lower in sodium and fat.

c. To assist the patient to eat foods that are more nutrient dense, you should:
   - Have the patient identify food preferences that have less sodium and fat.
   - Find a store nearby that has fresh fruits and vegetables. Determine if the store will deliver and if the patient can afford that service.
   - Find easy recipes for fresh food preparation.
   - Recommend the use of nonsodium spices and herbs for food flavoring.
   - Discuss with the patient the influence of sodium and fat on her cardiac status.
   - Review the labels for the prepared foods to identify the sodium and fat content.
   - Determine if Meals on Wheels is a good option.

- Investigate if there is a community center nearby where the patient can share at least one meal each day with others.
- Identify hobbies or activities the patient enjoys that may promote socialization and appetite.
- Discuss increasing fiber and water (within acceptable limits) to minimize possible constipation.
- Determine if the patient may benefit from vitamin and mineral supplements.
- Refer the patient for follow-up if there are issues with dentition, swallowing, pain, indigestion, or other problems that may be interfering with eating.

CHAPTER 31: COGNITIVE AND SENSORY ALTERATIONS

1. c	5. f	9. d
2. i	6. b	10. g
3. j	7. a	
4. h	8. e	

11. a. The frontal lobes of the cerebrum are the areas of the brain responsible for voluntary motor function, concentration, communication, decision making, and personality. A patient with a problem in this area will have difficulty speaking, focusing, completing ADLs, and possibly experience mood swings.

b. The occipital lobes process visual information. Damage in this area can result in the patient experiencing loss of vision or changes in visual fields.

12. Sensory changes that occur with aging include visual deficits/alterations (cataracts, presbyopia, macular degeneration); hearing deficits (presbycusis); reduced tactile and gustatory sensation.

13. Causes of delirium are drug or alcohol use, the side effects of medication, infections, fluid and electrolyte imbalances, low oxygen level, or pain.

14. a. Exogenous depression is triggered by a life situation, while endogenous depression is believed to be caused by chemical changes in the brain.

b. Treatment for depression includes elimination of the underlying cause, counseling, and administration of antidepressant medications.

15. Children are more prone to otitis media due to their shorter, more horizontal eustachian tube.

16. Patients with Meniere disease commonly experience b, c, e.

17. a. Presbyopia—decrease in the ability to focus on near objects

b. Cataracts—clouding of the lens with blurred vision

c. Glaucoma—loss of peripheral visual fields and possible blindness

d. Diabetic retinopathy—distortion of images leading to possible blindness

e. Macular degeneration—loss of vision in the central fields

18. This patient does not have metabolic syndrome as there are only two indicators noted.

19. A patient with a right-sided CVA is expected to demonstrate a loss of sensation and mobility on the left side of the body, along with visual and spatial problems.

20. The person with dementia suffers decline of cognitive functions, including reasoning, use of language, memory, computation, judgment, and learning.

21. Sensory overload can be caused by a patient being in an extremely busy environment, such as an intensive care unit (ICU), emergency department, or clinic. Sensory deprivation can occur if the patient is on isolation precautions or has sensory impairments (visual/auditory).

22. Lifestyle choices that put the patient at risk for sensory and cognitive problems include smoking, obesity, high-cholesterol diet, excessive alcohol use, cocaine use, and insufficient sleep.

23. This examination is simple and quick to administer and tests the patient's cognitive orientation, attention, calculation, recall, language, and spatial orientation.

24. Laboratory tests include complete blood count, electrolytes, blood glucose levels, urinalysis, and culture and sensitivity.

25. Patients who lose or have a reduction of their sense of taste may add too much salt to food or lose interest in food, which could lead to nutritional deficits.

26. Safety measures for the patient with dementia are:
- Checking that areas for ambulation are clear, clean, and dry
- Having the patient wear nonskid footwear
- Keeping the call bell within reach
- Making sure that lighting is sufficient
- Providing assistance for hygiene, grooming, dressing, and eating
- Considering social interaction and enjoyable activities
- Providing reality orientation and consistency in routine
- Maintaining supervision and observation

27. For a patient with tactile deficits, the nurse should check the temperature of bath water, monitor extremities for changes in range of motion and/or skin integrity, and make sure that the patient is not exposed to temperature extremes or prolonged pressure.

28. Safety concerns for the patient with an olfactory deficit include the inability to smell smoke or natural gas, along with the potential for eating spoiled food or suffering nutritional problems because of not being able to smell food.

29. a. Visual—
- Orient to the placement of items in the hospital room.
- Limit the amount of change in the environment. Furniture is kept in the same place.
- Keep items that the patient needs within easy reach, and let the patient know the location. The call light is placed within reach so that the patient calls for assistance with ambulating, especially in the first few days of hospitalization.
- Have glasses or other visual assistive devices, such as contact lenses, kept in good condition and available on the bedside table.
- Maintain adequate lighting, and minimize glare.
- Make sure the patient is wearing eyeglasses or contacts if prescribed.
- Use large print or clear handwriting when giving written instructions.
- Use photos, pictures, diagrams, or recorded instructions, if necessary.

b. Auditory—
- Encourage the patient to use an assistive device such as a hearing aid. Care is taken to keep the hearing aid in good working order and prevent it from getting lost.
- Be in position so that the patient can see the nurse's mouth, because many hearing-impaired patients read lips and watch facial expressions to assist hearing.
- Speak clearly and slowly without shouting.
- Keep background noise to a minimum.
- Ask the patient if hearing is better in one ear than the other, and stand on the patient's stronger-hearing side to converse.
- Use written instructions and information, if the patient is cognitively and visually able to read. Paper and pencil, a whiteboard, or a computer is kept at the bedside for use when the patient cannot hear a specific word or important instructions.
- Set up closed-caption television.
- Have a phone with a light that alerts the patient to an incoming call, if the patient is able to hear with an amplified receiver. Have access to a phone that allows for texting.

30. Home care considerations for the cognitively impaired person include:
- If 24-hour supervision and assistance with care are needed, provisions are made with loved ones or a day care service or placement is arranged in a long-term care facility.
- If the patient is cared for at home, information on day care and respite care is provided.
- Simple, calm environments help the dementia patient.
- Use of door locks that require a key may be necessary if the patient wanders.
- The environment is kept free of hazards such as sharp objects.
- Referral to home health agencies is made if assistance is needed with care.

 31. c    36. a    41. b
32. a   37. c   42. c
33. d   38. a   43. b
34. c   39. b   44. b
35. d   40. a

Practice Situations

a. For this patient after the CVA, possible nursing diagnoses are:
Impaired Verbal Communication
Risk for Injury
Impaired Mobility
- Goal/outcome examples—
Patient will be free of injury during hospital stay
Patient will be able to communicate needs effectively within 24 hours
Patient will perform passive range of motion to affected side twice daily
- Nursing interventions—

Obtain materials to promote communication, such as a picture/alphabet chart, white board, paper and pencil
Demonstrate/perform range of motion
Instruct patient to call for assistance—keep call bell within easy reach
Monitor status—vital signs, neuromuscular status, skin integrity, emotional response
Provide assistance in activities of daily living (ADLs), transfers, ambulating
- Assessment Data—
T 98.1° F, P 68 regular and strong, R 18 and unlabored, BP 128/76, pulse oximetry reading 96% on room air.
Alert and oriented to person but confused about place and time. Lungs are clear. Abdomen is soft and nontender, with bowel sounds present × 4. Denies pain. Mild weakness on her right side and is slightly unsteady on her feet, requiring the assistance of one person.
No redness or swelling at IV access in the left antecubital space.
Having mild difficulty finding some words—able to express needs. Speech clearer.
Strength on right side improved. Slight difficulty hearing conversational tone—no hearing aid.
Braden score is 21.

CHAPTER 32: STRESS AND COPING

1. Stress is defined by Kasl (1992) as a demand from the internal or external environment that exceeds the person's immediately available resources or ability to respond. Selye (1956) defines stress as "a non-specific response of the body to any demand made upon it."
2. Physiological stress is the body's potentially harmful reaction to a stimulus (Selye, 1976). Psychological stress comprises the emotional and cognitive factors involved in the appraisal of threat (Lazarus, 1966). When an individual interprets an event as a threat, the physiological stress response is activated. A third form of stress, sociocultural stress, occurs when social systems are challenged by factors such as racism, economic hardship, or political upheaval.
3. Some examples of stressors are the amount of work, situations at school, family responsibilities, financial concerns, and health issues.
4. The physiological responses are c, d, and e.
5. a. Alarm stage—Hypothalamic-pituitary-adrenal and autonomic nervous systems are activated, successively triggering responses in the sympathetic nervous system and the endocrine and immune systems.
   b. Resistance stage—The body attempts to adapt to the stressor, and some of the initial responses are attenuated as the parasympathetic nervous system reverses the sympathetic stimulation and stabilization occurs. The body begins to repair damage and restore resources.
   c. Exhaustion stage—When the stress is not relieved or the resources are inadequate to meet persistent demands.

200

Answer Key

6. a. Negative stress—distress
   b. Positive stress—eustress
7. General adaption syndrome (GAS) and local adaptation syndrome (LAS) are closely related, but the effects of LAS are most notably manifested by activities in the immune system, including inflammation, reflexive response to pain, or hypoxia.
8. This individual appears to have a strong sense of coherence.
9. Stress-related hyperglycemia may result from pregnancy, acute myocardial infarction, and postoperative state.
10. Stress appraisal is the individual's determination of the meaning of a stressful event. In the first stage the immediacy of the threat and the degree of ambiguity of the threat are factors. The person measures what is at stake in the stressful encounter. In the second stage coping options are evaluated. Primary and secondary appraisals determine whether the stressful situation or transaction is a threat or challenge.
11. Resilience (flexibility, resourcefulness), hardiness, and sense of coherence can buffer the impact of stress.
12. Anxiety is a response to stress that causes apprehension or uncertainty. Fear has an identifiable source of impending danger.
13. a. Mild anxiety can be motivational, foster creativity, and actually increase a person's ability to think clearly.
    b. Moderate anxiety narrows a person's focus, dulls perception, and may challenge a person to pay attention or use appropriate problem-solving skills.
    c. Severe anxiety results in the inability to make decisions or solve problems.
    d. Panic (the highest level of anxiety) is associated with a multitude of physiological symptoms, as well as feelings of extreme dread or terror.
14. Unresolved anger can lead to violent, abusive behavior and physiological changes, such as hypertension, GI distress, or depression.
15. The patient appears to be depressed.
16. Prolonged stress can result in irritable bowel syndrome, asthma, exacerbation of multiple sclerosis and other autoimmune diseases, a decreased immune response, and organ failure.
17. The accurate statements for stress are a, b, e, and f.
18. Nonverbal behaviors may be indicative of stress, including irritability, agitation, anxiety, and poor eye contact.
19. Examples of questions that would elicit information on physical symptoms are d and f.
20. a. A possible nursing diagnosis is Ineffective Coping related to information about the medical diagnosis as manifested by insomnia, nervous behavior, and negative attitude.
    Possible goals/outcomes are: *Patient will discuss possible coping strategies. Patient will participate in a support group. Patient will use relaxation techniques to focus on necessary activities. Patient will identify support network at home.*

    b. Nursing interventions include discussing the patient's feelings about the diagnosis, providing information on support groups or development of a support network, instructing the patient on ways to reduce anxiety via a holistic approach, and referring the patient to other members of the health care team (dietician, social worker, mental health therapist/advanced practice psychiatric nurse, clergy).
21. Strategies for stress management include progressive relaxation, mindfulness, nutrition, adequate sleep and rest, exercise, yoga, biofeedback, guided imagery, therapeutic touch, Reiki, massage therapy, and Eastern medicine.
22. Time management principles are prioritizing tasks, setting goals, increasing concentration skills, decreasing distractions, avoiding procrastination, setting boundaries, and maintaining self-discipline.
23. Increasing the intake of fruit, vegetables, legumes, fish, poultry, and whole grain enhances both psychological and physical responses to stress. Stress reduction may also be facilitated by taking multivitamins and herbal supplements.
24. Progressive relaxation has effectively been used to treat nausea and vomiting, pain, depression and anxiety, and sleep disturbances.

25. a	30. c	35. b
26. d	31. c	36. c
27. c	32. a	37. b
28. b	33. c	
29. b	34. d	

Practice Situations

a. You may suspect that your colleague is experiencing burnout or, more specific to his employment, compassion fatigue as the result of constant exposure to patients and families with many emotional needs.
b. To assist your colleague, you can do the following:
   • Recommend that he share his feelings with trusted co-workers, a counselor, and/or spiritual advisor/clergy.
   • Suggest relaxation activities outside of work, such as yoga and gardening.
   • Recommend an exercise plan, with a balance of rest.
   • Ask him to find a quiet place on the unit or in the hospital for him to relax on breaks.
   • Remind him to take breaks during his shift.
   • Recommend that he eat nutritious meals.
a. The patient's score on the Holmes-Rahe Life Stress Inventory is 168. This is associated with a chance of experiencing health issues within the next few years. The patient should begin to develop coping mechanisms and implement stress reduction strategies now to help her manage her current situation and prevent future issues.

CHAPTER 33: SLEEP

1. e
2. d
3. a
4. b
5. c
6. Examples of the changes that occur during sleep include:
    - Pulse, respirations, blood pressure, and muscle tone all decrease during sleep.
    - Rapid eye movement (REM) sleep is associated with memory storage, learning, increased cerebral blood flow, and epinephrine release.
    - Growth hormone is released to repair epithelial and brain cells, cell division for skin and bone marrow renewal occurs, and energy is conserved.
    - Body temperature, cortisol, and melatonin levels change.
7. Dreams and difficult arousal occur during REM sleep.
8. Nurses should allow for at least 90 to 120 minutes of uninterrupted sleep.
9. An individual who is blind may not be able to synchronize wake/sleep patterns with sunrise and sunset. His or her circadian rhythm could be disrupted.
10. The accurate statements are b, c, e, and f.
11. Physical problems that may occur with inadequate sleep include negative health effects on blood pressure (hypertension), glucose metabolism, and hormone regulation and to inflammation, increased frequency of seizures in patients with seizure disorders, and increased weight gain contributing to obesity.
12. Safety for infants includes placing them on their backs to sleep and keeping loose items out of the crib. For a toddler, keeping gates on stairs and locks on doors and cabinets prevents injury from waking during the night.
13. Toddler and preschool behaviors are a, b, and f.
14. Dyssomnias can be caused by excessive daytime sleeping, anxiety, depression, high levels of stimulation at bedtime, medication use, shift work, and hyperthyroidism.
15. For the patient with insomnia, the nurse should discuss stimulus control (using the bedroom for only sleep and sex), sleep restriction (staying in bed only if asleep), sleep hygiene, and cognitive therapy (relaxing and changing thought patterns). A combination of nonpharmacologic methods is often necessary to change sleep patterns. Treatment for hypersomnia is aimed at correcting any underlying conditions contributing to the hypersomnia.
16. Individuals with narcolepsy may fall asleep while driving or working with hazardous machinery, which could lead to injury.
17. The risk factors for obstructive sleep apnea (OSA) are c, d, and f.
18. Prolonged sleep apnea can lead to an increase in blood pressure, leading to cardiac arrest. Cardiac arrhythmias, pulmonary hypertension, and left-sided heart failure can also result.
19. Sleep deprivation is associated with b, e, and f.
20. Interventions based on this nursing diagnosis include:
    - Provide visual cues to decrease noise by dimming lights and closing curtains, but provide a night light for safety.
    - Provide privacy by drawing curtains between patients or closing room doors, if possible.
    - Negotiate times to mute television, radios, and music on hospital units.
    - Limit overhead pages to emergencies only at night.
    - Lower telephone ringtones.
    - Limit staff conversations in hallways and at nursing stations.
    - Conduct shift reports in areas away from patient rooms, unless the facility requires bedside reporting. If the patient is asleep during change-of-shift rounds, the nurses can check the patient and then step away and speak in soft voices.
    - Move equipment quietly, without hitting other objects.
    - Monitor equipment frequently to prevent alarm tones as much as possible.
21. The biggest safety factor is injury to self or others.
22. Sleep is influenced as follows:
    a. Exercise—Exercise can assist with weight-loss efforts and promote fatigue and relaxation, but excessive exercise, especially in the evening, interferes with sleep.
    b. Stress—Psychological stress decreases REM sleep and can prevent a person from getting enough sleep. Anxiety, including the stress associated with work, finances, illness, and family, can cause intrusive thoughts, muscular tension, and increased norepinephrine levels, which all interfere with being able to go to sleep and stay asleep.
    c. Family relationships—Difficulty in sleeping may occur for:
        - New parents adjusting to the parenting role and frequent nightly awakenings.
        - Caregivers of persons with chronic illnesses living at home.
        - A person going through the grief process following a loss.
        - Children away from home and suffering from homesickness.
        - Individuals with marital problems, both the involved adults and the children in the home.
        - Those who sleep with a partner who has a sleep disorder.
23. The nurse should recommend that this individual avoid tea with caffeine later in the evening. He can try decaffeinated herbal teas that have different flavors and may actually promote sleep. Other alternatives are fruit juices or milk or drinking caffeinated beverages earlier in the evening.
24. Polysomnography records eye movements, muscle movement and activity, heart and respiratory rate, oxygen levels, airflow, and brain activity while the patient sleeps. The results of polysomnography include the apnea-hypopnea index or the number of apneic or hypopneic episodes per hour. The normal number of these episodes for an adult is fewer than 5/hour; mild OSA is 5 to 15 episodes/hour; moderate OSA is 15 to 30 episodes/hour; and severe OSA is more than 30 apneic or hypopneic episodes/hour.
25. The equipment shown is a CPAP device (continuous positive airway pressure), which is used for patients experiencing OSA.

26. Examples of bedtime rituals include taking a warm bath or shower, reading, listening to music, and meditating or using relaxation techniques.

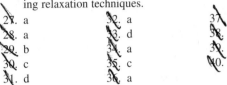

27. a
28. a
29. b
30. c
31. d

32. a
33. d
34. a
35. c
36. a

37. d
38. a
39. b
40. c

Practice Situation

a. To specifically minimize the effect of the change, you should try to:
- Eliminate overtime on a long shift.
- Complete challenging patient tasks early in the shift.
- Take responsibility for obtaining a minimum of 6 hours of sleep.
- Maintain a regular sleep schedule when working and on nights off.
- Include a 4-hour "anchor" sleep time during which sleep is scheduled whether on or off work. For example, after working, sleep from 8:30 A.M. to 4:30 P.M., and on days off, sleep from 4:30 A.M. to 12:30 P.M. The anchor sleep time is from 8:30 A.M. to 12:30 P.M.
- Wear dark glasses that block blue light when driving home after night work.
- Seek exposure to bright light (sunlight is best) as soon as possible after waking.
- Before the first night shift, power-nap 30 to 90 minutes before leaving for work.

In addition, other measures to maintain a more normal sleep pattern include:
- Taking a warm bath
- Eating a light snack that contains carbohydrates
- Drinking warm milk
- Avoiding caffeine, tobacco, and excessive alcohol
- Getting a back massage
- Relaxing using aromatherapy and music therapy
- Adjusting the environment for temperature, noise, and light
- Avoiding large meals and certain medications

b. You should be alert to difficulty in concentrating, fatigue, malaise, headache, nausea, increased sensitivity to pain, decreased neuromuscular coordination, irritability, and difficulty concentrating. Eventually, disorientation and hallucinations may occur.

CHAPTER 34: DIAGNOSTIC TESTING

1. i
2. h
3. g
4. j

5. c
6. a
7. f
8. b

9. e
10. d

11. The components of the CBC include the red blood cell count (RBC), hemoglobin level, hematocrit (HCT), red cell indices, white blood cell count (WBC), and differential WBC.

12. Tests for a patient on anticoagulants are platelets, bleeding time, prothrombin time/international normalized ratio (PT/INR), activated partial thromboplastin time, and fibrinogen.

13. Blood glucose is measured to determine the presence of diabetes mellitus.

14. High-density lipoprotein (HDL) is the "good cholesterol."

15. The expected findings for a urinalysis are a, e.

16. C-reactive protein (CRP) has been used in the past as a marker for inflammatory and autoimmune disorders, such as rheumatoid arthritis, lupus, and inflammatory bowel syndrome. High-sensitivity CRP (hs-CRP) is considered a marker for vascular inflammation. CRP is now used as a screening for coronary artery disease and as a predictor of future cardiac events.

17. Potential cardiac markers are b, d, and f.

18. For this patient, there appears to be bleeding in the upper GI tract.

19. A test for fecal ova and parasites is done, with the sample sent to the laboratory while still warm.

20. Culture and sensitivity is explained as follows: For a suspected infection, a specimen (urine, blood, sputum, etc.) is sent to the laboratory, where a section is placed on a culture medium. If bacteria are found to grow, it is a positive result. After identification of the bacteria, it is exposed to different antibiotics to see which one would be most effective in treating the infection.

21. A chest radiograph can be used to diagnose pulmonary disorders, such as TB, cancer, and pneumonia.

22. The nurse suspects that the patient is experiencing an allergic reaction, which may progress to anaphylaxis.

23. Fasting is required for b, and c.

24. Instruction provided to the patient before the MRI: It is contraindicated in patients with pacemakers, inner-ear implants, fragments from gunshot wounds, or any other metal object in the body. All jewelry is removed before the test. Some patients experience claustrophobia because the test is sometimes performed in a tunnel-like machine for 30 to 90 minutes. Rarely, people with a tattoo have reported burning and swelling in the area of the tattoo after MRI.

25. Screening for individuals older than age 50 includes:
- Fecal occult blood test annually
- Flexible sigmoidoscopy every 5 years or colonoscopy every 10 years (or double-contrast barium enema or computed tomography [CT] colonography every 5 years)

26. Ultrasound is used commonly for pregnant women to determine the status of the fetus. Abnormal organ growth, lesions or tumors, and structural damage can also be seen with ultrasound.

27. A critical question is to ask if there is any chance that they are pregnant and/or when the last menstrual period occurred?

28. Respiratory status is the most critical area to monitor.

29. a. Thoracentesis—nursing care:
- Position the patient to the unaffected side for at least an hour.
- Monitor vital signs until stable.
- Check the dressing frequently.
- Assess the puncture site for bleeding or crepitus.

203

- Assess respiratory status, including breath sounds and symmetry during respirations, and monitor for signs of distress.
  - Arrange for a chest radiograph if ordered.
  b. Lumbar puncture—nursing care:
  - Instruct the patient to lie flat for 4 to 8 hours.
  - Encourage fluids.
  - Perform neurologic assessment as ordered.
  - Assess the puncture site for drainage.
  - Administer analgesics prn.
30. Nursing diagnosis: Anxiety related to actual or perceived threat to physical health secondary to diagnostic testing as evidenced/manifested by fidgeting, pacing, facial expression, rapid heartbeat, insomnia.
Goals: Patient will use relaxation techniques while waiting for the testing and results.
Patient will sleep 6 to 7 hours on the night before the diagnostic procedure.
31. The tubes have stopper colors as follows: Blood culture—yellow, Blood chemistry—red, red/black, green (stat chemistry)
32. National Patient Safety Goals:
  - Identifying patients correctly continues to be a top National Patient Safety Goal.
  - Two patient identifiers are used when collecting blood samples and other specimens for clinical testing.
  - The patient's room number or physical location is not used as an identifier.
  - Containers used for blood and other specimens are labeled in the presence of the patient.
33. Standard precautions are as follows:
  a. Venipuncture—Hand washing is done before and after, gloves are worn throughout the procedure, and sharps are disposed of immediately after specimen collection.
  b. Urine collection—Hand washing is done before and after, gloves are worn during the procedure, and the specimen is stored in a plastic bag or biohazard container for transport to the laboratory.
34. During the procedure, the nurse can assist the patient to maintain a necessary position, pad bony prominences, explain what is happening, and offer emotional support, like holding the patient's hand.
35. Careful specimen collection and transfer requires that each one is placed in the appropriate container, correctly identified, handled with aseptic technique, and sent to the laboratory in a timely manner.
36. The correct procedure for the clean catch collection is d, c, f, a, e, and b.
37. a. The first voiding is discarded for the timed urine collection.
  b. If a voiding is discarded, the timed collection needs to be restarted.
38. Sputum collection is ordered when an infectious respiratory disease is suspected, such as pneumonia or tuberculosis. It can also be done to evaluate the effectiveness of antibiotic/antiviral therapy or identify the presence of abnormal cells (tumors).
39. The correct procedures for sputum collection are a, b, d, and e.
40. If the patient starts to gag during a throat culture, instruct the individual to sit upright and say "ahhh," place the swab off center, and swab quickly.

41. The nurse should monitor the patient's vital signs, airway, oxygenation status, and site of the procedure, if bleeding may occur.
42. The laboratory results indicate the following:
  a. RBC decreased—anemia, bone marrow suppression, chronic infection, hemorrhage, renal disease, vitamin B, or folic acid deficiency
  b. WBC increased—acute leukemia, infections, surgery, trauma
  c. Platelets decreased—anemias, transfusions of packed cells, HIV infection, chemo/radiation therapy
  d. BUN increased—acute glomerulonephritis, congestive heart failure, diabetes mellitus, high-protein diet, nephrotic syndrome, renal disease, severe dehydration, severe infection, shock.
43. CT scans of the brain can diagnose abscesses, cerebral infarctions (strokes), aneurysms, hemorrhage, hydrocephalus, and tumors.
44. To verify the presence of Crohn disease, a sigmoidoscopy or colonoscopy will be ordered.
45. For stool specimen collection:
  a. The nurse needs to:
  - Place a sign in the patient bathroom and on the patient's health record.
  - Remind the patient that samples are needed, and provide other procedural information.
  - Communicate information in the report and the patient's health record.
  - Ensure that valid samples are not discarded.
  - Remove the signs when the last sample has been obtained.
  b. If the sample is contaminated with toilet paper, bodily fluids, or toilet water, a new sample must be obtained.

46. c	49. b	52. d
47. b	50. c	53. b
48. a	51. a	54. a

Practice Situation

a. To make sure that patient safety and comfort are maintained, you should:
  - Check for the presence of an identification band. Ensure that the band is on the patient and is correct.
  - Review the medical record for a history of medical disorders that may signal a high risk for complications (bleeding disorders, hypertension, etc.).
  - Check for allergies to food or medications.
  - Check that the consent form has been signed and witnessed.
  - Obtain and document a complete set of vital signs. This provides a baseline for comparison during the procedure.
  - Consult with the health care provider as to whether regularly scheduled medications should be administered before the diagnostic test.
  - When appropriate, ensure that the patient has maintained NPO status.
  - Be sure that the IV access is patent and well secured.
  - Provide prescribed preprocedure sedatives or analgesics at the appropriate time.

b. Following the procedure, you should plan to:
- Assess the neurovascular status of the affected limb, including pain, pallor, paresthesia, paralysis, and pulse
- Monitor vital signs
- Elevate the extremity and apply ice
- Administer analgesics as needed (prn)
- Instruct the patient to avoid alcohol for 24 hours

c. You should anticipate that the patient will want pain relief. Analgesics should be available, as well as making sure that the leg is correctly positioned.

CHAPTER 35: MEDICATION ADMINISTRATION

1. i	5. a	9. j
2. g	6. h	10. e
3. d	7. c	
4. f	8. b	

11. A drug is any substance that either positively or negatively alters physiological function. A medication is a drug specifically administered for its therapeutic effect on physiological function.

12. a. Trade name
    b. Generic name
    c. Generic name
    d. Chemical name
    e. Trade name

13. The accurate identifiers are a, c, d, and e.

14. a. A woman who is pregnant—Take extreme care when administering medications throughout pregnancy, and especially in the first trimester, due to risk of harm to the developing fetus.
    b. An infant—Infants require small doses related to their body size and immature organs. A calibrated dropper is used for infants or very young children. Place the medication between the gum and cheek to prevent aspiration.
    c. An older adult—Increased fat deposits, decreased gastric mobility, decreased renal and liver function and changes in the blood-brain barrier can lead to increased side effects of medications.
    - Do not rush medication administration. Allow time for understanding of treatment and slower swallowing.
    - Crushed or liquid forms of medications may be easier to swallow.
    - Normal aging processes (decreased renal and hepatic function) may affect the dosage needed as drugs may be metabolized slower. Adverse effects may be increased in elderly individuals.
    - Patients may need instruction on medications to be taken at home. Focus on the name and purpose of the drug because the color may vary by manufacturer.
    - Loss of dexterity (and therefore the ability to open pill bottles), visual impairment, and cognitive impairment in elderly persons can affect safe medication administration.

15. a. Drug metabolism—liver
    b. Excretion—kidneys

16. The nurse should return at 8:30 a.m.

17. The nurse should determine if the patient has any known allergies to medications, especially antibiotics. The patient should also stay in the clinic for at least 20 to 30 minutes to observe if there is a reaction to the medication.

18. An example of a synergistic effect is alcohol with a narcotic (morphine)—both depress the central nervous system. An example of an antagonistic effect is a stimulant, such as cocaine taken with a depressant (e.g., codeine).

19. Examples of common over-the-counter medications are cough medicines, mild analgesics, sleep aids, and antacids.

20. a. The frequency of administration is missing.
    b. The route of administration is missing.

21. Special documentation is required on a computerized medication administration record (MAR) if the patient refuses a medication or it is held.

22. a. The sublingual route is being used.
    b. Nitroglycerin is a common example of a medication given this way.

23. Enteric-coated, time-release, sublingual, buccal, and medications with special coatings cannot be crushed.

24. The nurse can delegate to the UAP observation of the patient for changes in vital signs, patient complaints or discomforts, reporting of any medications found in the room, and sharing of any questions that the patient has about the medications. For IV infusion, the UAP can report on any issues at the access site, low volume in the IV bag, and pump alarms.

25. The topical administrations are b, c, e, and f.

26. a. IM injection—3-mL syringe, 1½-inch needle
    b. Subcutaneous injection—1-mL syringe (3 mL can also be used), ⅝-inch needle

27. a. Antihypertensive—vital signs, particularly the blood pressure, and other indications of lightheadedness or dizziness
    b. Bronchodilator—vital signs, particularly respiratory status and auscultation of lung sounds
    c. Narcotic analgesic—vital signs, particularly respiratory status and determination of level of consciousness and comfort level
    d. Anticoagulant—review of laboratory results for coagulant studies and observation for signs of bruising or bleeding
    e. Antipyretic—vital signs, particularly the temperature, and indications of reduced fever, such as cooler skin temperature

28. Examples of measures to reduce medication errors are taking time to read the orders carefully, being knowledgeable about the medications (e.g., dosages, side effects), recognizing prescription errors, following the Six Rights and performing triple checks before administration, and communicating with colleagues about questions or concerns.

29. Appropriate notations are a, d, e, and f.

30. a. 20mg/40mg x 1 mL = ½ mL (shaded on the syringe)
    b. 250 mcg/1000 mcg/mg = 0.25 mg
       0.25 mg/0.25 mg = 1/2 tablet

c. 750mg/500mg x 1 mL = 1.5 mL

d. 100 mg/50mg x 1 capsule = 2 capsules

e. 10,000U/20,000U x 1 mL = 1/2 mL (0.5 mL)

f. 30 U shaded on the U-100 insulin syringe

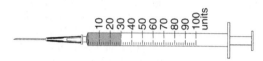

31. a. 90 degree, intramuscular (IM) or subcutaneous injection
    b. 45 degree, subcutaneous injection
    c. 5 to 15 degrees, intradermal (ID) injection

32. The "Six Rights" are the right:
    - Drug
    - Dose
    - Time
    - Route
    - Patient
    - Documentation

33. The nurse performs the three checks as follows:
    - Verifying that the medication matches the MAR, calculating the dosage, and checking the expiration date of the medication
    - Preparing the medication and checking the label again with the MAR
    - Rechecking the label of the medication before returning it to its storage area or right before opening the package at the bedside

34. Examples of questions include:
    - Do you have any food or drug allergies? If so, what was your reaction?
    - What prescribed medications are you currently taking? Do you have them with you?
    - Which over-the-counter medications and herbs do you take on a regular basis (e.g., antacids, laxatives, aspirin, creams or lotions)?
    - What is your alcohol intake? Caffeine intake? Use of home remedies?
    - What medications have you stopped taking recently?
    - Do you use any other methods to relieve your symptoms?

35. a. A nursing diagnosis can be *Knowledge deficit related to new diagnosis and prescriptions as evidenced by asking about the medications.*
    b. A goal for this patient can be:
       Patient will verbalize information about the prescribed medications before discharge or next clinic visit.
       Patient will state when the medications should be taken by next appointment.

36. Special considerations for children include:
    - Liquid forms of oral medications are preferred for children younger than the age of 5 years.
    - Parents or caregivers may need instruction, with pictures and written directions, on home medication administration.
    - A calibrated dropper is used for infants or very young children. Place the medication between the gum and cheek to prevent aspiration.
    - Uncoated tablets or soft capsules may be crushed and administered sprinkled over a small amount of food. Do not use a favorite food or formula as the child may avoid food associated with medicines in the future.
    - Give the child, if possible, a choice of how to take the medication, such as with water or juice.
    - Warn the child if the medication has an unpleasant taste; this helps to increase future trust in the nurse.
    - Praise the child after the medication is swallowed.

37. Oral medications are contraindicated if the patient is not able to swallow, has a diminished level of consciousness, no gag reflex present, nausea or vomiting, an NPO order, or procedures/treatment in the mouth or throat.

38. The types of oral medications that should be given last are sublingual, buccal, "swish and swallow" liquids, other oral or pharyngeal treatments, and cough medicines.

39. The correct techniques for enteral administration are a, d, and e.

40. a. pc—after meals
    b. bid—twice a day
    c. prn—as needed
    d. IV—intravenous
    e. qid—four times a day

41. The correct techniques for administration of transdermal patches are c, e, and f.

42. a. The nurse should use eardrops that are at room temperature.
    b. The pinna should be pulled up and back for an adult.

43. Have the patient blow his/her nose for the nurse before administering nasal medication.

44. a. The nurse should assess the patient's breathing, breath sounds, respiratory rate, and use of accessory muscles.
    b. The patient should rinse the mouth or receive oral care after receiving steroids by inhalation.
    c. The doses in a container are determined by dividing the total amount by the number of doses that the patient takes each day.

45. a. Positioning for vaginal suppository insertion is dorsal recumbent or Sims position (if necessary).
    b. Positioning for rectal suppository insertion is Sims position (left side with upper knee flexed).

46. Parenteral administration requires sterile technique.

47. The only way to cover the needle is to use a one-handed technique and slide the needle into the cap using a scooping motion, without contaminating it or using the free hand. When the needle is back on the cap, the syringe is held vertically and the cap is snapped back on by holding the sides of the cap.

48. The nurse uses a 2 x 2 gauze to cover the neck of the ampule to protect the hand while snapping off the top. Excess medication is discarded. A filter needle is used to remove the medication from the ampule and then changed for the injection.

49. The correct procedure is d, a, e, f, b, and c.

50. The sites for subcutaneous injections are shaded on the figure below.

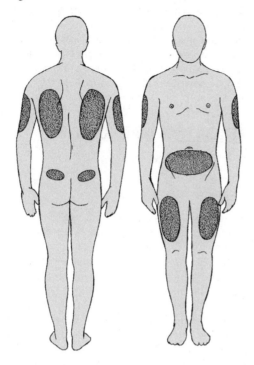

51. a. Intradermal injections are used to administer local anesthetics, test for allergies, and test for exposure to TB.
   b. The sites for the injection can be the inner forearm, upper arm, and scapular area.
52. False. Aspiration is not required for injections into the deltoid, vastus lateralis, or ventrogluteal sites.
53. a. Subcutaneous injections—0.5 to 1 mL
   b. Deltoid injection—1 mL or less
54. A Z-track injection is performed as follows:
   • Use the side of the nondominant hand to pull the skin tight below the injection site or to the side (Z-track).
   • Insert the needle quickly at a 90-degree angle.
   • Continue to pull on the skin with the side of the nondominant hand; use the thumb and index finger to stabilize the barrel of the syringe.
   • Move the dominant hand up on the barrel to the end of the plunger.
   • Administer the medication by slowly depressing the plunger—1 mL medication over 10 seconds. Hold the needle in place for 10 seconds after the medication is administered.
   • Perform the following steps in quick succession:
     • Withdraw the needle/syringe with the dominant hand.
     • Release the Z-tracked tissue from the nondominant hand.
     • Apply gentle pressure with the gauze with the nondominant hand. Do not massage the site.
55. True
56. IV medications can be administered by IV push, intermittent small-volume administration, or volume control administration set.

57. For administration of IV medications, the nurse must use caution and assess the following:
   • Patient allergies
   • Medication/IV solution compatibility
   • Amount and rate of the medication administration
   • IV access site—check for infiltration, phlebitis
   • Sterile technique is used consistently
58. The nurse can set up a pill reminder system with either a commercially made product that has the days of the week or homemade set of labeled containers. There are also automated reminder devices and phone calls. Calendars or journals may be used to reinforce the management of the medications, along with linking the medication administration with easy-to-remember times during the day (breakfast, lunch, bedtime).
59. The "Ask Me 3" program emphasizes questions patients should ask, including:
   What is my main problem?
   What do I need to do?
   Why is it important for me to do this?
60. The patient and nurse can check the blood glucose levels to see how the insulin is working, along with observation for signs and symptoms that would indicate an insufficient or excess amount of insulin.
61. The best routes for the patient are c and e.
62. Bar-code scanning is used to verify the patient's identification and medication.
63. The nurse instructs the patient not to swallow these medications but allow them to dissolve. Food and fluid are not administered along with sublingual or buccal medications.
64. The correct order for inhalation is e, c, a, d, f, and b.
65. Most medications in vials are mixed by rolling the vial in the hands. Shaking the vial can create excess air bubbles.
66. If the area has moles, scars, rashes, or breaks in the skin, the area should not be used for an injection.
67. The site to use for the injections is located at:
   a. Deltoid—Place the ring finger along the lower edge of the acromial process, with the middle finger (and possibly index finger) joined with the ring finger. The point of injection is midline immediately below the middle or index finger, in line with the axilla.
   b. Vastus lateralis—Place one hand below the greater trochanter of the femur, with the thumb pointing toward the knee to form an L or backward-L shape. Place the other hand above the knee, with the thumb pointing toward the hip to form an L or backward-L shape. The point of injection is in the center third of the lateral thigh between the hands and at the center of the side of the leg.
68. The steps for direct IV push of a medication are:
   • Prepare the medication in the syringe. A needleless port may be in place.
   • Use an alcohol wipe to clean the injection port of the saline lock.
   • Flush the IV per agency guidelines.
   • Inject the medication, adhering to safe medication guidelines.
   • Flush the IV.

207

Answer Key

69. c	78. a	87. c
70. b	79. d	88. a
71. a	80. c	89. b
72. b	81. c	90. b
73. d	82. b	91. d
74. a	83. b	92. d
75. b	84. d	93. c
76. c	85. d	94. c
77. a	86. c	95. a

Practice Situations

a. It is not good practice to administer medications that are prepared by another nurse. If the medications need to be given, it would be best to prepare them yourself. If the medications are all still in their packaging, they can be checked against the prescriber's order and MAR. If the nurse will be returning to the unit in a reasonable time frame, then it would be best if that individual administered medications to his or her patient.

b. After calculating a dosage that is unfamiliar, it is best to ask another nurse to check your work before giving the amount.

c. If you see that the two IV medications are incompatible, you will need to notify the prescriber/provider so that a different medication or route can be used.

d. For a liquid medication that is less than 10 mL, an oral syringe should be used for accuracy.

e. If the patient tells you that the pill looks different, it may be that the order has been changed or there is an error. Take the time to check and make sure that the medication order and MAR are accurate.

f. After recognizing that an error has been made, it is important to report it to your manager and the provider. There may be a need for follow-up care to counteract the medications given. The patient's health is your ultimate concern. You will need to follow agency policy for further reporting and possible remediation.

g. If the patient does not have an ID wrist band, you will need to make sure that one is obtained. An ID wrist band has critical information, such as the patient's hospital number, and is used as an identifier. If there is a photo of the patient, this can be used to verify the identity.

h. Medication administration should not be documented in advance, as the patient may refuse medications or they may need to be held and not given. This is especially important when giving controlled substances. You should speak with the fellow staff nurse about the hazards of this practice and make sure not to document in advance yourself.

i. If the label is not legible and cannot be cleaned effectively, it is unsafe to administer the medication. Another bottle of the medication should be obtained from the pharmacy.

j. If the pill is scored, it can be safely cut or cracked in half. Use of a pill cutter is preferable to breaking the pill apart by hand.

k. If a controlled substance needs to be discarded, a witness is required to verify that the medication was not used. This discard is usually documented in a record of the controlled substance inventory.

l. The patient's enteric-coated medication cannot be crushed. If the patient cannot tolerate this medication by mouth, then an alternative form, such as a liquid, will need to be investigated. You should contact the pharmacy to see if the medication is available in another form and then notify the provider about the situation.

m. Similar to the issue with the illegible label, the pharmacy needs to be contacted to get the correct and unexpired medications for the patient. Never assume that the medications in the patient's storage drawer are all correct.

CHAPTER 36: PAIN MANAGEMENT

1. h	5. b	9. a
2. i	6. d	10. g
3. c	7. e	
4. f	8. j	

11. Unrelieved pain is associated with a health care professional's failure to assess pain, failure to accept a patient's reported pain, and failure to initiate pain relief.

12. Nurses should assess pain along with other vital signs, before and after pain control interventions are performed or analgesic medication is administered.

13. The assessment findings are a, b, c, and e.

14. The skin is the area that is most sensitive to painful stimuli.

15. The four steps in the pain conduction process are transduction, transmission, modulation, and perception.

    Transduction—Conversion of the energy from the pain stimuli into electrical energy through nociceptors at the place of tissue injury.

    Transmission—The action potential, or electrical energy signal, is sent to the spinal cord and brain.

    Perception—Occurs when the brain translates the signals as pain.

    Modulation—Once pain is recognized, the brain can change the perception of pain by sending inhibitory input to the spinal cord to impede the transmission.

16. The pain threshold is the point at which the brain recognizes the stimulus as pain. Pain tolerance is the intensity or duration of pain that a patient is able or willing to endure.

17. The three major types of pain are acute pain, cancer pain, and noncancer pain.

18. The specific sensations for neuropathic pain include burning, aching, crushing, stabbing, shooting, tingling, or numbing.

19. Pathologies that can influence the pain experience are those that damage or create hypersensitivity along the pain pathway, such as spinal cord injuries (paraplegia/quadriplegia), peripheral neuropathy secondary to diabetes mellitus or peripheral vascular disease, and psychological dysfunction.

20. Physiological changes that occur with pain include:
    - Endocrine system: release of excessive amounts of hormones, leading to hyperglycemia.
    - Cardiovascular system: an increase in the heart rate, force of contraction, blood pressure, and coagulation.
    - Respiratory system: respiratory rate increases and becomes irregular.
    - Musculoskeletal system: impaired muscle function, muscle spasms, muscle tension, and fatigue.
    - Genitourinary system: an increase in blood pressure through activation of the renin-angiotensin system.

Urine output decreases, and urinary retention increases, with possible fluid overload and hypokalemia.

- GI system: a decrease in gastric emptying and motility, increased GI secretions, and smooth muscle tone. Metabolism is slowed, resulting in indigestion and constipation.
- Immune system: inflammatory mediators are released in an attempt to prevent and fight infection and to reduce the pain.

21. Pain is influenced as follows:
    a. Gender—Women have reported being in more pain, women seek help for pain more often than men do, but women are less likely to receive treatment. Women are more likely to be given sedatives for pain, and men are more likely to be given analgesics for pain.
    b. Disability—A patient with impaired cognition may not be able to communicate pain. Facial expressions, vocalization of noises, or changes in physical activity or routines may be signs of pain. Patients who are intubated may be able to write or point to a pain assessment tool to indicate their level of pain. Elevated blood pressure and/or pulse rate, as well as restlessness, may signal increased pain levels in patients who are intubated and sedated and unable to communicate verbally or in writing.
    c. Morphology—Obese people tend to experience more pain in more locations than individuals of more average weight, and pain medication dosages need to be adjusted on the basis of the height and weight of patients of all ages due to body surface area and metabolic differences.

22. The score for the infant = 6, which is indicative of pain.

23. Strategies that can be used to help a child include toys, video games, books, or other forms of entertainment.

24. Medications are given in lower doses to older adults.

25. The patient can be given a visual scale, such as the Wong-Baker Facial Grimace Scale or a scale of 0 to 10 that the patient can select from to indicate the level of pain. Pointing to the area can identify the location.

26. SOCRATES stands for:
    S = site (Where is the pain located?)
    O = onset (When did the pain start? Was it gradual or sudden?)
    C = character (What is the quality of the pain? Is it stabbing, burning, or aching in nature?)
    R = radiation (Does the pain radiate anywhere?)
    A = associations (What signs and symptoms are associated with the pain?)
    T = time course (Is there any pattern to when the pain occurs?)
    E = exacerbating/relieving factors (Does anything make the pain worse or lessen it?)
    S = severity (On a scale of 0 to 10, what is the intensity of the pain?)

27. Behaviors associated with pain include facial grimaces, clenched teeth, rubbing or guarding of the painful area, agitation, restlessness, and withdrawal from painful stimuli. A patient in labor may use effleurage and immobilization to help deal with uterine contraction pain. Vocalizations of pain may be expressed as crying, moaning, or screaming. Patients may exhibit psychological responses to pain, including anxiety, fear, depression, anger, irritability, helplessness, and hopelessness.

28. Delegation to the UAP can include back rubs, repositioning the patient, performing oral hygiene, changing the linens, talking to the patient, and darkening the room.

29. Legal risks can be reduced by:
    - Checking patient allergies and sensitivities before administering any medication
    - Administering medications using the Six Rights of Medication Administration
    - Following the steps of the nursing process
    - Monitoring for side effects or adverse effects of medication
    - Reporting uncommon patient responses to analgesia to the patient's physician or PCP
    - Communicating effectively to the patient
    - Teaching the patient about the use of medications and potential side effects
    - Evaluating the effect of medication on the patient, and document the patient's response. Use equipment such as patient-controlled anesthesia pumps properly
    - Documenting accurately and in a timely manner
    - Following the facility's policies and procedures
    - Arranging for appropriate referrals to meet the needs of the patient

30. Some herbal remedies may interact negatively with prescription analgesics.

31. Examples of distractions are having the patient watch television, listen to music, engage in conversation, participate in hobbies, or sing.

32. The advantages of the transdermal fentanyl system are that it can:
    - Eliminate having to program an intravenous pump.
    - Minimize preparation time, making it less time-consuming for nurses.
    - Eliminate medication errors.
    - Provide greater pain control for patients.
    - Enable patients to perform daily activities easier, due to the lack of an intravenous line.
    - Enable patients to move and ambulate earlier, due to improved pain control.

33. The opioid analgesics are b, c, e, and f.

34. The major side effect is respiratory depression.

35. For Patient-controlled analgesia (PCAs):
    a. Medications usually administered—morphine sulfate, fentanyl, or hydromorphone
    b. Frequency of assessment:
       - Assess the patient when he or she begins use of the PCA and again a half hour later.
       - Check the patient every hour for the first 8 hours of PCA use following the initial assessments.
       - After the first 8 hours, assess the patient as specified in the PCP order or every 4 hours at a minimum. (Assessment may be done more frequently in accordance with nursing judgment, depending on patient status.)
    c. Precautions:
       - Ensure that only the patient operates the PCA. Family members should never activate the pump for the patient.

209

- Keep naloxone, or another specifically indicated antagonist analgesic, immediately accessible in case of an overdose or emergency.
- Follow the PCP order for medications, dosage, and pump settings.

36. A nerve block is used for migraine headaches, dental work, back pain, herniated disks, and cancer pain.
37. False
38. The Joint Commission standards are:
- Recognize the right of patients to have appropriate assessment and management of their pain.
- Identify patients with pain in an initial screening assessment.
- Perform a more comprehensive pain assessment when pain is identified.
- Record the results of the assessment in a way that facilitates regular reassessment and follow-up.
- Educate relevant providers in pain assessment and management.
- Determine and ensure staff competency in pain assessment and management.
- Address pain assessment and management in the orientation of all new staff.
- Establish policies and procedures that support appropriate prescribing and ordering of effective pain medications.
- Ensure that pain does not interfere with participation in rehabilitation.
- Educate patients and their families about the importance of effective pain management.
- Address patient needs for symptom management in the discharge planning process.
- Collect data to monitor the appropriateness and effectiveness of pain management.

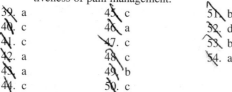

39. a	45. c	51. b
40. c	46. a	52. d
41. c	47. c	53. b
42. a	48. c	54. a
43. a	49. b	
44. c	50. c	

Practice Situation

a. You expect that the patient will have signs and symptoms of chronic pain associated with osteoarthritis. In addition to the joint discomfort and stiffness, there may be changes in the patient's vital signs, such as a decrease in blood pressure, pulse, and thoracic expansion; fatigue; malaise; and an inability to perform ADLs. Bowel and bladder function may decline with discomfort and difficulty in getting to the bathroom.

b. A potential nursing diagnosis is:
Chronic pain related to arthritic joint changes as evidenced by limited mobility and inability to manage ADLs.
Possible goals are:
- Patient will perform ADLs on a daily basis, reporting chronic pain at a level of 1 or less within 1 week of starting on nonpharmacologic interventions and nonopioid medications.
- Patient will report increased ability to perform routine activities within 2 hours of receiving the prescribed dose of analgesia.

Nonpharmacologic interventions include:
- Positioning for comfort and proper body alignment
- Massage to promote relaxation and decrease muscle tension
- Alternative/complementary therapies—progressive relaxation techniques, guided imagery, yoga, biofeedback, meditation, hypnosis, Reiki, therapeutic touch, Chinese medicine
- Distraction—television, music, conversation, singing

c. It is anticipated that the patient will be advised to take acetaminophen or a nonsteroidal anti-inflammatory drug (NSAID) for his or her level of pain. Patients on these medications need to be taught to maintain the recommended dosage (acetaminophen, NSAIDs) or take the medication with food (NSAIDs). Proton pump inhibitors (PPIs) or histamine receptor blockers (H2 blockers) are often prescribed for patients who are on long-term NSAID therapy to help reduce the incidence of stomach ulcers.

CHAPTER 37: PERIOPERATIVE CARE

1. d
2. f
3. e
4. a
5. b
6. c
7. a. Preoperative phase—This is the time when the patient decides or needs to have surgery, depending on the circumstances. Patient teaching is done, along with laboratory/diagnostic tests, and determination of risk factors and baseline vital signs. Preoperative forms and consents are completed.
   b. Intraoperative phase—This is the time when the patient enters the operating room and is anesthetized, monitored, prepped, and draped, and then the surgical procedure is performed. Patients are closely monitored for their respiratory, circulatory, and neurologic responses.
   c. Postoperative phase—This begins when the patient is admitted to the postanesthesia care unit (PACU) and ends when the patient has completely recovered from the surgical procedure, which in some cases is several months.
8. The "time-out" during surgery is when everyone in the operating room stops what they are doing to communicate. This will allow for a final assessment to verify the correct patient, procedure, and surgical site. The time-out is documented.
9. a. Gynecologic surgery—lithotomy or dorsal recumbent
   b. Cardiac—supine or dorsal recumbent
   c. Renal—lateral
   d. Rectal—lithotomy or jacknife
10. The scrub nurse prepares the surgical setup for handling instruments, maintains surgical asepsis while draping, and assists the surgeon by passing instruments, sutures, and supplies. The circulating nurse acts as the patient's advocate and a liaison between scrubbed personnel and the surgical team and coordinates the needs of the surgical team by obtaining supplies and carrying out the nursing care plan.

11. For the obese patient, a towel can be positioned under the right lower back and hip. This will correct the inferior vena cava occlusion by causing the patient to shift to the left side.

12. Skin preparation includes removing the hair, cleansing the skin, and using an antimicrobial agent. Whenever possible, the hair is left intact. Clippers can be used when the removal of hair is needed.

13. Hand-off communication between the intraoperative and PACU nurse should include an update on the status of the patient (vital signs, responsiveness, etc.) and medications given during the procedure.

14. The priority assessments for this patient in the PACU are respirations, circulation, neurologic status—level of consciousness, and pain level. Additional assessments include:
    - Skin color and temperature
    - Patency of IV lines, IV fluids, and rate
    - Patency of drains
    - Urinary output
    - Surgical site
    - Drainage on dressing (type, amount, and color)
    - Drainage under the patient
    - Ability to move all extremities
    - Nausea
    - Emesis
    - Laboratory results

15. Examples of surgeries are as follows:
    a. Elective—hysterectomy, cholecystectomy
    b. Urgent—hip pinning, bowel resection
    c. Emergency—control of internal bleeding, appendectomy for a ruptured appendix
    d. Minor—cataracts, small biopsies
    e. Major—bowel resection, transplants

16. a. Infants—Infants have an immature sympathetic nervous system, which could increase the risk of developing bradycardia during surgery. They have lower blood volume, so blood loss could contribute to dehydration and the inability to respond to an increase oxygen demand. The renal system in the infant metabolizes drugs slower and the immature liver could lead to lengthened effects of narcotic medications. Shivering reflexes are not well developed, and they have a relatively large body surface area, which leads to difficulty maintaining a stable body temperature resulting in hyperthermia or hypothermia. The immune system is immature, which compromises the ability to resist infection.
    b. Older adults—Older adults may have unique physical, physiological, and pharmacologic changes that potentially impact preoperative and postoperative care and could influence how the body responds to anesthesia. Many older adults have a decreased physiological reserve that can result in a reduced ability to compensate for changes that take place during the surgical procedure. Infection, anemia, and hemorrhage are some of the complications that can occur. There is potential for a fluid and electrolyte imbalance because older adults have a smaller percentage of body water, a decreased thirst response, and decreased kidney function.
    c. Obese individuals—Obesity can cause significant mechanical difficulty for the surgeon. This could lead to excessive blood loss and problems exposing, accessing, and retracting tissue of the surgical site. During the postoperative phase, the patient may have difficulty with lung expansion, leading to the development of pneumonia and wound infections. The increase depth and size of the surgical wound could cause wound infections and poor wound healing. Individuals have higher risks for delays in metabolizing medications, hypertension, cardiovascular, respiratory, and GI complications. Hypoxemia is often associated with obesity due to increased respiratory effort, ventilation-perfusion mismatch, closure of small airways, and reduced total lung capacity.
    d. Patient with schizophrenia—The illness could interfere with the patient's ability to follow instructions and care for the surgical wound. Some individuals may be prescribed antipsychotic or anticonvulsant medications, which could interact with anesthetic agents. In addition, surgery is a major psychological stressor.
    e. Patient with cardiac disease—These patients have an increased risk for infarction or potential life-threatening dysrhythmias. If hypertension is not controlled, the risk for anesthesia and complications significantly increases.
    f. Patient with diabetes—Diabetes can increase the risk for delayed wound healing. If NPO for surgery, glucose levels need to be monitored closely and insulin doses adjusted accordingly. Glucose levels may fluctuate in people with diabetes because of the stress of surgery resulting in hypoglycemia or hyperglycemia.

17. Malignant hyperthermia is characterized by a and d.

18. The immediate treatment for malignant hyperthermia is to stop the surgery, discontinue the anesthesia, administer oxygen and IV fluids, and cool the patient. Dantrium can be given for muscle spasms.

19. a. The major postoperative problem related to the anesthesia is a spinal headache.
    b. The headache can be alleviated with a blood patch placed over the dura hole. This is accomplished by removing blood from the patient's arm and injecting the blood into the epidural space at the level of the dura hole. Many patients receive immediate relief. The patient must remain flat for approximately 2 hours following this procedure.

20. Critical questions to ask are:
    Do you have any medication or food allergies?
    What surgeries have you had in the past and when were they performed?
    Have you or any family members had problems with anesthesia?
    What prescription medications are you currently taking?
    Do you take any over-the-counter medications?
    Do you take any herbal medications or vitamin supplements?
    Do you take any narcotic medications?
    Do you smoke?
    Is there a possibility you may be pregnant?
    How often you do smoke and how long have you smoked?
    How much alcohol do you drink in a typical day or week?

21. Baseline information to obtain before surgery should include vital signs, pain level, level of consciousness, orientation, the ability to maintain thought patterns, follow

commands, respond to questions and tactile simulation, and the results of diagnostic preoperative tests.

22. False

23. a. The patient is using an incentive spirometer.

    b. The device is used to prevent respiratory complications, such as atelectasis and pneumonia.

24. Goals for the nursing diagnosis (*Anxiety* related to concern over the surgery as evidenced by pacing, tachycardia, diaphoresis, and verbalization of anxiousness) are:

    Patient will express feelings about the upcoming surgical procedure.

    Patient will implement relaxation techniques before the procedure.

    Interventions include demonstrating and reinforcing relaxation techniques, such as deep breathing.

    Sitting with the patient and providing information on the usual preoperative procedures to expect.

25. The key nursing interventions in the preoperative phase are patient assessment and education.

26. The order for deep breathing is f, e, b, a, d, and c.

27. Areas for preoperative teaching are:
    • Perioperative care and routines
    • Preoperative testing
    • Preoperative skin preparation
    • Postoperative exercises—leg, respiratory
    • Postoperative positioning, ambulation
    • Pain management
    • PACU, discharge

28. a. The informed consent discloses the following:
    • Medical diagnosis and reason for treatment
    • Procedure to be performed
    • The name of the person performing the procedure
    • Qualifications of the person performing the procedure
    • Name of individual(s) assisting with the procedure
    • Risks and benefits of the procedure/surgery
    • Alternative treatments
    • The right to refuse or withdraw consent at a later date

    b. The nurse witnesses the signing of the form, provides information about nursing care, facilitates preoperative teaching, and reinforces information about the procedure. If the nurse finds that the patient does not understand the procedure or is unsure of whether to sign the consent, the nurse informs the physician of the situation and asks the physician to talk to the patient.

29. Patients are NPO in order to prevent aspiration of gastric contents.

30. a. Pain assessment is done at least every 2 hours postoperatively.

    b. Assessment is done with a pain scale or other tool.

    c. Providing pain relief to the patient makes him or her more likely to participate in important postoperative activities to prevent complications, such as ambulating, coughing, and deep breathing.

31. a. Airway obstruction—Intervention includes manual opening of the airway with a jaw-thrust or chin-lift maneuver and determination if there is an obvious obstruction such as the tongue, vomit, blood, secretions, loose teeth, or a foreign body that needs to be removed. Suctioning can be performed to remove vomit, blood, and secretions. The patient may need the assistance of an anesthesiologist. An ambu bag with oxygenation may be used to help facilitate obtaining a patent airway.

    b. Thrombophlebitis—Prevented with leg exercises, ambulation, hydration, antiembolic stockings, and sequential compression devices. Treatment consists of the administration of anticoagulants and analgesics, bed rest, elevation of the affected extremity, and measuring the circumference of the affected extremity every shift. Laboratory values for clotting times are monitored, and the patient is instructed not to rub or massage the affected extremity.

32. Atelectasis is characterized by diminished lung sounds in the affected lobe, along with cough, dyspnea, anxiety, chest pain, cyanosis, and crackles.

33. Care for an evisceration includes placing the patient in semi-Fowler position, placing sterile saline-soaked gauze over the incision, and notification of the surgeon.

34. Postoperative healing can be delayed by infection, blood clots, tissue hypoxia, trauma, advanced age, abnormal laboratory values, malnutrition, immunosuppression, and systemic disease.

35. The nurse should make sure that the patient is stable and pain is controlled, the top side rails are raised, the bed is in the lowest position, and the call light is placed within reach.

36. The complications are dehiscence and evisceration.

37. The nurse should use a bladder scanner to determine if there is residual urine. As able, patients should be provided with some privacy and assisted to a normal position for urination. If a bathroom is available, the patient may be assisted to go there to attempt to urinate. Running water in the sink and/or placing the hands in warm water can stimulate the urge to void.

38. The correct actions are b, d, and e.

39. The order for removing surgical attire is c, a, d, and b.

40. Wound assessment includes:
    • Size (current size; size may decrease with healing)
    • Type of closure (e.g., transverse, midline, horizontal)
    • Edges (well approximated with staples, sutures, Steri-Strips, or surgical glue)
    • Presence of drains (type of drain, amount, and type of fluid in drains)
    • Drainage (type, consistency, color, odor) for the type of drainage
    • Signs of infection (redness in the surrounding skin, yellow wound bed, purulent drainage, and malodorous)

41. If the nurse observes that a break has occurred in sterile technique, it must be brought to the attention of the physician and the operating room staff. Contamination could result in an infection for the patient, which could seriously jeopardize the recovery process. This communication is done in a professional manner, rather than accusatory tone.

42. c	50. a	58. b
43. c	51. a	59. d
44. d	52. d	60. c
45. b	53. a	61. a
46. d	54. c	62. d
47. c	55. d	63. a
48. b	56. a	64. c
49. b	57. a	65. d

212

Practice Situations

a. Using understandable terminology, you should instruct the patient's wife about indications for contacting the surgeon, hospital, or possibly 911, such as a:

- Large amount of drainage on the dressing, especially if it is deep red blood or purulent.
- Change in the respiratory status or level of consciousness of her husband.
- Significant increase in pain.
- Distention and extremely rigid feel to the abdomen.
- Problem with elimination.

You should make sure that they have the phone numbers for the surgeon and hospital, and that they have necessary prescriptions and instructions from the surgeon (keeping the area dry, when to remove the dressing, return to regular diet, etc.). There should also be an appointment date for the follow-up visit. You can also tell her that there is usually a follow-up call from the surgery center within 24 hours.

a. Assessment data:

Patient information: Mrs. Logan is a 72-year-old

Admitting diagnosis/chief complaint: abdominal pain and cholecystitis

Preoperative assessment data: no known drug allergies (NKDA), full code status

States that she is "afraid of surgery and nervous about being under anesthesia." Has never had surgery before and states she "doesn't know what to expect."

T 37° C (98.6° F), P 104 and regular, R 24 and shallow, BP 150/88, pulse oximetry—94% on room air, pain 4 out of 10

b. Medication and treatment orders:

Medication/fluid orders include:

IV Dextrose 5% and 0.9% sodium chloride at 100 mL/h

Ancef 2 gm IVPB q8h

hydrochlorothiazide 25 mg PO daily

Potassium 20 PO mEq daily

Lovenox 40 mg subcut daily

Tylenol #3, 2 tabs PO q4h prn for moderate pain

Morphine 10 mg IV q4h prn for severe pain

Zofran 4 mg IV q8h prn for nausea

Treatment includes:

Vital signs with O_2 sat q4h

Incentive spirometry

BRP with assistance

Sequential compression devices (SCDs) while in bed

I and O every shift

Assess voiding, bladder scan if unable to void in 6 hours

Abdominal dressing change every shift

Advance to clear liquid diet when bowel sounds return

CHAPTER 38: OXYGENATION AND TISSUE PERFUSION

1. e
2. d
3. b
4. a
5. c

6. The normal heart rate is 60 to 100 beats per minute.

7. Oxygenation can be influenced by atherosclerosis, arterial spasm or malformation, blood clots, dysrhythmias, valvular issues, failure, and trauma.

8. a. Emphysema—caused by smoking, exposure to pollution, or family history
   b. Pneumonia—caused by an infectious agent or aspiration
   c. Atelectasis—caused by decreased diaphragmatic movement and hypoventilation

9. Scoliosis and kyphosis are curvatures of the spine that limit thoracic movement and result in hypoventilation, retention of carbon dioxide, and reduced oxygenation.

10. The nurse should ask about chest pain, shortness of breath, dyspnea, weight gain/loss, dizziness, blood clots, weakness/fatigue, persistent cough, and a history of smoking or cardiopulmonary disease.

11. For the physical assessment, the nurse should obtain vital signs, auscultate heart and lung sounds, evaluate peripheral pulses, and observe for changes in the skin (hairless, shiny extremities) or structure (barrel-chest) that would indicate alterations.

12. a. Cyanosis—bluish discoloration of the skin related to deoxygenation of hemoglobin
    b. Hemoptysis—blood in the sputum
    c. Hypercapnia—an abnormally high level of carbon dioxide in the blood
    d. Arrhythmia—abnormal rhythms of the heart
    e. Necrosis—tissue death
    f. Hypoxemia—low level of oxygen in the blood

13. a. Lower/less than normal.
    b. Higher/more than normal.

14. a. Decreased (dilution from excess fluid)
    b. Decreased (hypokalemia related to diuretics)

15. Abnormal findings on a chest radiograph are rib fractures, tumors, pneumothorax, pneumonia, pleural effusion, pericardial effusion, enlarge heart, and atelectasis.

16. For the cardiac catheterization, the patient will have a contrast dye injected, which could result in an allergic reaction. The nurse also has to monitor for bleeding and circulation to the extremity used for access.

17. Examples of nursing diagnoses are:

Impaired Gas Exchange related to destruction of alveolar walls as evidenced by SpO_2 of 90% and patient complaints of inability to breath.

Ineffective Airway Clearance related to bronchoconstriction, increased mucus production, and cough that is ineffective as evidenced by thick sputum, rhonchi in lung fields, and prolonged coughing incidents.

Activity Intolerance related to low oxygen levels and need for more oxygen with activity, as evidenced by complaints of fatigue with activity, slow gait, and dropping O_2 saturation levels with activity.

Ineffective Breathing Pattern related to ineffective movement of air into and out of the lungs, as evidenced by difficulty breathing with activity and at rest, use of pursed lip breathing.

Ineffective Peripheral Tissue Perfusion related to decreased oxygen levels in the blood, as evidenced by fatigue with exercise and cyanosis when inspired oxygen is decreased.

213

18. Examples of goals/outcomes are:

Patient will maintain SpO_2 at 92% or greater by the end of the shift.

Patient's lungs will be clear to auscultation within 24 hours.

Patient will maintain SpO_2 at 92% or greater with activity within 48 hours.

Patient will report decreased fatigue during hospitalization.

Patient will demonstrate a breathing cycle that returns to a normal pattern after aerosol treatments.

Patient's extremities will be pink and warm to touch after supplemental oxygen is applied.

Patient will verbalize an increase in psychological and physical comfort within 8 hours.

Patient's respirations will return to 16 to 20 breaths per minute after pain medication is administered before cardiac catheterization.

19. Measures to promote oxygenation include positioning in semi- or high-Fowler position, providing oxygen, maintaining airway clearance, instructing the patient in respiratory exercises (deep breathing, coughing, incentive spirometer use), providing adequate hydration, and administering medications to improve cardiovascular and pulmonary function.

20. Oxygen saturation should be at 90% or higher.

21. The patient needs to have an order from the PCP, be instructed in the proper use and storage of the oxygen, have signs for "No Smoking," and determination of the type of delivery device and tubing.

22. The health team members involved will most likely be the nurses, respiratory therapist, PCP, speech therapist (aspiration risk), and physical therapist (increase activity tolerance).

23. The nurse should tell the patient's wife that the higher levels of oxygen may create respiratory depression. In patients with emphysema who have high levels of carbon dioxide, low oxygen levels drive respiration. Higher amounts of oxygen will drop the respiratory rate.

24. a. Nasal cannula:

Correct application involves placing the prongs in the patient's nares with the curved side at the top and the prongs pointing toward the back of the head; looping the tubing around the patient's ears (gauze or special tubing covers may be used as a cushion where the tubing rests on the ears to prevent sores and protect the skin); and tucking the tubing under the patient's chin and securing it with the sliding adjustment piece. Encourage the patient to breathe through the nose. Do not administer oxygen through a nasal cannula at greater than 6 L per minute. Consider humidification at all levels, especially at flow rates of 4 L per minute and higher.

b. Simple face mask:

If there is a bag reservoir, ensure it is filled before placing the mask on the patient. Always humidify oxygen delivered via mask. If the patient is able to eat, obtain an order for a nasal cannula during meals. Correct application involves the following: Place the mask over the patient's nose and mouth. Secure the mask around the back of the head with the adjustable strap, pulling evenly from both ends of the strap to secure it in place. If the straps are around the ears where they may chafe, cushion the ears with gauze. Adjust the nosepiece by

pinching it to provide for comfort and to ensure fit. There are several types of oxygen masks but no reservoir bag is used for a simple face mask.

25. a. CPAP is used for treating obstructive sleep apnea and to prevent atelectasis.

b. Barriers to compliance are dry nares, skin irritation, claustrophobia, perception of an inability to breathe, and noise of the device.

c. BiPAP provides two pressures—higher during inhalation and lower during exhalation, whereas CPAP maintains the same pressure throughout.

26. A bag-valve-mask (BVM) or Ambu bag is used to ventilate and oxygenate a patient who needs ventilatory support in an emergency situation.

27. For airway insertion:

	Oropharyngeal Airway	Nasopharyngeal Airway
Size	90 mm	28 French
Insertion	Insert the airway while directing the curve of the airway at the roof of the mouth, and then rotate the airway 180 degrees once it reaches the back of the throat.	Lubricate the airway before attempting insertion. The airway is inserted gently; if resistance is encountered, try the other nostril.
Nursing Care	Secure the airway in place with a holder or tape. Remove the airway every 4-8 hours. Provide oral care.	Secure the airway in place with a holder or tape. Remove the airway every 8-24 hours, and alternate nares. Provide oral and nasal care.

28. The following equipment should be in the room of a patient with a tracheostomy:
    - Ambu Bag
    - Endotracheal and oropharyngeal suction equipment
    - Waterproof adhesive tape
    - An extra tracheostomy care kit
    - Two extra inner cannulas (one the same size as worn by the patient, and one a size smaller)
    - Two extra outer cannulas (one the same size as worn by the patient, and one a size smaller) with obturators
    - Scissors
    - Extra tracheostomy ties
    - Oxygenation equipment

29. Interventions to assist patients with cardiopulmonary function include:
    - Diets high in fiber and low in fat
    - Exercise
    - Medications
    - Chest physiotherapy
    - Antiembolism stockings
    - Sequential compression device
    - Smoking cessation
    - Immunizations
    - Chest tubes, tracheostomies, airways, suctioning

30. Medications to be expected are:
  a. Pulmonary disease—bronchodilators, anticholinergic agents, corticosteroids, vaccines, antibiotics, mucolytic therapy, leukotriene modifiers
  b. Cardiovascular disease—diuretics, angiotensin-converting enzyme inhibitors, angiotensin II receptor antagonists, beta blockers, calcium channel blockers, vasodilators, antiarrhythmics, anticoagulants
31. The UAP is instructed to report on the following:
  • Changes in vital signs, respiratory status, or level of consciousness
  • Pain or discomfort noted by the patient
  • Skin breakdown
  • Excessive secretions
  • Difficulties encountered with any of the treatments
32. For a patient with excessive secretions, presuctioning ventilation is done with a tracheostomy oxygenation mask set for 100% FiO$_2$ for several respiratory cycles.
33. This suctioning is contraindicated for a, c, d, and e.
34. Sterile normal saline solution is used to clear and check the suction catheter.
35. a. Tracheostomy suction: 80 to 120 mm Hg continuous
  b. Oropharyngeal suction: 120 to 150 mm Hg continuous
36. The sequence for tracheostomy cleaning is c, e, a, d, and b.
37. a. Semi-Fowler position is used for a pneumothorax.
  b. Notify the PCP if bubbling is occurring in the water-seal system.
  c. Lift the tubing up to clear the drainage. Do not lift the system above chest level.
  d. Every 4 hours is a minimum period of assessment.

38. d	43. b	48. c
39. c	44. a	49. c
40. b	45. c	50. d
41. d	46. d	51. b
42. b	47. a	

Practice Situation

a. You anticipate that the patient will have the following interventions:
  • Diuretics
  • Antiarrhythmic
  • Potassium supplements (depending on the diuretic ordered)
  • Reduced sodium diet
  • Oxygen—2 L/min via nasal cannula

• Possible fluid restriction
• Possible stool softeners to decrease straining
b. You can assist the patient by:
  • Elevating the head of the bed
  • Assessing vital signs and activity tolerance
  • Evaluating response to oxygen therapy
  • Elevating the lower extremities when the patient is out of bed
  • Monitoring daily weights and intake and output
  • Providing rest periods between activities
  • Assist with ADLs as needed
  • Assessing peripheral edema and providing skin care
  • Administering medications and observing response
  • Instructing in respiratory exercises to clear pulmonary secretions, as tolerated

CHAPTER 39: FLUID, ELECTROLYTE, AND ACID-BASE BALANCE

1. f	5. j	9. c
2. d	6. g	10. h
3. i	7. a	
4. e	8. b	

11. a. 0.9% NaCl—isotonic
  b. 5% Dextrose/water (D$_5$W) —isotonic
  c. 0.33% NaCL—hypotonic
  d. Lactated Ringer (LR) —isotonic
  e. Dextrose 5% in lactated Ringer (D$_5$LR)—hypertonic
12. Two of the body's compensatory mechanisms are the respiratory and renal systems. Carbon dioxide can be reduced with a change in ventilatory rate and depth, and bicarbonate can be retained or excreted by the kidneys.
13. a. A person with type A blood can receive type A and type O.
  b. A person with type O blood can receive type O.
14. The criteria for blood donation are being at least 17 years of age, weighing at least 110 pounds, and having not donated blood within the past 8 weeks. The blood is then tested for ABO and Rh typing and antibodies to several viruses including hepatitis B and C, HIV, syphilis, human T-cell lymphotropic virus (HTLV), and, in some cases, cytomegalovirus.
15. The signs of a hemolytic reaction are a, c, and e.
16. A 2% loss in total body weight is mild dehydration.
17.

Electrolyte Imbalance	Underlying Causes	Nursing Interventions
Hypokalemia	Loss of excess potassium due to: • Vomiting, gastric suction, diarrhea • Laxative abuse, frequent enemas • Use of potassium wasting diuretics • Inadequate intake seen in anorexia, alcoholism, debilitated patients • Hyperaldosteronism	Monitor vital signs, especially heart rate and rhythm. Monitor cardiac rhythm via ECG. Monitor laboratory results: serum potassium levels. Assess for signs of digitalis toxicity. Encourage foods high in potassium. Administer potassium supplements as ordered; IV potassium is diluted properly and administered slowly, usually by infusion. *Never administer potassium as an IV bolus or IV push.*

Continued

Electrolyte Imbalance	Underlying Causes	Nursing Interventions
Hyperkalemia	Renal failure, massive trauma, crushing injuries, burns, hemolysis, IV potassium, potassium-sparing diuretics, acidosis, especially diabetic ketoacidosis	Monitor vital signs, especially heart rate and rhythm. Monitor cardiac rhythm via ECG. Monitor laboratory results: serum potassium levels. Limit potassium-rich foods. Administer cation-exchange resins (Kayexalate) as ordered. Administer glucose and insulin as ordered.
Hypocalcemia	*Hypoparathyroidism* Pancreatitis, vitamin D deficiency, inadequate intake of calcium-rich foods *Hyperphosphatemia* Chronic alcoholism Monitor heart rate and rhythm.	Monitor cardiac rhythm via ECG. Take fall and seizure precautions. Administer oral and/or IV calcium supplements as ordered. Encourage calcium- rich foods.
Hypercalcemia	Prolonged bedrest, hyperparathyroidism, bone malignancy, Paget disease, osteoporosis	Monitor heart rate and rhythm. Monitor cardiac rhythm via ECG. Encourage increased fluid intake. Increase patient activity.

18. Alterations in sodium can occur with severe vomiting, administration of hypertonic IV fluids, excessive sweating, congestive heart failure, renal failure, increased/decreased sodium intake, or hormonal imbalances.
19. Infants, young children, and older adults are most susceptible to imbalances.
20. Diuretics will promote fluid output, and they can enhance the excretion of electrolytes, such as sodium and potassium. Some diuretics are potassium sparing.
21. The potassium-rich foods are c, d, and e.
22.

Acid-Base Imbalance	Underlying Causes	Nursing Interventions
Respiratory acidosis	Result of hypoventilation due to: Chest injury Asthma attack Pulmonary edema Brainstem injury Medications: • Anesthetics • Opioids • Sedatives	Assess vital signs, especially rate and depth of respirations, pulse oximetry. Assess breath sounds. Assess cardiac rhythm. Administer oxygen as ordered. Monitor ABG results. Have mechanical ventilation available. Encourage deep breathing and coughing. Encourage fluid intake.
Metabolic alkalosis	Vomiting Nasogastric suctioning Overuse of bicarbonate antacids Hypokalemia Loop and thiazide diuretics Monitor ABGs and serum electrolytes, especially potassium.	Assess vital signs, especially cardiac rate and rhythm, respiration rate and depth, pulse oximetry, blood pressure. Assess level of consciousness. Administer oxygen as ordered. Take seizure precautions. Treat hypokalemia if appropriate.
Metabolic acidosis	Shock Trauma Cardiac arrest Diabetic ketoacidosis Chronic renal failure Salicylate overdose Sepsis Chronic diarrhea	Assess vital signs, especially respiratory rate and rhythm, blood pressure, and pulse oximetry. Monitor cardiac rhythm. Monitor ABGs and serum electrolytes, glucose, BUN/creatinine. Monitor level of consciousness. Have mechanical ventilation available as needed. Administer sodium bicarbonate as ordered.

23. The signs of dehydration are a, b, and f.
24. For an isotonic fluid volume excess:
    a. Clinical manifestations are weight gain, edema in dependent areas, bounding peripheral pulses, hypertension, jugular vein distension, dyspnea, cough, and abnormal lung sounds.
    b. The nursing interventions are to monitor vital signs, monitor intake and output, assess for edema and jugular vein distention, auscultate lung fields, and monitor laboratory results, especially hematocrit, BUN, and urine specific gravity.
25. a. Neurologic assessment—Assess for Chvostek sign, Trousseau sign, deep tendon reflexes, tremors, confusion, agitation, and coma.
    b. Cardiovascular—Assess for jugular vein distension, ECG waveforms, pulses, and blood pressure.
26. Examples of medical conditions that can lead to fluid and electrolyte imbalances are diabetes mellitus, renal disease, heart failure, thyroid or parathyroid disorders, burns, infections, and GI problems (gastroenteritis, Crohn disease, vomiting, diarrhea).
27. If the blood volume decreases, the blood pressure decreases.
28. Fluid intake includes all fluids and anything that becomes fluid at room temperature, such as ice, gelatin, popsicles, ice cream, IV fluids, liquid medications, blood products, enteral feedings, and large-volume irrigations and enemas.
29. A baby's urinary output is measured by weighing the wet diaper and subtracting the weight of the unused diaper.
30. Skin turgor is assessed at the forehead, anterior chest, and medial forearm.
31. With a loss of fluids and sodium, sport drinks are a good choice. For children, Pedialyte provides replacement.
32. The Six Rights for IVs are:
    • Right patient: Use two unique identifiers.
    • Right solution (medication): Make sure the correct solution is infusing.
    • Right rate (dose): Verify that the IV is infusing at the ordered rate.
    • Right route: Certain IV fluids cannot be administered through a peripheral site.
    • Right time: The IV should finish at a designated time.
    • Right documentation: IV therapy documentation includes the IV site, solution, rate, and patient tolerance.
33. When administering potassium IV, it is always diluted, usually in 1000 mL, and the maximum rate of infusion is 40 mEq/hour.

34.

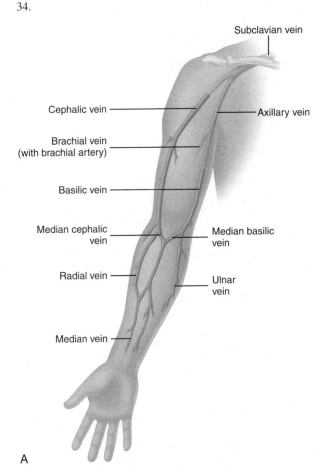

Subclavian vein
Cephalic vein
Axillary vein
Brachial vein (with brachial artery)
Basilic vein
Median cephalic vein
Median basilic vein
Radial vein
Ulnar vein
Median vein

A

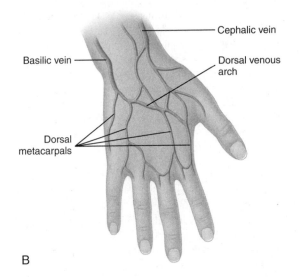

Cephalic vein
Basilic vein
Dorsal venous arch
Dorsal metacarpals

B

35. Scalp veins—newborns and infants. Veins of the feet—infants and children.
36. The vein to select for the IV site should be:
    - The most distal location
    - Away from the joints
    - Away from an extremity that has been compromised (i.e., surgery)
    - Soft and full feeling, easily palpated
37. a. A central venous catheter (CVC) is used for administration of large amounts of fluid, irritating medications, and hypertonic solutions, such as TPN. Central venous pressure can also be monitored.
    b. Placement is confirmed with a radiograph.
    c. Sterile technique is used for care.
38. Advantages of a PICC line are that it does not have the risk of a pneumothorax and it is associated with less catheter-related infections.
39. The correct sequence for care of the Mediport is d, b, e, c, f, and a.
40. The solution should be checked to make sure that it is the fluid ordered by the provider, it is clear and there is no evidence of contamination or leakage, and it is not expired.
41. The infusion device should be set at 125 mL/hour.
42. The nurse must use sterile technique, cleanse the port with antiseptic or alcohol, flush the intermittent device (saline lock), and then connect the infusion.
43. a. Intake = 1200 mL, Output = 925 mL
    b. Positive fluid balance
44. a. Catheter occlusion—Assess tubing and site for obstructions such as kinked tubing or arm position. Attempt to flush catheter with normal saline. *Do not force.* Forcing the flush could dislodge the clot to become an embolism. If peripheral IV, discontinue the site and restart a new site. If a central venous catheter (CVC), notify the PCP or IV team.
    b. Air embolism—Place patient in Trendelenburg position on left side, locate source of air and close off, notify PCP immediately, administer oxygen as needed, and have emergency resuscitation equipment available.
45. Documentation should include the IV site, solution, rate, and patient tolerance. It may also be policy to indicate the type of catheter and date of insertion.
46. The correct actions for the CVC are a, c, e, and f.
47. a. Before administration, two nurses identify the patient, blood group and type, ID number of the blood product, and the expiration date of the blood.
    b. The infusion rate should be 25 to 50 mL/hour.
    c. The blood must be infused within 4 hours after leaving the laboratory.
    d. The most common cause of a reaction is inappropriate identification of the patient.
48. For TPN, the nurse should:
    - Monitor the infusion carefully.
    - Apply the Six Rights.
    - Monitor the patient's vital signs, intake and output (I&O), and weight.
    - Check laboratory results.
    - Use a pump for infusion.
    - Ensure that vitamin K is ordered.
    - Maintain sterile technique.
    - Discard solutions over 24 hours old.
    - Collaborate with the dietician and pharmacist, as needed. There should not be any other substances infused through the line for the TPN, and the infusion should never be discontinued suddenly.
49. The correct sequence for IV insertion is b, c, e, a, d, and f.
50. a. If the IV solution is discolored, it should be discarded immediately, and a new solution obtained.
    b. If the IV will not infuse, the tubing should be checked for kinks and the IV site assessed for signs of infiltration, phlebitis, or extravasation.
51. On the dressing/dressing label should be written the nurse's initials, and the date and time of the dressing change. The label should not be placed in a way that the site is occluded.

52. a	64. b	76. c
53. a	65. c	77. c
54. c	66. a	78. a
55. b	67. c	79. a
56. c	68. b	80. c
57. b	69. c	81. c
58. a	70. a	82. d
59. a	71. c	83. b
60. c	72. b	84. c
61. a	73. b	85. a
62. d	74. d	86. c
63. b	75. b	

Practice Situation

a. You anticipate that the patient will also have the following signs and symptoms:
   Confusion, thirst, dry mucous membranes, orthostatic hypotension, tachycardia, weak and thready pulse, decreased skin turgor, prolonged capillary refill, weight loss, and decreased urinary output.
b. You will expect the following results:
   - Urine specific gravity > 1.030
   - Hematocrit increased
   - BUN > 20
c. Nursing diagnosis—*Deficient Fluid Volume* related to vomiting and fever as evidenced by the S/S.
   Patient goal/outcomes—Fluid volume will be reestablished within 2 to 3 days.
   Weight will return to baseline within 2 days.
   Urine specific gravity will be within expected limits at next testing.
   Mucous membranes will be pink and moist within 24 hours.
   Vital signs, especially temperature, will return to expected range within 24 hours.
   Nursing interventions—Administer fluids; monitor vital signs; monitor intake and output; monitor daily weights; assess for neurologic changes; monitor laboratory results, especially hematocrit, BUN, and urine specific gravity; and establish safety measures to prevent injury from orthostatic hypotension.

CHAPTER 40: BOWEL ELIMINATION

1. Bowel elimination can be influenced by food and fluid intake, various illnesses and diseases, trauma and surgery, medications, immobility, and psychological issues (anxiety, depression, eating disorders).

2. Hemorrhoids are swollen and inflamed veins in the anus or lower rectum.

3. Diarrhea is associated with abnormal frequency and fluidity of fecal evacuations, hyperactive bowel sounds, urgency, abdominal pain, and cramping.

4. The causes of diarrhea can be: b, e.

5. Straining during defecation can stimulate the Valsalva maneuver, which could lead to bradycardia and death.

6. a. Cause/etiology of *Clostridium difficile*—occurs after use of antibiotics
   b. Common symptoms—watery diarrhea three or more times a day for 2 or more days, abdominal cramping, and tenderness

7. A primary concern for an incontinent patient is skin breakdown from exposure to urine and feces. Prompt cleansing and protecting of the skin is critical.

8. In preparation for the fecal occult blood test, the nurse tells the patient to avoid beets; broccoli; cantaloupe; carrots; cauliflower; cucumbers; fish; grapefruit; horseradish; mushrooms; poultry; radishes; red meat; turnips; and vitamin C–enriched foods and beverages.

9. A cardinal sign of a fecal impaction is continuous oozing of liquid stool with no normal stool.

10. The patient with "gas" or flatus may be helped by moving around in bed or ambulating, rocking, or insertion of a rectal tube, if necessary.

11. For the double-barrel colostomy, the stoma on the left (proximal) will produce fecal material, while the other (distal) may have mucous discharge.

12. The accurate statements about bowel elimination are b, d, and e.

13. Possible causes of constipation are:
    - Irregular bowel habits
    - Ignoring the urge to defecate
    - A low-fiber/high-fat diet
    - Hemorrhoids
    - Reduced fluid intake
    - Nerve blockage (spinal cord injury/damage)
    - Metabolic issues (hypothyroidism)
    - Psychiatric issues
    - Prolonged bed rest
    - Lack of exercise
    - Medications (anticholinergics, depressants, iron supplements)
    - Surgery and anesthesia
    - Cognitive or physical impairment with decreased ability to respond to urge

14. These foods affect bowel elimination as follows:
    a. Pasta and cheese—constipation
    b. Spicy foods—diarrhea and flatus
    c. Figs—promote defecation
    d. Chocolate—promotes defecation

15. The factors that will promote bowel elimination are c and f.

16. Patients taking iron supplements usually have stool that is black and tarry.

17. The inspection of the GI system starts in the patient's mouth with the condition of the teeth, tongue, gums, and mucous membranes. For the abdomen, the nurse looks at the contour, the appearance of any distention, scars, stomas, or lesions, and signs of umbilical displacement, hernia or bulging masses.

18. For the patient with persistent diarrhea, the nurse expects that a stool culture will be ordered.

19. The major side effect of the GI series is constipation from the barium.

20. a. The patient is instructed to not eat anything for at least 8 hours before the examination.
    b. Medication that can cause drowsiness, relaxation, amnesia, and possible light-headedness will be given. The throat will be sprayed with a numbing medicine, which works for 30 to 45 minutes. The patient may be asked to swallow during the initial insertion of the endoscope. The procedure usually lasts only about 10 to 20 minutes. A feeling of fullness may be felt afterward if air is injected into the stomach.
    c. After the procedure, the patient's gag reflex will be checked before anything to eat or drink is provided. Driving is not permitted for 12 hours while the sedative wears off, so the patient needs someone to drive him or her home.

21. a. Preparation for the colonoscopy includes bowel preparation: clear liquid diet for 1 to 3 days, no foods or beverages with red or purple dye, and a laxative/enema the night before.
    b. Similarities to an endoscopy are NPO before the examination, use of conscious sedation, minimal possibility of complications, and driving not permitted afterward.
    c. The American Cancer Society has recommended the following examinations for early detection of colorectal cancer for people of average risk who are asymptomatic:
       - Fecal occult blood test annually starting at age 50. (If the test is positive, a colonoscopy should be performed.)
       - Flexible sigmoidoscopy every 5 years starting at age 50 (if the test is positive, a colonoscopy should be performed) *or* colonoscopy every 10 years starting at age 50 *or* double-contrast barium enema every 5 years, *or* CT colonography every 5 years.

       Patients considered at higher risk undergo the examinations at more frequent intervals.

22. Overuse of laxatives can lead to increased/rebound constipation and impaction, predisposition to colorectal cancer, dependency on their use, and electrolyte imbalances.

23. For the patient who is immobile or cognitively impaired, the nurse needs to set up a regular schedule for defecation, such as in the morning after breakfast. Patient requests for toileting need to be responded to promptly. Warm liquids, adequate hydration, high-fiber foods, and proper positioning will aid in the process. The patient should also be monitored for constipation and impaction. Stool softeners may be ordered, as indicated, to prevent these problems.

24. Enteral tubes that are used for gastric lavage are Salem sump, Levin, and Ewald tubes.

25. Principles for use of a bedpan to incorporate into the teaching of the UAP are:
    - Always wear gloves when assisting a patient with elimination.
    - Place a waterproof pad on the bed.
    - The patient must be properly positioned, with buttocks centered on the bed pan.
    - If the patient is unable to assist with lifting/movement, roll the patient to one side and place the bedpan on the bed, then roll the patient onto the bed pan.
    - Elevate the head of the bed, using Fowler position if it can be tolerated by the patient.
    - Do not leave the bed pan in place for longer than 10 minutes; doing so will promote or exacerbate pressure ulcers and/or skin breakdown.
    - After bedpan removal, provide pericare and skin care (a skin protectant/barrier cream may be used to prevent breakdown).
    - Remove gloves and perform hand hygiene. Protective equipment may be necessary for emptying and cleaning of the bedpan, if splashing may occur.
26. Use of a laxative/cathartic is contraindicated for a patient with nausea, vomiting, dehydration, or abdominal pain.
27. Enemas are used to relieve constipation, remove impacted feces, empty the bowel before diagnostic tests, and instill medications.
28. The correct steps for suppository insertion are c, d, and f.
29. The nurse will specifically want to include the patient and family as much as possible in the care of the ileostomy. Attention needs to be paid to the following: body image, self-esteem/sexuality, skin care, elimination/site management, nutritional needs, and support group referral.
30. The nurse recommends that the patient avoid beans, beer, broccoli, Brussels sprouts, cabbage, sodas, eggs, fish, garlic, onions, some spices, and deep-fried or fatty foods.
31. a. An enema is contraindicated for patients with increased intracranial pressure, glaucoma, or recent rectal or prostate surgery.
    b. The procedure can be delegated to the UAP after the nurse has assessed the patient, unless delegation is not within the agency's or state's guidelines.
    c. If the patient cannot assume the usual position, dorsal recumbent position can be used.
    d. The procedure should be stopped immediately if the experiences abdominal distention or rigidity.
    e. For adults, the tube is lubricated and inserted slowly 3 to 4 inches toward the umbilicus.
    f. The solution bag should be held or positioned 12 to 18 inches above the patient's hip.
32. The correct sequence for ostomy care is b, d, a, f, c, and e.
33. a. The pouching system can stay in place for 3 to 7 days. Frequent changes can contribute to skin breakdown.
    b. If skin barrier fragments remain on the patient's skin, an adhesive remover should be used. Cleansing can be done with warm water, patting the site dry with a towel. Alcohol-based products are to be avoided.
    c. The ostomy bag should be emptied when it is one-third to one-half full.

34. For the patient who has episodes of constipation, the nurse recommends exercise, a high-fiber diet, at least six to eight glasses of fluid daily (hot liquids and fruit juices stimulate peristalsis), heading the urge and allowing time for defecation, and avoiding overuse of laxatives.
35. The expected appearance of the stoma is c, d, and f.

36. a	42. c	48. c
37. b	43. c	49. a
38. a	44. a	50. a
39. c	45. a	51. b
40. a	46. c	52. a
41. d	47. d	

Practice Situation

a. For the conceptual care map, nursing diagnoses should include:
   Disturbed Body Image related to bowel diversion as evidenced by statements made, such as "My husband will not want to look at me."
   Knowledge deficit related to newly created colostomy as evidenced by inability to perform self-care and statements made, such as "I have no idea how to manage this."
b. Patient goals:
   - Acceptance of change in body image with colostomy.
   - Ability to independently manage colostomy care.
   Patient outcomes:
   - Patient will verbalize feelings about change in body image and coping mechanisms before discharge.
   - Patient and husband will discuss feelings regarding body image and intimacy.
   - Patient will contact support group and identify meeting times or appointment with support person within 24 hours.
   - Patient will verbalize procedure for colostomy care within 24 hours.
   - Patient will demonstrate, with guidance, colostomy and skin care within 24 hours of instruction.
   - Patient will independently demonstrate colostomy care before discharge or after first home care visit or physician appointment.
c. Nursing interventions:
   - Spend time with the patient to talk about her feelings.
   - Recommend that the patient speak with her husband about her concerns.
   - Provide information on how to manage sexual intimacy with the colostomy, referring as needed to counseling.
   - Allow time for patient to adapt to looking at the colostomy—providing information on how it will look and that the size of the stoma will shrink in 6 to 8 weeks.
   - Take time to explain colostomy care and show the patient the equipment needed. If an ostomy care nurse/team is available, refer the patient and follow up on information provided.
   - Demonstrate/reinforce colostomy and skin care. Have the patient return demonstrate the procedure.
   - Refer for home care nursing follow-up and make sure that the patient has necessary prescriptions, appointment with surgeon, and information on where to obtain supplies.

CHAPTER 41: URINARY ELIMINATION

1. d	5. h	9. c
2. g	6. a	10. e
3. j	7. b	
4. i	8. f	

11. 1440 mL (minimum of 30 mL/hour)
12. Factors that influence urinary output include psychosocial factors, food and fluid intake, surgical and diagnostic procedures, pathologic conditions, and urinary tract infections.
13. a. Hemodialysis takes the patient's blood and has it flow through the filters of a machine and ultrafiltrate. Peritoneal dialysis uses the abdominal cavity as the membrane for exchange of fluid and molecules.
    b. The goal of dialysis is to remove toxins and maintain fluid, electrolyte, and acid-base balance.
14. Cautious monitoring of the patient includes strict I&O and daily weights, along with assessment of vital signs, neurologic status, and overall condition.
15. Dysuria is associated with bladder or urinary tract infection, cystitis, sexually transmitted disease, yeast infection, kidney or bladder stones, prostatic enlargements, malignancy, allergic or irritant reaction to soaps, vaginal lubricants, spermicides, contraceptive foams and sponges, tampons, and toilet paper.
16. Individuals most prone to urinary incontinence are a, d, and e.
17. Conditions that contribute to urinary retention include vaginal childbirth; infections of the brain or spinal cord; diabetes; stroke; neurologic disorders; heavy metal poisoning; pelvic injury or trauma; prostate enlargement; infection; surgery; medications such as antihistamines, anticholinergics, antispasmodics, and tricyclic antidepressants; bladder stones; rectocele; cystocele; constipation; or stricture.
18. The patient with an enlarged prostate may have urinary frequency, hesitancy, retention and a feeling of bladder fullness, pressure, or pain.
19. a. Dehydration—reduced urinary output
    b. Diuretics—increased urinary output and loss of electrolytes
    c. Paraplegia—loss of sensation and muscle control to the lower part of the body with resultant urinary retention
    d. Renal calculi—possible obstruction of urinary flow
20. The female urethra is significantly shorter than that of the male and is located near sources of bacteria from the anus and vagina. The shorter urethra also contributes to the risk of infection associated with sexual intercourse.
21. To determine renal and bladder status, the nurse will inspect the abdomen for color, contour, symmetry and distention. The renal arteries should be auscultated. Palpation and percussion of the bladder are performed.
22. Normal findings of the physical assessment include d and f.
23. a. Beets and blackberries—can turn the urine pink or red
    b. Warfarin—can turn the urine orange
    c. Liver failure—can turn the urine brown to tea colored
24. Normal characteristics of urine are a, d, and f.
25. Blood tests to evaluate renal function include blood urea nitrogen (BUN) and creatinine levels.
26. a. For an intravenous pyelogram, the patient is NPO 8 to 12 hours before and may need a laxative or enema to empty the bowels.

b. The use of radiographs and contrast dyes are contraindicated for pregnant patients.
27. For a cystoscopy, the following are accurate: a, b, d, and f.
28. To promote urinary elimination and prevent infection, the nurse should:
    - Instruct patients and families on safe transfer techniques for individuals with limited mobility needing voiding assistance.
    - Instruct patients to respond promptly to urge to avoid urinary retention and reduce infection risk.
    - Emphasize the importance of maintaining fluid intake to help flush the urinary system.
    - Instruct patients to promptly report pain or burning on urination; changes in urine color, odor, or clarity; or changes in voiding patterns.
    - Reinforce with female patients proper aseptic technique, including washing front to back to maintain perineal cleanliness. Remind male patients to retract foreskin, if present, to thoroughly wash the urinary meatus. Be sure to stress the importance of drying the area thoroughly to prevent skin breakdown or irritation.
    - Teach proper care of indwelling catheters and the perineal area, including emptying and cleaning the device, maintaining a closed system, and bladder irrigation, or flushing, if necessary.
    - Arrange for a wound ostomy continence nurse to teach patients with a urinary diversion appropriate care for the stoma, drainage devices, and skin.
    - Teach patients the importance of taking medications as prescribed. Instruct patients and families in desired or adverse side effects that may influence the patient's urinary elimination pattern. Stress the importance of maintaining fluid intake or restrictions based on medication requirements.
29. For the patient in the acute care environment, the nurse should:
    - Provide privacy as possible—closing the bathroom door, pulling the curtain closed around the bed, facing away from the patient.
    - Warm the bedpan before use.
    - Assist the patient to as normal a position as possible—standing, sitting, or with the head elevated, if possible, when using the bedpan.
    - Run water to stimulate the urge to void.
    - Respond promptly to patient requests for assistance, and treat the patient with dignity.
30. The commode is used for patients who are weak or unsteady on their feet or become short of breath upon ambulation. It is not used for the patient who cannot stand or transfer safely.
31. An example of an initial toileting schedule is upon awakening, q1-2h during the day, before bedtime, q4h during the night, with the time intervals gradually increased.
32. To minimize nocturia, the patient should not drink fluids within 2 hours before bedtime.
33. Urinary tract infections (UTIs) can be prevented by b, c, and d.
34. Catheterization is the primary cause of UTIs, so the nurse needs to follow sterile technique during insertion, employ asepsis during routine care, maintain a closed system, keep

the drainage bag below the level of the bladder, and recommend removal as soon as possible. The smallest-size silver alloy or silver-impregnated catheter should be used.

35. Lumen # 3 is used for balloon insertion.
36. Straight catheterization is done for a, b, and f.
37. Routine catheter care includes cleansing the urinary meatus with soap and water one to two times daily, keeping the drainage system intact and below the level of the bladder, and cleansing the catheter proximally to distally if it becomes encrusted.
38. Condom catheters are kept in place with an adhesive at the base of the penis.
39. Soap and water or no-rinse cleansers should be used to provide perineal care. Moisture barrier cream may be used to prevent/heal breakdown.
40. The correct sequence for catheterization is c, e, a, b, f, and d.
41. Bladder irrigation is performed to maintain patency of the catheter, postoperatively for GU surgery, and to decrease complications, such as infections.
42. a. Resistance is encountered.
    - Pull back the catheter, and attempt a gentle reinsertion/repositioning.
    - Ensure proper lubrication has been applied to the catheter.
    - Ensure insertion is into the urinary meatus if the patient is female.
    - With gentle pressure, grasp and straighten the male penis, holding it at approximately a 45-degree angle from the abdomen, if resistance is met.
    - Check that the smallest catheter size is being used.
    - It may be necessary to contact the patient's physician or urologist, per facility policy, to insert a coudé catheter if resistance is persistent.
    b. No urinary drainage occurs.
    - Assess the catheter, its placement, and the urinary system.
    - Verify correct placement.
    - Check the quantity and time of the last void or catheterization, and check the volume of intake.
    - Ask the patient to cough; this increases pressure, which may promote urine flow.
    - Ask the patient to take a deep breath in and out to relax the abdominal muscles.
    - Check the catheter itself for kinks or other possible obstruction.
    - Assess the bladder for distention; perform a bladder scan if necessary and equipment is available.
    - Push the catheter in slightly and rotate it; the catheter may not quite be fully inside the bladder, or the opening may be up against the bladder wall.
    - Pull the catheter out slightly and rotate it; the catheter may be above the level of urine, or the opening may be blocked.
    c. Lidocaine 2% gel is available to use as a lubricant.
    - Check for patient allergy to lidocaine. If none, obtain and substitute lidocaine 2% gel in place of the lubricant in the kit for male catheter insertion.
    d. Contamination of the equipment is suspected.
    - Stop the procedure, obtain new materials, and restart the procedure.

43. d	51. d	59. b
44. a	52. a	60. c
45. b	53. c	61. c
46. d	54. a	62. d
47. c	55. b	63. b
48. a	56. c	64. d
49. c	57. a	65. a
50. d	58. c	

Practice Situations

a. With paraplegia below T-12, the patient will probably have a flaccid bladder and have lost the ability to empty the bladder naturally. The patient will then be required to perform self-catheterization to remove residual urine. This is important to prevent complications, such as infection.
b. You will specifically want to assess whether the patient has a distended bladder, determine the urinary output and characteristics, and evaluate the patient's ability to understand the procedure, manipulate the equipment, and self-catheterize. You will also want to investigate if the patient has the necessary supplies and access to soap and water for hygienic care of the hands and perineal area. You will also assess the patient's understanding of how to evaluate his output and contact his provider if there are problems.
   Intake = 2725 mL (remember to count Jell-O and liquid medication)
   Output = 1930 (includes wound drainage)
   Positive fluid balance of 795 mL

CHAPTER 42: DEATH AND LOSS

| 1. d | 3. e | 5. c |
| 2. a | 4. f | 6. b |

7. a. Loss—Often defined as the absence of something or someone that a person has formed an attachment to and can include people, places, and things.
   b. Grief—The emotional response to a loss.
   c. Mourning—The outward, social expression of loss.
   d. Bereavement—Can be described as the inner feelings and outward expressions that people experiencing loss are demonstrating over a period of time.
8. The nurse can help the person who is grieving by assisting that individual to go through the stages or tasks, communicating regularly, recognizing cultural/personal practices, sharing information for decision making, referring him or her to community resources, providing emotional support, and encouraging health behaviors (rest, sleep, nutrition, etc.).
9. The possible practices for a Jewish family are a, d, and f.
10. Worden identifies that the first task is to accept the reality of the loss, as the feelings of shock and disbelief that occur during the initial stage of grieving are the most common emotions felt by those experiencing a loss. Kubler-Ross also identifies the first stage as denial of the loss.

11. a. Physical—tightness in the chest and throat, oversensitivity to noise, breathlessness, muscular weakness, lack of energy, fatigue, sleep disturbances, changes in appetite
    b. Emotional—numbness, loneliness, sadness, sorrow, guilt, shock, anxiety, depression, anger, agitation, lack of interest or motivation, lower level of patience or tolerance
    c. Cognitive—preoccupation with the deceased, forgetfulness, preoccupation with the loss, inability to concentrate, inability to retain information, disorganization, feeling confused
    d. Behavioral—crying, insomnia, restlessness, withdrawal, irritability, apathy, impaired work performance
12. Examples of ethical issues related to end-of-life care include patient self-determination and options for continuing or withdrawing care, futile medical care, assisted suicide, and euthanasia.
13. a. Relationship of the deceased—The relationship of the survivor to the deceased and the type and quality of the relationship that they had affects the grieving process. Examples of difficult losses with the potential for complicated grief include miscarriage, loss of a child, or loss of a first-degree relative or spouse.
    b. Available support systems—Social support is essential during the process of grieving. Sources of support include family members and friends, members of a religious or spiritual community, and support groups for those who have experienced a similar loss.
    c. Other stressors—Stressors in daily life are numerous and can include family issues, caregiving concerns, financial problems, workplace demands, and lack of a support system. Multiple stressors can complicate the grieving process and result in a crisis situation.
    d. Type of loss—Loss related to a suicide leads survivors to feel shame, fear, guilt, rejection, and anger. When a loss is related to a murder, the survivor's personal sense of security is threatened and a sense of control is lost. Grief reactions are usually severe, intense, exaggerated, and complicated.
14. Dysfunctional grieving can be assessed by asking the patient the following:
    • Do you feel that your support system is inadequate?
    • Are you using more alcohol, tobacco, drugs, or prescribed medications?
    • Do you have more difficulty sleeping than usual?
    • Have you lost or gained weight?
    • Has your grief subsided or intensified in the past few weeks?
    • Are you able to carry out your day-to-day activities including work, social commitments, and household responsibilities?
    • Do you have any new health concerns?
15. The nurse should assess the following for the caregiver:
    • General health checkup
    • Focused assessment of any physical, mental, or emotional symptoms
    • Assessment of nutritional status
    • Sleep evaluation
    • Examination of the caregiver's ability to maintain work and family roles
    • Maintenance of dental and visual health
    • Assessment of social network
    • Evaluation of support systems
16. a. Algor mortis—cooling after death
    b. Livor mortis—skin becomes pale, then bluish
    c. Rigor mortis—stiffening of the joints of the body
17. The specific signs associated with imminent death are a, b, and c.
18. Hospice is a program that provides comfort and supportive care for terminally ill patients and their families, either directly or on a consulting basis with the patient's physician or another community agency. Palliative care emerged in response to the needs of patients who were not terminally ill but needed quality symptom control for a serious or life-threatening illness. This type of care is appropriate for anyone who has a chronic, debilitating condition.
19. Pronouncement of death includes:
    a. Identification of the patient
    b. General appearance of the patient—lack of reaction to stimuli, no vital signs
    c. Death has not occurred under "unusual circumstances"
    d. Documentation—time of death, patient's name, time the call was made to the provider, findings of physical examination
    e. Notification of physician and other health care providers
20. The correct actions for postmortem care are c and d.
21. Key elements in nursing care for individuals and families going through the grieving process are communication and caring.

22. d	28. c	34. a
23. d	29. b	35. b
24. a	30. a	36. b
25. c	31. d	37. c
26. d	32. c	38. a
27. b	33. d	

Practice Situations

a. Your assessment may indicate that the woman's mother is close to death. She also appears to be having discomfort, as evidenced by the crying and moaning when touched.
b. You can assist the daughter by offering analgesia (morphine drops, fentanyl patch or alternative per the prescriber/provider). The daughter can also be instructed about the other signs of imminent death and what the expectations will be for this time. One of the most important things for you to do is to be present for the daughter, offer emotional support, and help her to manage this experience.

For the daughter or UAP, the following actions are appropriate: gentle bathing, oral care, turning and positioning, decreasing environmental stimuli (especially with the seizure activity), playing soothing music, and having oxygen and suctioning available (as indicated/desired).

a. For this complicated loss, you may expect to see a greater intensity of denial, anger, or shock, verbalization of helplessness or hopelessness, panic attacks, substance abuse, or chronic depression. Complicated loss/grief can lead to long-lasting physical problems and serious mental health issues.

Answer Key

b. *Complicated grieving* related to an unexpected loss of a family member as evidenced by fatigue and minimal verbal response.

Goal—Mother will be able to talk about the loss and the meaning the loss has on the family during your visit and/or a therapy session.

Mother will identify coping mechanisms and support systems during the visit.

c. To assist this individual to deal with complicated loss/grief, you should:

- Listen while the mother/family talks about the loss. Let the mother and family know that they are heard and understood as they are trying to make sense of the loss and the emotions of grief.

- Offer information about the stages of grief and that how she and others are feeling is expected.
- Encourage healthy behaviors, such as exercise, rest and sleep, adequate diet, journaling, stress-relieving techniques, and other healthy coping mechanisms.
- Including the entire family or significant others.
- Use community resources and make appropriate referrals. The mother and/or other family members may need more formal counseling.

Illustration Credits

CHAPTER 1

Question 12 from Potter PA, Perry AG, Stockert P, Hall A, and Castaldi P: *Study guide for essentials for nursing practice,* ed 8, St. Louis, 2015, Mosby.

CHAPTER 3

Question 21 from Sorrentino SA: *Mosby's textbook for nursing assistants,* ed 8, St. Louis, 2012, Mosby.

CHAPTER 19

Questions 14 and 15 from Potter PA, Perry AG, Stockert P, Hall A, and Castaldi P: *Study guide for essentials for nursing practice,* ed 8, St. Louis, 2015, Mosby.

CHAPTER 20

Questions 6, 25, 27, 31, and 38 from Potter PA, Perry AG, Stockert P, Hall A, and Castaldi P: *Study guide for essentials for nursing practice,* ed 8, St. Louis, 2015, Mosby.

Question 12a from Habif TP: *Clinical dermatology,* ed 4, St. Louis, 2004, Mosby.

Question 12b from Goldman MP, Fitzpatrick RE: *Cutaneous laser surgery,* St. Louis, 1994.

Question 12c from Weston WL, Lane AT, Morelli JG: *Color textbook of pediatric dermatology,* ed 2, St. Louis, 1996, Mosby.

Question 12d from Farrar WE, Wood MJ, Innes JA, Tubbs H, et al: *Infectious diseases,* ed 2, London, 1992, Gower.

CHAPTER 26

Questions 28 and 29 from Potter PA, Perry AG, Stockert P, Hall A, and Castaldi P: *Study guide for essentials for nursing practice,* ed 8, St. Louis, 2015, Mosby.

CHAPTER 29

Questions 20 and 21 from Potter PA, Perry AG, Stockert P, Hall A, and Castaldi P: *Study guide for essentials for nursing practice,* ed 8, St. Louis, 2015, Mosby.

CHAPTER 35

Questions 30, 31, and 50 from Potter PA, Perry AG, Stockert P, Hall A, and Castaldi P: *Study guide for essentials for nursing practice,* ed 8, St. Louis, 2015, Mosby.

CHAPTER 40

Question 11 from Phillips N: *Berry & Kohn's operating room technique,* ed 12, St. Louis, 2013, Mosby.

CHAPTER 41

Question 35 from Potter PA, Perry AG, Stockert P, Hall A, and Castaldi P: *Study guide for essentials for nursing practice,* ed 8, St. Louis, 2015, Mosby.